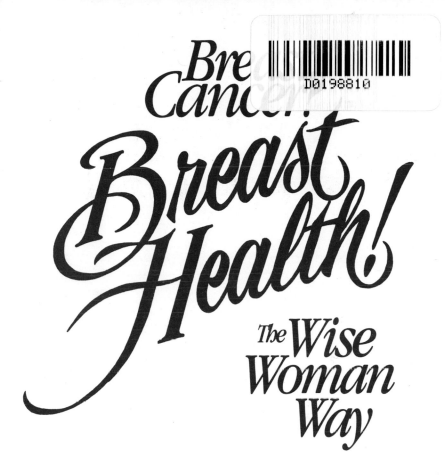

# Breast Cancer?

# Breast Health!

## The Wise Woman Way

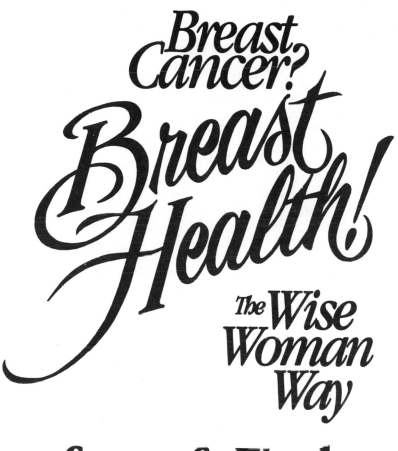

# Breast Cancer? Breast Health!

## The Wise Woman Way

## Susun S. Weed

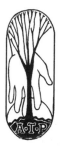

**Ash Tree Publishing**
Woodstock, New York

*All information in this book is based on the experiences and research of the author and other professional healers. This information is shared with the understanding that you accept complete responsibility for your own health and well-being. You have a unique body, and the action of each herbal medicine and home remedy is unique. Health care is full of variables. The result of any treatment suggested herein cannot always be anticipated and can never be guaranteed. The author and publisher are not responsible for any adverse effects or consequences resulting from the use of any remedies, procedures, or preparations included in this Wise Woman Herbal. Consult your inner guidance, knowledgeable friends, and trained healers in addition to the words written here.*

© 1996 by Susun S. Weed
**Ash Tree Publishing**
PO Box 64, Woodstock, NY 12498; 914-246-8081

Illustrations pages 58, 70, 103, 106, 124, 130, 136-7, 138, 160, 165, 167, 176, 182, 189, 190, 196, 222, 242, 244, and 307 © 1995 by Kimberly Eve.
Illustrations pages 28, 30, 32, 35, 36, 40, 41, 43, 62, 85, 86, 158, 217, 236, 252, 266, and 275 © 1995 by Alan McKnight.
Illustrations pages 2, 128, 130, and 262 © 1995 by Susun Weed.
Cover design and calligraphy by Scott Fray.
Inanna cover photo © 1995 by Star River Productions

### Publisher's Cataloging-in-Publication Data
#### *(Prepared by Quality Books Inc.)*

Weed, Susun S.
    Breast cancer? breast health! : the wise woman way / Susun S. Weed.
    p. cm. -- (Wise woman health series)
    Includes bibliographical references and index.
    Preassigned LCCN: 94-71323
    ISBN  09614620-78

    1. Breast--Cancer.    2. Women--Health and hygiene.    3. Alternative medicine.    I. Title.

RC280.B8W44 1996                         616.99'4'49
                                         QBI96-20036

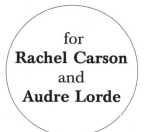

for
**Rachel Carson**
and
**Audre Lorde**

When Rachel Carson wrote *Silent Spring,* publicly expos-ing the detrimental effects of agricultural chemicals, I was still a teenager. Her work motivated me to base my diet on organically grown food. If herbicide and pesticide residues in our food do promote breast cancer then Rachel—who died of breast cancer—has helped me avoid her fate. I dedicate this work to her memory.

Audre Lorde, poet laureate of New York State, was a woman who dared to speak the truth of her life as a black lesbian with breast cancer. She taught me that every woman's voice is important and that each woman's truth is vital to us all. As I wrote the first draft of this book, I heard of her death. I dedicate this work to her memory, too.

To them I offer my breasts on my open palms, in an an-cient gesture of gratitude, woman to woman.

# Acknowledgments

This book comes to you from the hearts and hands of many beings.

To the women who have shared with me some part of their dance with cancer, I offer thanks: *Robin Birdfeather, Joan Bolga, Joy Craddick M.D., Elaine Geouge, Pamela Getner, Deborah Ann Light, Raven Light, Deena Metzger, Roslyn Reid, Betsy Grace Sandlin,* and *Nicki Scully.*

To those who eased my work load by researching, filing, confirming, reading, and offering nourishing assistance, I offer thanks: *Candace Cave, Alberta Darlau and the Herb Research Foundation, James Duke, Barbara Feldman, Keyawis Kaplan, Penny King, Morna Leonard, Amy Sophia Marashinsky, Monica Meyer-Cook, Sylett Strickland, Carole Tashel, Cynthia Werthamer,* and *Corinna Wood.*

To those remarkable beings whose lives are spent helping those dancing with cancer and who freely shared their wealth of clinical expertise, I offer my thanks: *Bobbi Aqua, Carolyn Dean M.D., Holly Eagle, Deborah Maia, Suresh B. Katakkar M.D., Dr. Ingrid Naiman, Monica Miles, Marie Summerwood, Callie Weston FNP,* and *Donny Yance.*

To my editor, *Clove Tsindle* , who lavished attention on every word, thought, and nuance, I offer bosom bouquets and my heartfelt thanks. To my friend and editor, *Betsy Sandlin,* who saw to all the details, I offer my ongoing, liver-deep blessings and thanks.

To my beloved consort, *Michael Dattorre,* who has cosseted and coddled me, tended fires and goats while I attended to computer keys, and in every way possible aided, abetted, assisted, encouraged, nurtured, and supported the manifestation of this book, I offer my thanks.

To all of you, and to all the trees whose fiber we use here, I offer my deepest respect and my ecstatic gratitude for all the pleasure and support you have given, and continue to give, to me.

# Table of Contents

## Section One:  For All Women

## Section Two: For Women Dancing with Cancer

# Section Three: Help

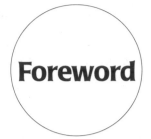

# Foreword

My wake up call from my healer within came to me through my breasts; I think of it as my "Amazon awakening." Fourteen years ago, while feeding my first child exclusively with my breast milk and working 60-100 hours a week outside my home attempting to heal others, I developed a large breast abscess, resulting in complete destruction of that breast's duct structure, making it impossible for me ever to nurse a baby on that side. I realized that I had halved my physical nourishing ability by worshipping too long and too steadily at the altar of outer achievement and authority figure approval. I had ignored my own physical needs and my inner wisdom completely. No wonder I sustained a wound in my breast that dissected right into the muscles of my chest wall!

From this experience I learned my first lesson of breast wisdom: We cannot nurture others fully or well unless we also nurture ourselves. Our breasts know this. And they will not be silenced in their attempts to bring this to our attention.

With my awakening, I joined all the women whose breasts have told them of the need for balance in their lives, the need for heeding inner wisdom, the need for pleasure, the need for passion. Sometimes these needs are subtle, sometimes they are urgent. Either way, we've been taught to ignore them. So we lose touch with the wisdom and power of our breasts.

So many of the women who come to me tell me they don't know how to examine their breasts, they don't know what normal feels like, and they're afraid of what they might find. So many women choose implants because their breasts aren't "big enough." So many have surgery because they're too big.

How can it be that our breasts, these beautiful centers of nurturing, fullness, and pleasure, are looked upon by so many as inadequate at best, or breeding grounds for cancer, pain, and fear at worst? In what kind of culture can this happen? A culture that has been out of touch with women's wisdom for too long. A culture in which the women's wisdom in each of us, what Susun calls the Wise Healer Within, has been silenced, ignored, and ridiculed both outside of ourselves and within each of us for the last several millennia. And so our breasts become a cultural battleground where a war is waged between our fear of living fully and our fear of dying before we've ever lived fully.

But what if each of us were to remember her woman's wisdom? What if we remembered that every cell of our breasts could be nurtured and rejuvenated and healed by the energies of touch, pleasure, love, whole food, and green healing plants? What if we collectively discovered that our healer within has never gone away, that she has simply waited, biding her time until it was safe to come out and speak her truth?

I'm certain that the time for acknowledging and collectively acting upon our inner wisdom has now arrived. This wisdom and truth have never been more crucial for our personal and planetary health. Women's wisdom is the balance that modern technological medicine needs. She is the balance that brings healing back to medical care. She is the voice that says, "I'm going to be all right"—even when all the lab reports and doctors say otherwise. And sometimes she is the voice that says, "My time on Earth is now at an end"—even when all the lab reports and doctors say otherwise. She is the voice of the heart, the same voice whose energy heals our breasts, regardless of their current state of health. Her voice sings on every page of this magnificent book.

As you read these pages, let this voice sweep you along with it, let it wrap you in its warmth, and let it challenge you when you need that, too. Allow its whispers to help you remember your own wise voice within. Here is the information and spirit that our hearts and breasts have needed for a very long time.

Christiane Northrup, M.D.
Yarmouth, Maine, March 15, 1995

Fellow of the American College of Obstetrics and Gynecology,
co-founder of Women to Women Healthcare Center,
author of *Women's Bodies, Women's Wisdom.*

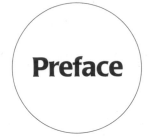

# Preface

Winter lies piled at my door; winter is leaking in through my roof; winter has stopped my water and is holding it in a frozen grip.

I'd like to leave this all behind, go visit friends who live on tropical isles. A vacation would be fun. But breast cancer doesn't go on vacation, so I'm crafting my collection of information on preventing and dealing with breast cancer—a collection that spans twenty-five years—into a book.

It's hard to write about breast cancer. It's frightening to read about it, to listen to women's stories, and to speak with oncologists (experts on cancer). Like winter, the facts pile up at my door, leak in through my dreams, stop my thoughts and hold them in a frozen grip, a grip of dread, of deep unease.

What feeds my fear of cancer? I keep hearing, and have been hearing all my life, that the incidence of breast cancer is increasing. That no one knows what causes it or how to prevent it. That I could have breast cancer even if I feel incredibly well. That cancer is silent and deadly and my only hope is to expose my breasts to radiation in hopes of finding it when small. That I need be prepared to fight viciously—slashing and burning and poisoning to within an inch of my life—should cancer ever be found.

I feel myself tightening in fear, clutching my breasts to my chest, shoulders hunched over. But I know that won't help. I breathe out and allow my hands to relax and open. I breathe out with a sigh and let my head come up and my shoulders fall back. I breathe out and sigh audibly as my arms relax and my unbound breasts fall into the warm hollows of my palms.

My right hand, palm open, is under my right breast. And my left hand, palm open, is under my left breast. This is an ancient gesture. A gesture of offering and a gesture of power.

I invite the Ancient Ones with this gesture. I open my heart and silently cry: "I don't want to die of breast cancer! I don't want my sister, my lover, my mother, my daughter, my aunt, my friends to die of breast cancer."

The Ancient GrandMothers are humming. Their hands are under their breasts. Their breasts are cupped in their open palms in an ancient gesture of power.

"Breast cancer is a paradox, GrandDaughter, for cancer is life itself: soaring, unstoppable life. Yet cancer seems to threaten life. Just so, your wild, untamed, unpredictable parts are the living core of your life but seem to threaten the stability of your life. Cancer is an invitation to dance with them in wild abandon. A chance to reclaim and nourish passion and a greedy zest for life. An opportunity to nurture and tend to the dark, the hidden, the inner child, the shadow. A reason to bare your breasts, literally and figuratively.

"And breast cancer is a dance of initiation, for no woman who dances with cancer is ever the same. She has visited the source and tasted the waters of life and death, savored the sweetness and the sharpness of her own mortality, and tasted her desire to survive.

"We have no right answers, no rules to follow, no promises of life eternal. Death is certain for every living thing. But there are many ways to prevent and reverse cancerous changes in your cells. We ask that you observe the consequences, to your inner ecology and to the outer world, of reliance on supplements and drugs made by petrochemical corporations. We ask you to question the ever-growing use of chemicals on farms, and electricity, whose humming wires sing the cancer song, and uranium, the mutater, the changer, now invisibly vibrating with greater and greater intensity from more and more places.

"And we insist that you trust your inner sense of rightness and be willing to act on your own convictions. Walk with truth and beauty, GrandDaughter. There are no wrong answers. There are no wrong paths. Each woman is unique. We are here to support you, no matter what confronts you. And to remind you that you can leave a trail of wisdom, a trail of beauty, no matter which path you choose. That is the Wise Woman Way the world 'round."

"I thank you, Ancient Ones," I whisper, my heart beating more easily in my breast. But surely there is much that is wrong about breast cancer. It can't be right that any woman has to hear the words: "You have breast cancer." It can't be right that breast cancer seems to increase every decade. It can't be right to cut into ten women's breasts to find one or two cancers. I feel so much rage and frustration about breast cancer. How could anything about breast cancer not be wrong?

The Wise Woman Way demands that I be willing to see the perfection in every problem, that I be willing to allow breast cancer to have its own beauty, its own truth, and its own ways of offering health/wholeness/holiness. The Wise Woman Way offers me a vision of completeness—with things just as they are—if I am brave enough to accept the possiblity that any so-called problem is already absolutely perfect.

How ironic that I feel called to find the rightness of breast cancer even as I collect ways to prevent and eliminate it. Is it that breast cancer, like childbirth or menopause, is an initiation where one's former self dies, and a new self emerges? Yes. But we're talking about an epidemic. Surely what's right about breast cancer can't be limited to personal transformation, no matter how profound for the individual, no matter how much difference that one person can make to the whole. What's right about breast cancer must be a larger answer, a meta-story, an archetypal resonance, a story that reveals the power of breast cancer.

During the past three decades women have repeatedly tried to come together around a focus that leads to cohesiveness rather than divisiveness. But every effort has seemed to fail. Could it be that what's right about breast cancer is that it finally gives us all a focus, a common enemy?

Breast cancer doesn't care what color your skin is. Breast cancer doesn't care who you love or sleep with. Breast cancer can't be prevented by being rich (although money can buy more care and more free time to take care of yourself). Breast cancer doesn't care whether you are single, monogamous, swinging or celibate. Breast cancer concerns us all, men as well as women, and it will surely concern more and more of us as we grow older.

Perhaps breast cancer can bring us together, can unite our voices into a chant that vibrates with respect for women, for our breasts, and for the Earth's sweet breast. Perhaps our solitary grief and our public wailing will stop the poisoning of our bodies and our planet. Perhaps we will find a song that will ease our way through chaos and cancer and into the depths of our selves. Perhaps the act of considering, even for a moment, that cancer can be an ally of wholeness will help us nurture health/wholeness/holiness inside and out, healing the Earth as we heal ourselves. This is the Wise Woman Way the world 'round.

Susun S. Weed
February 26, 1995
Laughing Rock Farm

# My Anti-Cancer Lifestyle

An anti-cancer lifestyle is not a rigid set of rules to follow, but a safe space to be filled with your favorite ways of nourishing health and discouraging cancer. Since cancer thrives in a too-ordered situation, relax and let chaos give a hand now and then in the execution of your plan. I include all the following elements in my anti-cancer lifestyle. Were I to be diagnosed with cancer, I would continue to do these things in addition to any other remedies I might choose.

• Stay in touch with my own daily and seasonal rhythms.
• Sleep in total darkness or moonlight; get into the sun daily.
• Eat one meal at the same time each day.
• Have emotional outlets.
• Choose friends who support me and my truth.
• Have artistic outlets.
• Receive lots of appreciation and approval (a.k.a. love).
• Exercise one hour three times a week.
• Get a massage once a month or more.
• Do my yoga practice once a week or more.
• Have sexual outlets.
• Take a quiet time of beingness daily.
• Make full use of all sources of joy available to me.
• Eat a Mediterranean-style diet of mostly organically grown foods including daily use of cabbage family plants, raw and cooked greens, whole grains, beans, sunflower seeds, soy products, olive oil, garlic, seasonal fresh fruit, seaweed, yogurt and cheese, herbal infusions, herbal vinegars, and antioxidant seasonings. Plus, at least four times a month, seafood, nuts, mushrooms, dried fruit, and eggs; and, less than four times a month, meat, alcohol, white sugar, and coffee.
• And I avoid: Vitamin/mineral supplements, chlorine, nitrates, tobacco, prescription hormones, TV, white flour, processed foods, and non-organic animal products.

# The Six Steps of Healing
*(with a few of the modalities available at each step)*

### Step 0: Do Nothing
(sleep, meditate, unplug the clock or the telephone)

### Step 1: Collect Information
(low-tech diagnosis, books, support groups, divination)

### Step 2: Engage the Energy
(prayer, homeopathy, ceremony, affirmations, laughter)

### Step 3: Nourish and Tonify
(herbal infusions and vinegars, hugs, exercise, food choices, gentle massage, yoga stretches)

*Note: Healing with Steps 4, 5, and 6 always causes some harm.*

### Step 4: Stimulate/Sedate
(hot or cold water, many herbal tinctures, acupuncture)
For every stimulation/sedation, there is an opposite sedation/stimulation, sooner or later.
*Addiction is possible if this step is overused.*

### Step 5a: Use Supplements
(synthesized or concentrated vitamins, minerals, and food substances such as nutritional yeast, blue-green algae, bran)
*These substances may do as much harm as good.*

### Step 5b: Use Drugs
(chemotherapy, tamoxifen, hormones, high dilution homeopathics, and potentially toxic herbs)

### Step 6: Break and Enter
(threatening language, surgery, colonics, radiation therapies, psychoactive drugs, invasive diagnostic tests such as mammograms and C-T scans)
*Side effects, including death, are inevitable.*

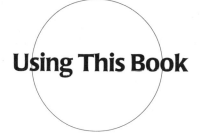

# Using This Book

The remedies gathered here are generally considered effective ways to promote breast health, reverse *in situ* cancers, and moderate the side effects of orthodox cancer treatments.

• To maintain breast health, read Section One. If you've recently been diagnosed with breast cancer, read Section Two. To prevent recurrence, go back and read Section One. To help you take action on the remedies discussed in each section, most chapters conclude with a section of resources.

• The remedies are presented in the framework of the Wise Woman Tradition and the Six Steps of Healing.

     The Wise Woman Tradition offers a view different from that of both alternative and orthodox medicine. In the Wise Woman Tradition, illness is viewed as an opportunity for greater health/wholeness. Death is seen as an initiation, a graduation, the last act, the climax. While death is acknowledged as the ultimate outcome of all lives, accepting this does not mean relinquishing the desire to stay alive. The Wise Woman Way offers us prevention and treatment options that benefit us and help maintain the health of our families, our communities, and the Earth.

     The Six Steps of Healing give us a way to use all available healing options as safely as possible. (*See* chart opposite.)

• All Step 0 suggestions are interchangeable for all problems.

• Steps 0, 1, 2, and 3 can prevent *and* help you deal with breast cancer. Daily doses of deep relaxation (Step 0), varied intellectual and sensory information (Step 1), energetic engagement (Step 2), loving nourishment, and adequate exercise (both Step 3) are important parts of maintaining or reclaiming breast health.

• Remedies from Steps 0, 1, 2, and 3 are considered safe even if you are using orthodox treatments. When Step 4 and 5a remedies work well with orthodox treatments they are called *complementary medicines.* Seek expert advice before using Steps 5b or 6.

• The Six Steps of Healing can be used incrementally and globally:
   **Incremental Approach**: Start with Steps 0 and 1, setting a time limit for yourself. (It can be three seconds or three months or . . .) When the time limit is up, you can extend it (and continue with Steps 0-1) or add on Step 2, setting another time limit. Again, when time's up, you can extend it or add Step 3. Continue this way, adding remedies from Steps 4, 5a, 5b, and 6 as needed. *When the problem is resolved, don't stop.* Go back through the steps, in reverse order, letting go of each one before returning to Step 0. (When you return to Step 1, it becomes *share information.*)
   **Global Approach**: If you know you are going to use orthodox treatments such as surgery, radiation, or chemotherapy (Steps 5 and 6), use all six steps together: Surrender to the mysteries of life and death (Step 0), collect information (Step 1), explore energy work (Step 2), nourish all aspects of yourself (Step 3), stimulate your immune system (Step 4), and take supplements for a brief interval (Step 5a). Healing from surgery is amazingly rapid when the global approach is used. Side effects of chemotherapy and radiation are kept to a minimum with the global approach.

• Consult the Materia Medica for cautions, dosage range, botanical name, and other helpful information about the herbs mentioned most frequently in this book. Consult the Herbal Pharmacy for instructions on making specific preparations such as infusions and infused oils. Different preparations of herbs can produce very different effects. Unfamiliar word? Look in the glossary, page 327.

• The ★ indicates remedies recommended by many women.

• Trust your own sense of what's right for *you.* Seek second and third opinions. Respect the uniqueness of *your* body, *your* intuitions, and *your* feelings.

*May it be in beauty; may it be in a sacred way.*

# Using Herbs Safely

Plants feed us, clothe us, house us, heal us, and can help us keep our breasts healthy, yet they can harm or kill us. Here's how to use them safely.

• When you buy herbs, check that they are labeled with the botanical name (e.g., *Trifolium pratense*). Common names for plants often refer to several plants; botanical names are specific to one plant. "Marigold" refers to two plants with different uses. *Calendula officinalis*, or pot marigold, is a medicinal herb; *Tagetes* is the marigold usually sold for flower borders.

• Learn about the weeds of your doorstep. Become more aware of the vitality and abundance of Nature. Eat or use as a remedy one wild plant that grows near you this year. When you make your own medicines and healing foods, you control one of the major ways you can come to harm from using herbs: mistaken identity (or right label, wrong herb). Not that you can't make mistakes, but you're more likely to catch your own mistake than someone else's. When you make your own medicines and healing foods, they are fresh, full of energy, and in tune with you and your environment. Making your own herbal remedies is simple and fun; directions begin on page 293.

• The results and safety of any remedy are dependent on the way it is prepared and used. Notice that I prefer infused herbal oils (not essential oils) and powerful herbal infusions (not herbal teas).

• Different people can have different reactions to the same substance, whether drug, food, or herb. If you take lots of herbs mixed together and have distressing side effects, how can you know which one is the cause? For safety, I use one herb (sometimes two, and only rarely three) at a time. Limiting the number of herbs I use in one day helps me discern my response to the plant allies I've chosen. If I have an adverse reaction, I can tell which herb caused it, avoid that herb, and try other herbs with similiar properties.

• Side effects from herbs are less common than side effects from drugs and usually less severe. If an herb disturbs your digestion, it may be that your body is learning to process it. Give it a few more tries before deciding it's not for you. An herb that really doesn't agree with you may cause nausea, dizziness, sharp stomach pains, diarrhea, headache, or blurred vision, and these effects will generally occur quite quickly. Stop taking the herb or reduce the dose dramatically. Slippery elm is an excellent antidote to poisons; *see* Materia Medica.

• When a dosage range is given, start with the smallest recommended dose and increase as needed. Note: 25 drops is 1 ml.

• Respect the power of plants to change the body and spirit in dramatic ways, even when taken in minute doses.

• Increase your trust in the healing effectiveness of plants by trying remedies for minor or external problems (side effects of orthodox cancer treatments, for instance) before, or while, working with your major and internal problems.

• Gather—in person or in books—with others interested in herbal, homeopathic, and home remedies. Call on them as well as professionals when you feel uncertain. Develop ongoing relationships with knowledgeable healers who are as interested in helping you maintain health as in helping you cure problems.

• Respect the uniqueness of every plant, every person, every situation.

• Remember that you become whole and healed in your own unique way, at your own speed. People, plants, and animals can help in this process. But your body/spirit does the healing/wholing. Don't expect plants to be cure-alls.

• If you are allergic to any foods or medicines, it is especially important to check out the side effects of *any* herb you are considering using.

Herbs comprise a group of several thousand plants with widely varying actions. Some are nourishers, some tonifiers, some stimulants and sedatives, and some are potential poisons. To use them wisely and well, we need to understand each category, its uses, best manner of preparation, and usual dosage range.

**Nourishers** are the safest of all herbs; side effects are rare. Nourishing herbs are taken in any quantity for any length of time. They are used as foods, just like spinach and kale. Nourishers provide high levels of anti-cancer vitamins, minerals (especially selenium), antioxidants, carotenes, and essential fatty acids.

Nourishing herbs in *Breast Cancer? Breast Health!* include: alfalfa herb, amaranth, astragalus root, calendula flowers, chickweed, comfrey leaves, dandelion herb, fenugreek, flax seeds, honeysuckle flowers, lamb's quarter, marshmallow root, nettle herb, oatstraw, plantain leaves and seeds, purslane herb, raspberry leaves, red clover blossoms, seaweeds (kelp), Siberian ginseng, slippery elm bark, violet leaves, and wild and exotic mushrooms.

**Tonifiers** act slowly in the body and have a cumulative, rather than immediate, effect. They build the functional ability of an organ (like the liver) or a system (like the immune system). Tonifying herbs are most beneficial when they are used in small quantities for extended periods of time. The more bitter the tonic tastes, the less you need to take. Bland tonics may be used in quantity, like nourishing herbs. Side effects occasionally occur with tonics, but are usually quite short-term. Many older herbals mistakenly equated stimulating herbs with tonifying herbs, leading to widespread misuse of many herbs, and severe side effects.

In Traditional Chinese Medicine, potentially poisonous herbs are used as tonics by women at high risk of developing breast cancer. (The herbs are taken daily, for one week only out of every six months.)

Tonifying herbs in *Breast Cancer? Breast Health!* include: barberry bark, burdock root, chaga, chaste tree berries, cronewort (mugwort), dandelion root, echinacea root, elecampane root, fennel seeds, garlic, ginkgo leaves, ginseng root, ground ivy, hawthorn berries, horsetail herb, lady's mantle herb, lemon balm, milk thistle seeds, motherwort herb, mullein leaves, parsley, pau d'arco, peony root, raspberry leaves, redroot, schisandra berries, self-heal, sundew, St. Joan's wort, turmeric root, usnea, wild yam root, and yellow dock root.

**Sedatives and stimulants** cause a variety of rapid reactions, some of which may be unwanted. Some parts of the person may be stressed in order to help other parts. Strong sedatives and stimulants, whether herbs or drugs, push us outside our normal ranges of activity and may cause strong side effects. If we rely on them and then try to function without them, we wind up more agitated (or depressed) than before we began. Habitual use of strong sedatives and stimulants—whether opium, rhubarb root, cayenne, or coffee—leads to loss of tone, impairment of functioning, and even physical dependency. The stronger the herb, the more moderate the dose needs to be, and the shorter the duration of its use.

Herbs that tonify and nourish while sedating/stimulating—especially oatstraw, motherwort, and peppermint—are among my favorite herbs. I use them freely as they do not cause dependency.

Sedating/stimulating herbs that also tonify or nourish are used frequently in *Breast Cancer? Breast Health!* including: boneset flowers, catnip, citrus peel, cleavers, ginger, hops, lavender, marjoram, motherwort, passion flower, many mints (e.g., lavender, rosemary, sage, and skullcap), and sheep sorrel.

Strong sedating/stimulating herbs used in this book include: angelica, bayberry, blessed thistle root, cancerweed, cinnamon, cloves, licorice root, marijuana, oak, osha root, passion flower herb, shepherd's purse, sweet woodruff, turkey rhubarb root, uva ursi leaves, valerian root, Venus's flytrap, wild lettuce sap, willow bark, and wintergreen leaves.

**Potentially poisonous herbs** are potent medicines. They activate intense effort on the part of the body and spirit. Potentially poisonous herbs are taken in tiny amounts and only for as long as needed. Unexpected side effects are common when potentially poisonous herbs are used without regard for their power. To increase your sense of security when contemplating the use of a potentially poisonous herb, consult other herbal references and several experienced herbalists.

Potentially poisonous herbs in *Breast Cancer? Breast Health!* include: arbor vitae, arnica, autumn crocus root, belladonna, bloodroot, celandine, chaparral, comfrey root (not leaf), foxglove, goldenseal root, henbane, iris root, Jimson weed, lobelia, May apple (American mandrake) root, mistletoe, poke, poison hemlock, stillingia root, turkey corn root, wild cucumber root.

**Green blessings.**

# section one
# For All Women

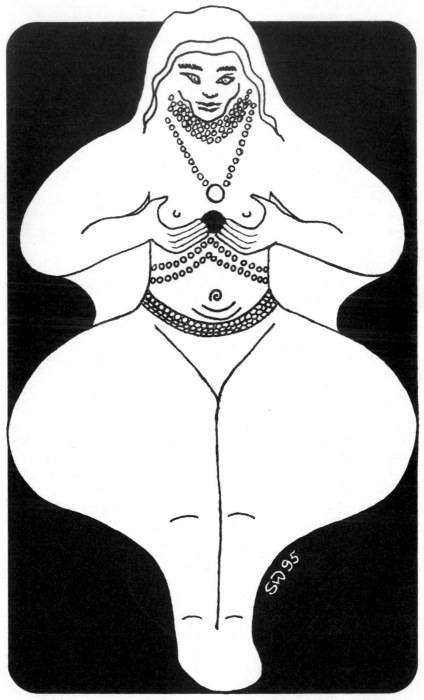

Inanna · 2500 B.C.E.

# 1.
# Can Breast Cancer Be Prevented?

Sometimes it seems that every magazine, newspaper, radio show, and piece of mail has a headline declaring that every woman's risk of developing breast cancer is increasing. There is a numbing feeling of inevitability in these pronouncements. More and more women think about breast cancer as a *when* rather than an *if.*

It's true that there's more breast cancer now than ever before, that between 1979 and 1986 the incidence of invasive breast cancer in the United States increased 29 percent among white women and 41 percent among black women, and incidence of all breast cancers doubled. It's true that the percentage of women dying from breast cancer has remained virtually unchanged over the past 50 years, and that every 12 minutes throughout the last half of the twentieth century another woman died of breast cancer. And it's true that breast cancer is the disease that women fear more than any other, that breast cancer is the biggest killer of all women aged 35 to 54, and that of the 2.5 million women currently diagnosed with breast cancer, half will be dead within ten years.

These facts frighten me, and they also make me angry. My studies spanning 25 years and many disciplines have convinced me that the majority of breast cancers are causally related to the high levels of radiation and chemicals released into our air, water, soil, and food over the past 50 years. United States government researchers estimate that 80 percent of all cancers are environmentally linked.

What can be done? The answer isn't as simple as a yearly mammogram. That may help detect breast cancer, but it won't prevent it. To prevent breast cancer we need to take individual and collective action.

Effective action requires understanding the causes of breast cancer and what decreases breast cancer risk. But there are few conclusive answers to these queries, partly because most research focuses on eliminating breast cancer after–not before–it occurs. Science has validated so few risk factors for breast cancer that 70

3

percent of the women diagnosed with breast cancer have "no iden-
tifiable risk factors."

---

### Scientifically accepted risk factors for breast cancer

1. **Sex** (Women get a lot more breast cancer than men.)
2. **Age** (Seventy-five percent occurs in women over 50.)
3. **Lifetime exposure to estrogen** (Early menarche, no pregnancies, late menopause, hormone pills increase risk.)
4. **Family history** (Two close relatives with premenopausal breast cancer increases risk.)
5. **Lifetime exposure to radiation** (The greater the exposure, up to a threshold, the greater the risk.)
6. **Race** and **culture** (White, European-extraction women are at greater risk than other women.)
7. **Height** and **weight** (Larger women are at greater risk.)

---

Unfortunately, our sex, age, reproductive history, family history, exposure to radiation (such as fallout from above-ground atomic bomb tests), race, culture, and height are beyond our control. When we're told these are the only risk factors, we can be left with feelings of hopelessness and panic.

But when we include risk factors that are considered "not well substantiated"—but which are clearly contributing to breast cancer incidence—including ingestion of and exposure to prescription hormones, hormone-mimicking organochlorines, prescription drugs, petrochemicals, and electromagnetic fields, as well as unwise lifestyle choices such as smoking tobacco, drinking alcohol immoderately, wearing a bra, or not exercising, then we can find many ways to lower breast cancer risk. No need to panic.

---

### Not accepted, but likely, risk factors for breast cancer

8. **Organochlorines** (Exposure increases risk.)
9. **Electromagnetic fields** (Exposure increases risk.)
10. **Tobacco smoke** (Exposure increases risk.)
11. **Alcohol** (Greater use increases risk.)

# Breast Cancer Prevention

We can help prevent breast cancer on an indi
by buying organically grown food, filtering our wate
powerful immunity, living wisely and vigorously, bein
with our breasts, using natural remedies for menopau
lems, and by paying attention to our Wise Healer Within.

But there's a limit to the control that any one woman has
over her exposure to petrochemicals, radiation, and other environmental cancer-inciters. Limiting the production and discharge
of substances that initiate and promote cancer is collective work.
When our individual acts are combined with the acts of others, we
can achieve the envisioned social change. For example, as I saw
more and more evidence that chlorine residues from papermak-
ing contribute to breast cancer, I began to ask for chlorine-free
paper from my book printer. They went from amazement and
puzzlement at my request to contracting with a new paper sup
plier who can provide them with elemental chlorine-free paper.
(I'm not the only one asking, you see.)

Whether you think your risk of breast cancer is high, low,
or average, there are things you can do, individually and with
others, to help yourself stay free of breast cancer and to help stop
the epidemic of breast cancer, too. (What *is* your risk of breast
cancer? See "Risk Assessment," page 317, to educate your guess.)

*Since 1950 the incidence of breast cancer in the U.S. has increased by 53
percent, according to Nancy Brinker, chair of President Clinton's Special
Commission on Breast Cancer.*

# Reproductive Factors

• **Giving birth before the age of 20** confers powerful protection against breast cancer. In general, the shorter the period between the onset of your menses and your first full-term pregnancy,
the less your risk of breast cancer. Why? Breast cells begin a matu-
ration process each month, but don't complete it unless you become pregnant (and carry to term). Partially matured breast cells
have unstable DNA and are easily involved in a cancer cascade.
But breast cells that are completely matured by pregnancy (and
lactation) become stabilized, less affected by menstrual cycle hormones, and actually resistant to breast cancer. This protection
ceases with menopause.[1-3]

# Breast Health!

• Herbalist Juliette de Bairacli Levy writes: "In my experience, it is very rare for the nomadic Gypsy women to have breast cancer. I attribute this to the long periods of time they allow their children to suckle at the breast."

A University of Nottingham Medical School study found a decrease in breast cancer risk in women under 36 who **breast fed** as little as three months, but other studies found risk reduction only when nursing continued beyond three months. All agree that the longer you nurse, the less your risk of breast cancer. A 1994 study found that breast feeding for at least six months before the age of 20 cut risk by half. Women who nursed for at least six months after the age of 20 cut their risk by 25 percent. Nursing reduces risk only before menopause and has little effect on the likelihood of developing postmenopausal breast cancer.[4, 5]

# Estrogenic Factors

• Estrogens (there are many) do not initiate cancer, but some of them, especially estradiol, do promote it. The risk factor for breast cancer most validated by science is **estradiol exposure**. The greater your exposure, the greater your risk.[6] Where does estradiol come from? Some women take it in pills to relieve menopausal symptoms, but most of it is produced by our own ovaries during each menstrual cycle. (After menopause the ovaries stop producing estradiol, but other estrogens continue to be made.)

The more menstrual cycles you have, the more estradiol you'll produce and the greater your likelihood of breast cancer. Late onset of menses, early menopause, pregnancy, lactation, and some birth control pills reduce the number of menstrual cycles and thus the risk of breast cancer.

• Most women, if asked for the usual age of the onset of menses, would say 11 or 12 years old. This is true only for the past century in industrialized countries. Historically the normal or average age of **menarche** is **16-17 years** of age.[7] Five extra years of estradiol production during the teen years (when breast tissue is very sensitive to cancer initiators) significantly increase breast cancer risk, especially for women who never carry a pregnancy to term.

Want to help your daughter begin her menses later rather than earlier? Encourage her to engage in regular vigorous athletic activity, to eat only hormone-free animal products, and to get less exposure to electric light at night.[8]

• Menstruating women can reduce their risk of breast cancer by maintaining regular **menses at 25-30 day intervals**. Since shorter menstrual cycles mean more menstrual cycles and more doses of estrogens—which are produced in greatest abundance at midcycle—it is not surprising that women whose cycles are shorter than 25 days have double the risk of breast cancer. It is astonishing, however, that women with cycles longer than 30 days are also at twice the risk.[9, 10] An easy way to regulate the onset of your periods to 28 days: Sleep in total darkness for 14 days, then with a small light on for three nights, then in a repeating cycle of total darkness for 25 days and light for three nights.

• Another way to moderate your risk from exposure to estradiol is to interfere with your breasts' ability to absorb it. How? Paradoxically, by **consuming plants rich in hormones**. Plant hormones (phytosterols or phytoestrogens)—found in foods and herbs such as lentils, dried beans, tofu and fermented soy products, burdock roots, parsnips, sweet potatoes, pomegranates, red clover, hops, ginseng, and wild yam—stop breast cells from absorbing estradiol. (The action is similiar to tamoxifen but without its side effects.) Estradiol absorption is also blocked by an enzyme available from cooked dried beans and a phytochemical (indole-3-carbinol) found in cabbage and broccoli.[11, 12]

    Estrogens are metabolized by one of two pathways: the short (safe) path or the long (cancer-promoting) path.[13] Phytoestrogens and other estrogens which don't promote cancer take the quicker short path. Estradiol, estrogen replacement therapy, and organochlorine estrogen-mimickers must take the slower long path. When there are plenty of short path estrogens in the blood, carcinogenic estrogens arrive at the breast cells only to find themselves blocked from entry, thus unable to promote cancer.

• Menopausal and postmenopausal women: Doesn't it make sense that taking **estrogen pills** would increase breast cancer risk? Eight percent of breast cancers are attributed to the use of prescribed estrogens.[14] Using estrogen or hormone replacement for more than five years can nearly double your risk of breast cancer and increase your risk of dying from it.[15] The lowest risk increase for women using estrogen replacement is one percent yearly. A

20-year nationwide study of 70,000 nurses published in the June 1995 *New England Journal of Medicine* confirms that combining progestin with estrogen (hormone replacement therapy) still leaves women at greatly increased risk of breast cancer.[16] Risk decreases rapidly once you stop taking hormones, however.

• **Phytoestrogens** also protect menopausal and post-menopausal women from the cancer-promoting effects of fuel combustion, and agricultural, industrial, and household chemicals.[17-20]

• Women who took **DES** have a 44 percent greater risk of breast cancer. And their daughters face greater risk as well.[21]

• What about **birth control pills**? Don't they increase breast cancer risk? Yes. And no. Current birth control pills reduce estradiol absorption and lower risk slightly. But if you used pills in the 1960s and 1970s, you may have increased your risk. Breast cancer risk is lowered if birth control pills are used after pregnancy, but doubled or tripled if used before pregnancy or before the age of 20, or if used for more than five years before the age of 35. After the age of 45, pill users are at no more risk for breast cancer than women who never used them.[22, 23]

## Hereditary Factors

• The risk of breast cancer, if it is "in your family," is probably the breast cancer risk most **overestimated** by women.[24] Previous studies reported genetic links for 10-14 percent of breast cancers, but more recent, more thorough, studies have found only 2-5 percent of breast cancers linked to inherited genetic faults such as those on genes BRCA-1 and BRCA-2.[25, 26]

• Women whose mothers had breast cancer are not quite twice as likely to have breast cancer as women with no maternal history of breast cancer. Women whose mothers were diagnosed with breast cancer before the age of 40 are at exactly double the usual risk. *The older the mother when diagnosed, the lower the risk for the daughter.* A woman whose 70-year-old mother has breast cancer is only at one-and-a-half times greater than average risk of developing it herself.

• Your **siblings' health** has a greater relationship to your risk than your mother's. If your only sister has breast cancer, you're two-and-a-half times as likely to develop it as a woman with a cancer-free sister. If your mother and sister have breast cancer, you're also two-and-a-half times as likely to develop it as a woman with no family history. If your brother has prostate cancer, your risk of breast cancer increases an incredible fourfold.[27]

• Women with a **genetic fault** don't always get breast cancer, although as a group they have a 59 percent chance of developing it by age 50 and an 80 percent chance by age 65. If you are one of the .5 percent of all women with a genetic fault, you do start out one step closer to breast cancer than usual. But the same factors influence the promotion and progression—and reversal—of these cancers as any others. Building powerful immunity (*see* page 79) and developing an anti-cancer lifestyle (*see* page xv) may help as much as prophylactic mastectomy, which can't guarantee freedom from cancer. Indeed, since genetic faults are expressed in the ovaries as well as the breasts, if the breasts are removed, ovarian cancer (which is harder to detect and treat) may be the result.

• At every age, **light-skinned women** are more prone to breast cancer than dark-skinned women. Healthy lifestyle choices can mitigate this risk.

• **Large women** who weigh more than 154 pounds and are over 5 feet 6 inches tall have 3.6 times the risk of a woman under 132 pounds and below 5 feet 3 inches.[28] To counter this, build powerful immunity and exercise regularly.

• You are seven times more likely to get breast cancer if your **waist-to-hip ratio** is over .81 than if it's under .73. Determine your ratio by dividing your waist measurement by your hip measurement.[28] More seaweed in the diet can decrease this risk.

• Postmenopausal women who are 50 pounds or more **overweight** are one-and-a-half times more likely to develop breast cancer. Women who are physically active and eat a cancer-preventing diet lower their risk, no matter how much they weigh.

*From 1985 to 1995 in the U.S., breast cancer took more lives than AIDS.*

## Environmental Factors: Organochlorines

• A great many researchers believe that organochlorines–from sources such as agricultural chemicals, chlorinated water, and plastics–are a major factor in the current epidemic of breast cancer. Organochlorines initiate and promote breast cancer in many ways: They mutate genes, alter breast cells so they absorb more estradiol, suppress the immune system, and mimic the bad effects of estrogen. Despite much evidence, organochlorines are not accepted as a risk factor by orthodoxy.[29] Could this be due to the presence of petrochemical and pharmaceutical corporation executives on the boards of major cancer research institutions?[30]

Organochlorines are chlorine-based chemicals. Herbicides, pesticides, chlorine bleach, most disinfectants, and many plastics, especially vinyl chloride are organochlorines. They enter our bodies in many ways: from drinking water polluted with them, from food grown with agricultural chemicals, from drinking (even more so from showering or swimming in) chlorinated water, from plastics migrating into canned and microwaved foods, and from food or body contact with chlorine-bleached paper products (coffee filters, tampons, paper cups, toilet paper).

## How I Avoid Organochlorines

• I buy only organic butter, dairy, grains, beans, meats.
• I avoid non-organic produce from places where pesticide standards are lax (e.g., Mexican tomatoes, Spanish olive oil).
• I buy and store food in glass, not plastic.
• I don't eat microwaved food; I don't buy canned food.
• I don't drink chlorinated water.
• I avoid showering or swimming in chlorinated water.
• I buy peroxide-bleached or unbleached paper products.
• I use non-chemical cleaning supplies and no bleach.
• I am part of a coalition of publishers urging mills to find ways to produce paper without chlorine-bleaching.

• **Dioxin**, a by-product of chlorine-bleaching, is now present in the water supplies of most industrialized nations. Dioxin has been consistently implicated as a breast cancer promoter. A German study of dioxin-exposed workers showed an 87 percent increase in breast cancer rates after 20 years. Repeated minute exposures can increase risk by 100 percent. (Recent studies offer some hope that breast cancers caused by dioxin are milder than those triggered by other carcinogenic chemicals.)

• Organochlorines are metabolized by the liver and by helpful phytochemicals (especially saponins and indole-3-carbinol). Because they are large and complex, this isn't easy. The majority wind up **stored in fat cells** and breast tissues. Some are eliminated in tears, breast milk, and egg cells (or sperm). What a legacy for our offspring! The tendency of organochlorines to stay in the body is evidenced by the fact that recent samples of fat and breast milk collected from women in the USA and Canada contained organochlorines banned for over three decades (DDT, chlordane, and deldrine) as well as those in current use (DDE and PCBs).

• Here are a few more facts: Women with high levels of agricultural organochlorines in their blood are 4 to 10 times more likely to develop breast cancer than women with low levels.[8] Women with breast cancer have 50–60 percent more PCBs, DDE, and other pesticides and organochlorines in their tissues than women without breast cancer.[31, 10] For each 10-part-per-billion increase in tissue levels of **PCBs** and **DDE** (over 0) there is a 1 percent increase in breast cancer. Women in the United States and Canada currently have 300 ppb PCBs and 1000 ppb DDE in their breast tissues.[32] In New Zealand these rates are 2–4 times higher.[8] These two organochlorines (PCBs and DDE) alone could cause the 1–2 percent yearly increase in breast cancer seen in industrialized nations each year for the past 50 years.

• Two years after **Israel banned the organochlorine pesticides** DDT, y-BHC (lindane), and a-BHC (benzene hexachloride), Israeli women's breast cancer mortality (which had been double that of American women) began to drop, and was ultimately reduced by one-third in women under 44. This research has stood up to severe scrutiny and is a landmark showing the potent ability of environmental chemicals to increase breast cancer.[1]

• **Atrazine**, one of the most widely used herbicides in North America and Europe, causes mammary cancer in laboratory animals and has been linked to elevated risk of ovarian cancer in women.[9]

• Eating only **organically produced animal products** (eggs, milk, cheese, meat) will reduce your dietary exposure to organochlorines by 80 percent. (Meat contributes 55 percent of the chemical residues in most diets; milk, 23 percent.) Eating a completely chemical-free diet is even safer. Supporting organic farmers protects the environment, and pays you back with cleaner water supplies, more wildlife, and healthier offspring.

Collectively, we can let it be known that we want safe food and water. We can let our town boards and city councils know that there are ways to disinfect water without chlorine. We can ask for organic food at our supermarkets and restaurants. We can write and call our legislators when factories pollute. Collective and individual action can make a difference in your risk of breast cancer.

*Worldwide production of organochlorines in 1994 was 40 million tons.*[1]

## Dietary Factors

• Some researchers attribute as much as a quarter of all breast cancers to **dietary fat**.[2] I agree, but not for the reasons you may think. The fats in meat and milk, and the oils of plants, are dietary sources of concentrated agricultural organochlorines. I believe that breast cancer risk is increased not so much by the *amount* of fat in one's diet, but by the *kind* of fat eaten. Low-fat diets prevent breast cancer by reducing organochlorine exposure, not by reducing fat.

• Most of the fats commonly available in Western countries contain large amounts of organochlorines.

• Worse yet, when fats are **hydrogenated**—as in margarine—they form trans-fatty acids which are also carcinogenic.

• Linoleic acid—found in nuts, **corn oil**, and most **margarines**—speeds up both the rate of growth of breast cancers and the rate of metastases in mice when fed at levels ranging from 8 to 50 percent of total dietary fat.[33]

• A diet rich in **olive oil** and **butter** from organic sources can reduce the risk of breast cancer. Olive oil and butter contain phytochemicals that stop the initiation and promotion of breast cancer. Greek women who ate olive oil more than once a day lowered their risk of breast cancer by 25 percent.[34]

• Although women in most countries where fat intake is high do have a greater incidence of breast cancer, women in countries where the diet is high-fat but even-caloried (that is, the total calories do not exceed the individual's needs and the set-point weight is easily maintained) have very low rates of breast cancer, lower even than women from areas where the traditional diet is very low in fat, such as Japan. Women of Crete get 60 percent of their calories from fat, yet have the lowest incidence of breast cancer in the world.[36] Even-caloried diets also boost night-time production of **melatonin**, a hormone that inhibits formation of breast cancer.

• I use **organic fats**, especially olive oil, local butter, and goats' milk cheese, with a lavish hand. Women on low-fat diets who switch to a healthy-fat diet often have less arthritis, insomnia, infertility, hot flashes, irregular menses, and premenstrual symptoms. Organic butter and goat cheese are usually twice as expensive as agribusiness products, but olive oil doesn't have to break your budget. Olive oil produced in Crete, Greece, and Italy is usually organic, whether it says so or not, and—like all olive oil—is extracted by pressing, without the use of any chemicals. (Spanish olive trees are often heavily sprayed, and Spanish oil can be packed in Italy and labeled as Italian oil.) Good quality olive oil, packed in a can to exclude light (and thus preserve the essential fatty acids) is available in my area for a very reasonable price.

• Don't let all the information on organochlorines get you down. Here's the good news: An abundance (5 servings a day) of cooked, canned, frozen, dried, and raw **fruits** and **vegetables** in your diet can lower your breast cancer risk by 46 percent.[12, 34-36] And members of the cabbage family—including broccoli, kale, turnips, radishes, cabbage, and cauliflower—do even more. They contain a phytochemical which helps you metabolize organochlorines, increasing the production of benign metabolic by-products over potentially carcinogenic ones.

*About 45,000 women die annually from breast cancer in the U.S.*

• How do fruits and vegetables prevent cancer? With concentrated amounts of antioxidants, carotenes, folates, selenium, indole-3-carbinol, and other anti-cancer phytochemicals and nutrients in synergistic combinations impossible to duplicate in a pill. I eat some from every category every day:

**Raw** ones for antioxidant vitamin C.

**Oily** ones, such as avocado or purslane, for antioxidant vitamin E.

**Green**, **yellow**, and **orange** ones for antioxidant carotenes (which become vitamin A in the liver).

**Leafy green** ones for anti-cancer folates.

**Garlicky** ones for selenium, the mineral that lowers risk of breast cancer. (Non-organic garlic may be low in selenium.)

**Cabbagey** ones for indole-3-carbinol, to reduce estrogen-related, organochlorine-related, and age-related breast cancers.

*See* "Anti-Cancer Foods," page 29.

• In a Harvard School of Public Health survey, women who ate less than one serving per day of **vitamin A-rich food** (such as cooked greens, carrots, cantaloupe, sweet potatoes, winter squash, stinging nettle) had 25 percent more breast cancer than those who ate two servings a day. (There didn't appear to be any advantage to eating more than two servings though.)

• Foods from the **bean family**, including red clover blossoms, lentils, and all soy products, can decrease breast cancer risk. Legumes contain enzymes which reduce the production of estradiol, and plant hormones which help keep estradiol out of breast cells. The more estradiol in your body, the greater your benefit from eating legumes, especially if you are premenopausal, taking replacement hormones, or regularly ingesting organochlorines.[11, 31]

• Women who eat **red meat** at least once a day have twice the risk of developing breast cancer as women who eat fish, poultry, and dairy products daily.[37] Calorie-balanced diets (where intake balances requirements) lower risk of breast cancer whether they include meat or not. Diets which provide optimum nutrition with the fewest possible calories often include small amounts of meat.

• A Canadian study found women whose diets were high in **fiber** had 30 percent less breast cancer than those with fiber-poor diets. Whole grains, beans, fruits, and vegetables supply fiber.

• **Plastics** used to line cans migrate into food and mimic cancer-promoting estrogens.[38] So do the plastics used when food is heated in microwave ovens. Buy fresh, not canned, produce and avoid microwaved food for greatest protection from breast cancer.

*In 1900, cancer was responsible for 4 percent of deaths worldwide. By 1958, it was responsible for 15 percent of all deaths. By the end of the twentieth century, if trends continue, 40 percent of all adults will have cancer and cancer will be responsible for 25 percent of all deaths.*

## Health-Care Factors

• Regular use of **prescription drugs** can increase breast cancer risk. Beta-blockers treat high blood pressure, but suppress production of anti-cancer melatonin. Prozac and Elavil, both anti-depressants, promote the growth of initiated cancers.[39] Cimetidine, an ulcer medication, acts paradoxically: It blocks the short safe path for estrogens, but it has put some cancers into remission. Long-term use of steroids and cortisones increases risk. Seek out practitioners of Traditional Chinese Medicine, homeopathy, naturopathy, or medical herbalism for alternatives to drugs.

• In a study of 34,000 people who were at normal or low risk of developing cancer, those who had **allergies** were one-third more likely to develop cancer than those who reported freedom from allergies. Those with **asthma** were one-fifth more likely to be diagnosed with cancer. Antihistamines such as Claritin (loratadine), Hismanal (astemizole), and Atarax (hydrocyzine) are known to incite existing cancers to grow more quickly and more aggressively.[39] Do they promote initiated cancer cells too?

• **Chronic viral infections** increase breast cancer risk. Breast cancer in mice can be initiated by a virus passed through the dam's milk. Human cervical cancer is known to be initiated by a virus, and recent studies have shown that Epstein-Barr virus can trigger breast cancer (but only when the immune system is not functioning well.)[39a] Even a chronic bacterial infection can weaken the immune system and increase breast cancer risk. Donnie Yance, a health care provider who works with many women diagnosed with breast cancer, believes that a genetic predisposition to a weak immune system is a very strong risk factor for breast cancer.

• **Iodine** and **thyroid hormones** (both natural and synthetic) generally reduce risk of breast cancer. Max Gerson, M.D., an acclaimed (and controversial) cancer specialist, believed that iodine was critical to the process of countering cancer. Some researchers speculate that the low rate of breast cancer in Japan is due to the iodine-rich diet. **Iodine deficiency** during puberty produces changes (hyperplasia) in breast tissues which can lead to breast cancer later in life. But when supplemental iodine–such as in iodized salt–exceeds need in the adult diet, breast cancer rates increase. Seaweed is an excellent, safe, source of iodine.

   Low iodine levels directly impair thyroid functioning. It is fairly well established that women with **underactive thyroids** are more prone to breast cancer. The incidence of breast cancer is higher in regions where soils are low in iodine. British medical doctors report that large doses of synthetic thyroid can be used with success to treat women with advanced breast cancer.[40]

• Ready for more good news? Having **fibrocystic breasts** won't increase your risk of developing breast cancer. Really. Even if you have lots of lumps. Numerous cysts can make a tiny cancer difficult to feel, but cystic breasts are no more likely to develop cancer than non-cystic breasts. Nine out of ten women will find a benign cyst in their breasts at some time in their lives.[41] Clinically, most women could be diagnosed with fibrocystic breast disease; microscopic examination of breast cells finds signs of this "disease" in 90 percent of all women.[42] Regular mammograms of women with fibrocystic breast disease are as likely to initiate cancer as find it. An anti-cancer lifestyle and regular breast self-massage or self-exam, on the other hand, can actively prevent cancer, as well as providing early detection.

• Although sclerosing adenosis, apocrine metaplasia, duct ectasia, lipoma, fat necrosis, and mastitis are scary sounding, they aren't serious and do not increase risk of breast cancer.[41]

• Having a **biopsy** does not increase your risk of being diagnosed with breast cancer. Almost all biopsies (90 percent) are negative for cancer. There is a risk that the biopsy may leave scar tissue, however, which can later mask a small cancer.

• Regular, **screening mammograms** are dangerous for premenopausal women. For postmenopausal women, they can increase the time between the detection of cancer and death (from any cause), but they don't reduce actual risk of cancer, nor do they prevent cancer. (For more on mammograms, *see* pages 93-103.)

• In a ten-year trial in England, breast cancer deaths were reduced by 20 percent among women who did a monthly **breast self-exam**. (To learn how, *see* pages 68-74.)

## Environmental Factors: Radiation

• According to researcher John Gofman, 75 percent of breast cancers are caused by radiation.[43] Breast tissue is quite sensitive to radiation, especially during the fertile years. High-level radiation is more damaging than low-level (diagnostic) radiation, but low-level radiation does initiate cancer when you accumulate enough of it.[44] Risk of breast cancer increases with increasing exposure to radiation. Radiation-induced cancers may appear ten years after exposure, but incidence doesn't peak until 40 years after exposure.[45]

• One-and-a-half percent of the women in North America (one million women) carry the **gene for ataxia-telangiectasia** (AT), a rare nervous system disorder. While only one out of 20 of them will develop AT, the difficult-to-detect gene makes them all six times more likely to develop breast cancer after exposure to x-rays—such as mammograms. Researchers at the University of North Carolina say the gene may account for up to 14 percent of all U.S. breast cancer cases.[1]

*Breast cancer diagnosis is the most expensive (and second most common) cause of medical litigation in the U.S.A., accounting for 27 percent of cancer-related claims at a cost of over $2 million per claim in 1994.*

• Some doctors claim that the **amount of radiation** in a mammogram is so small that it's more dangerous to fly coast to coast. Not true. One mammogram is not a large amount of radiation, but it is much more than a plane ride. And a mammographic series consists of *four* mammograms. Furthermore, radiation focused

## How Much Radiation?

- One week at a high altitude (Denver) = less than 1 millirad
- Jet flight of 6 hours = 5 millirads
- Chest x-ray = 16 millirads (about 1 millirad reaches breast tissue)
- Smallest possible dose from a screening mammogram done with the best possible equipment = 340 millirads

closely and directly on the breast tissues is far more likely to initiate cancer than whole-body radiation (such as at high altitudes).

• Between 1951 and 1963, over 200 nuclear bombs were detonated in the deserts of Nevada in the U.S.A. In addition, 109 nuclear bombs were detonated in the South Pacific between 1946 and 1958. **Radioactive fallout** from these tests contaminated milk, meat, fish, and vegetables throughout Canada and the U.S.A. during much of this time. Exposure to nuclear fallout substantially increases risk of breast cancer, especially if that radiation is absorbed by the developing breast tissues of women 8-20 years old.[46] More seaweed in the daily diet and an anti-cancer lifestyle can help mitigate this risk.

• Exposure to low-level contamination from **nuclear waste** and nuclear "accidents" (including intentional discharges disguised as accidents) may account for a significant amount of the rise in breast cancer during the past 50 years.[47] Breast cancer mortality in the area surrounding the Millstone nuclear power plant on Long Island has risen 40 percent in the 17 years since it was started up. Since 1950, breast cancer deaths among women living within 50 miles of nuclear plants have increased ten-fold overall (twenty-five-fold in some locations—such as Rowe, Massachusetts near the Yankee nuclear power plant), according to the National Cancer Institute.

• I could not locate specific data on women living near medical or military nuclear facilities, but the Nuclear Regulatory Commission admits that 1 out of every 285 people exposed to the legal dose limit of 100 millirems per year of released radiation will get a fatal cancer as a result. (For x-rays, 100 millirems equals 100 millirads.)

## Environmental Factors: Petrochemicals

• Rigorous scientific proof that specific petrochemicals increase breast cancer is lacking, but the circumstantial evidence is quite clear. For example: Breast cancer rates are 60 percent greater among postmenopausal women living within a half-mile of a chemical plant in Syosset, Long Island, New York, than the rates in virtually identical communities farther away from the plant.[29]

Handling and breathing petroleum products such as **gasoline** and **kerosene**, or petrochemicals including **formaldehyde** and **benzene**, is inherently risky, as is living where they are stored, or where their manufacture or use allows them to contaminate water supplies, the soil, and the air.

• Benzene and other combustion by-products produced when oil, gasoline, or kerosene are burned are known to induce and promote mammary cancers in animals.

## Environmental Factors: Electromagnetic Fields

• Electric and electromagnetic fields are ubiquitous in our lives, but recent years have brought an ever-increasing stream of information on the detrimental effects of constant exposure to such fields. Both men and women regularly exposed to electrical fields at work have startling increases in breast cancer rates.[48-50] The rate of breast cancer among male electricians, power station operators, and telephone linemen is 6 times more than expected.[51, 52] Women employed in the **electrical trades** run a 38 percent greater risk of dying from breast cancer than other working women, while female electrical engineers' risk is 73 percent greater. Women who install, repair, or do line work with telephones are 200 times more likely than average to have breast cancer.[53]

• It isn't just high power electrical transmission lines, **microwave towers**, and **phone cables** that increase risk of breast cancer. Exposure to **extra low frequency electromagnetic fields** (EMFs) does, too.[48] EMFs disturb the normal growth pattern of cells by interfering with their hormonal, enzymatic, and chemical

signals, causing DNA damage and switched-on oncogenes (cellular codes that can begin a cancer cascade). EMFs also reduce production of melatonin; deficiencies of this brain chemical are linked
to increased breast cancer.

• The 60-hertz magnetic field of your **house wiring** and your
phone line produces EMFs. So do computer terminals, TVs, re-
frigerators, hair dryers, electric blankets, clocks, ovens, electric
fans, vibrators, and all other **electrical appliances**.

• EMFs go through lead; ordinary filters don't touch them. But
they don't travel far. Within 28 inches of the source, they are less
than 80 percent as powerful. Hair dryers and bedside clocks do
more damage than TVs because they are close to the head (and
the pineal and pituitary glands) for regular, extended periods of time.

## Lifestyle Factors

• Tobacco smoke contains aromatic amines that initiate breast cancer. Pre-menopausal women who smoke **commercial cigarettes**
daily are twice as likely to get breast cancer as nonsmoking women.
Smoking two packs a day for ten or more years doubles the risk
again. And the longer one smokes, the greater the risk.[54] Worse
yet, women who smoke cigarettes heal more slowly after surgery,
have more side effects from chemotherapy, and are more likely to
die of breast cancer once they develop it. Women who smoke more
than 40 cigarettes a day are 75 percent more likely to die of their
breast cancer than women who don't smoke. *Important*: Once you
quit smoking, your risk slowly returns to normal.

• When ordinary chemical phosphate fertilizers are used to grow
tobacco, radon is liberated from the soil. It outgasses and sticks to
the undersides of the resinous tobacco leaves, where it quickly
breaks down, leaving behind high concentrations of radon-daughters (radioactive lead-210 and polonium-210). Many researchers
implicate these radon-daughters, not tobacco itself, in the epidemic
of lung and breast cancers among smokers of commercial tobacco.
Moderate use of organically grown plants, even if you inhale, is
unlikely to increase your risk of breast cancer. (It increases your
risk of heart disease, however, which kills far more women than

breast cancer does.) Combustion by-products from chlorine-bleached cigarette papers are carcinogenic; use a pipe.

• Some studies show increased risk of breast cancer with as few as four **alcoholic** drinks a week, others that the risk is not increased unless you're drinking daily, others that you have to start drinking before the age of 30, still others that the greatest risk comes from regular drinking before the first pregnancy. For breast health, drink only organic wines and beers in moderation.

• A recent National Institutes of Health study found a 100 percent increase in risk of breast cancer when women under 55 drank 9 drinks a week. The risk increase was 250 percent for women who drank 2 or more drinks daily.

• Alcohol in the blood temporarily blocks the safe short path for estrogen utilization, allowing long path (carcinogenic) estrogens more time to get to the receptor sites. The longer the short path is blocked, that is, the greater the amount and duration of alcohol consumption, the greater the risk for breast cancer, but more so for premenopausal than postmenopausal women, and even more so before a first full-term pregnancy.[55-56] Daily use of alcohol increases breast cancer risk by blocking the short path for extended periods. In addition, daily use hinders the liver's ability to break down hormones and chemicals, and reduces production of melatonin, a brain chemical that inhibits proliferating breast cancer cells and increases levels of naturally occurring antioxidants in breast cells.

• Strangely enough, daily consumption of alcohol does not appear to increase the risk for women who are already at high risk.

• The Centers for Disease Control examined the death certificates of nearly three million women (1979-1987) to see how many had died of breast cancer and whether they clustered in any occupations. They did: **teacher, librarian,** and **religious worker**. These jobs are not inherently risky, but women so occupied may have common characteristics, such as delayed childbearing, that put them at increased risk.

• A National Cancer Institute report done by Suzanne Haynes found **lesbians** three times likelier than heterosexual women to get breast cancer.[57] She speculates that the increase is due to greater alcohol consumption and body fat, fewer pregnancies, and limited access to health care, not to sexual orientation.

• The pineal gland reacts to **light at night** by reducing production of breast cancer-inhibiting melatonin. Constant exposure to illumination at night (even from a night light or street light through your window) reduces the production of melatonin as much as daily use of alcohol, and may increase breast cancer risk by as much.[13] According to John Ott, pioneer researcher into the health effects of light, this risk can be countered by working under full-spectrum lighting or by getting direct sun on your closed eyes (minus contacts or glasses) for 5–15 minutes daily, as well as by sleeping in a totally darkened room.[58]

• **Sunscreen** is promoted for preventing skin cancer, but it also prevents the formation of vitamin D, an antioxidant which inhibits the initiation phase of breast cancer. Habitual sunscreen users have unusually low levels of vitamin D. **Mineral oil**, found in many skincare products, also blocks production and absorption of vitamin D.

• The belief that **shaving the underarms** and applying **antiperspirants** promotes cancer has never been put to the test. Shaving does abrade the skin, making it more open to infection and more porous to the irritating effects of aluminum in antiperspirants (even those "natural" clear stones). Habitual irritation stresses the underlying lymph vessels, and can hinder the immune system's ability to deal with cancer cells.

• Many women have told me they eliminated the lumpiness of their breasts and reduced their premenstrual tenderness by banning their **bra**. In a study of 5,000 women, those who reported irritation and red marks from wearing a bra were twice as likely to develop breast cancer as those who did not. Women who wore bras for more than 12 hours a day increased their risk by a factor of six.[59] Women who generally go braless reduce their risk by a factor of 20. The elastic of the bra encircling the chest effectively hinders immune response, slows lymph fluid circulation, and traps energy in the breasts. Underwire bras magnify these problems.

*About 175,000 U.S. women receive a diagnosis of breast cancer each year.*

• Women who exercise regularly are 35 percent less likely to get breast cancer. An intense period of exercise or training during the teen years seems to confer lifelong protection, but regular exercise begun at any age decreases breast cancer risk (up to 72 percent for women who bear children, and by 27 percent for those who don't).[60] Exercise directly decreases estradiol absorption and also stops the formation of carcinogenic metabolic by-products from the breakdown of estrogens. Exercise improves the functioning of the immune system and relieves stress. Even five minutes, three or four times a day, counts as exercise. Do it.

• Do some women get cancer instead of getting angry? Do some women get cancer because their inner children are starved for attention? Do some women get breast cancer because they are **constantly going, going, going** like a cancer cell that can't stop growing, growing, growing? Maybe.[61]

• The few studies done on the connection between emotions and cancer found that "difficult" cancer patients (those who don't do as they are told, who are demanding, and who express their uncomfortable feelings) live longer after diagnosis and have less recurrence of cancer. The "typical" woman with cancer is overwhelmingly **eager to please others** and generally puts others' needs and feelings before her own (as many women are encouraged—or forced—to do).

• Two medical doctors, women with years of experience, sought me out when I was in New Zealand to tell me that the unexpected death of a loved one was the single greatest cause of breast cancer they'd seen. The Simontons, Bernie Siegel, and William LeShan—healers with decades of experience helping those dancing with cancer—have also observed that emotional distress can promote a cancer that has been initiated but is lying dormant. (And that emotional healing, self-love, and forgiveness can be instrumental in sending cancer into remission.)

*Breast cancer is the leading cause of death among women 35-54 (in the U.S.). For women over 55, breast cancer is second only to heart disease as the primary cause of death.*

# Breast Cancer?

These things are strongly implicated in the initiation, promotion, or growth of breast cancer.

**Hormones**, especially estrogens such as estradiol.
• Sources: Your ovaries, your fat cells, commercial meat and milk, hormone pills, steroids, cortisone.
• Reduced by: Strenuous physical activity, pregnancy and lactation, balanced-calorie diet, menopause.

**Organochlorines**, pesticides, herbicides, bleach, plastics.
• Sources: Chemical farming practices, drinking and bathing in chlorinated water, bleached paper, water pollution.
• Reduced by: Eating organically grown food, filtering drinking water, filtering bathing water, using unbleached paper, using less plastic, buying fresh (not canned) food.

**Radiation**, especially when young.
• Sources: Mammograms, fallout, x-rays.
• Reduced by: Avoidance. Doses are cumulative.

**EMFs** (Electromagnetic Fields)
• Sources: TVs, hair dryers, microwave towers and ovens, computer monitors, all electrical appliances and lines.
• Reduced by: Distance rather than shielding.

**Agribusiness tobacco**
• Sources: Smoking cigarettes, living with someone who does.
• Reduced by: Avoidance. Smoke organic tobacco or herbs in a pipe.

**Excessive use of alcohol**
**Excessive calories in the diet**
• Sources: Easy availability, peer pressure, convenience.
• Reduced by: Wise food choices, herbal infusions, hugs.

**Growing older**
• Source: Living long.
• Reduced by: Dying young. (Not worth it.)

# Breast Health!

These things offer ways to counter and reverse the initiation, promotion, and growth of breast cancer.

## Consumption of phytoestrogens
• Sources: Tofu, red clover infusion, pomegranates, roots.

## A diet rich in cabbage family plants, grains, and beans.
• Source: Semi-vegetarian diet.

## High dietary intake of carotenes
• Sources: Dark leafy greens, orange and yellow produce.

## High dietary levels of vitamin C complex
• Sources: Fresh, raw fruits and vegetables.
• Reduced by: Oxidation from washing, heating, aging.

## High dietary levels of vitamin E
• Sources: Sunflower seeds, freshly ground wheat, freshly pressed oils, olive oil, flax oil.
• Reduced by: Heat, light, time.

## High dietary levels of selenium
• Sources: Organically grown garlic, onions, mushrooms.

## Sufficient production and absorption of vitamin D
• Sources: Sunlight, 10 minutes daily; sardines, tuna.

## Adequate levels of melatonin production
• Sources: Darkness, low-calorie diet.
• Reduced by: Alcohol, beta-blockers, lights on at night.

## Regular, significant exercise throughout one's life.
• Sources: Active lifestyle, yoga, dance, moving!

**Note**: Supplements in pill form do not have the cancer-preventive effects of vitamin and mineral complexes found in whole foods, weeds, and herbs. In fact, some supplements can promote cancer.[62]

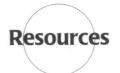

# Resources

• National Cancer Institute **Risk Assessment Test**: 1-800-4-CANCER

• *Breast Cancer: Reducing Your Risk*, Mary Eades, Bantam, 1991

• **"Pesticide–Breast Cancer Link**," articles and bibliography for $5 from New York Campaign Against Pesticides, PO Box 6005, Albany, NY 12206-0005

★ Reprints of **"The Breast Cancer Cover-Up"** from Mother Jones, May/June 1994 issue are available for $1.95 from M.J. Reprints, 731 Market St., Suite 600, San Francisco, CA 94103.

• Food & Water, National Citizens' Campaign to Stop Pesticides, 1-800-EAT-SAFE

• "Public Testimony Before Texas Officials: Breast Cancer and Radiation," 1994, six videotapes; available from Foundation for a Compassionate Society, 1-800-852-9741

• Environmental Research Foundation, PO Box 5036, Annapolis, MD 21403

• My favorite **non-chemical household cleaners**: vinegar, baking soda, sweet birch twig tea, bay leaf infusion.

• **Full-spectrum lights** from Ott-Lites, 1-800-842-8848

• **Unbleached paper products** and **shower filters** from:

Seventh Generation, 49 Hercules Dr., Colchester, VT 05446; 1-800-456-1177

Real Goods, 966 Mazzoni St., Ukiah, CA 95482; 1-800-762-7325

# 2.
# Can Foods Prevent Cancer?

Absolutely, without a doubt, eating certain foods can prevent breast cancer. Analysis of 156 studies linking diet and cancer found extraordinarily consistent evidence that some foods actively protect cells from undergoing cancerous changes, especially breast, cervical, ovarian, and prostate cells.[1] While these foods don't guarantee freedom from cancer, they are vital elements of an anti-cancer lifestyle.

The United States National Research Council states that 35-70 percent of all U.S. cancer deaths are related to diet and that 60 percent of the cancer incidence in women is related to diet.

Fruits, vegetables, whole grains, and beans contain phytochemicals that are active against cancer initiation in many direct and indirect ways. They neutralize carcinogenic compounds. They capture and neutralize free radicals. They protect DNA from environmental damage. They prevent the activation of oncogenes. They nourish anti-cancer enzymes in the digestive tract and strengthen the immune system cells which search out and eliminate cancer cells. [2-5]

If cancer has already begun to grow, phytochemicals can disrupt the processes necessary for the growth and spread of the tumor. They block metastasis by checking the growth of blood vessels to the tumor. Some foods can even reverse damage to the DNA and turn oncogenes off. [6-8]

Here's the rub: It doesn't work as well if it isn't organic.[9, 10] An apple a day may even promote breast cancer if it's been heavily sprayed with pesticides. Eating anti-cancer foods as the mainstay of your diet will improve your chances of living a long life even if they aren't organic, but choosing organic foods pays the extra dividend of knowing you're investing in the health of future generations as well as your own.

# Anti-Cancer Foods

These foods are wonderful preventive medicines for all women who love their breasts and want to keep them, as well as trustworthy complementary medicines for women dancing with cancer. (Glossary of anti-cancer phytochemicals begins on page 46.)

**ALMONDS** (*Prunus dulcis*)
"Eat three almonds a day," was the first cancer prevention remedy I heard. They were believed to work because of their relation to apricot pits (a source of laetrile).[11] Now we know it's their phytochemicals—protease inhibitors, phytate, genistein, lignans and benzaldehyde—that are anti-cancer. *See* nuts; *see* apricots.

**AMARANTH** (*Amaranthus retroflexus* and other species)
All wild and cultivated species of amaranth give us a double dose of cancer prevention by producing both greens and grain. The greens are a superb source of antioxidants, folic acid, carotenes, calcium and other vital minerals. The seeds are high in protein, and rich in lignans and protease inhibitors.

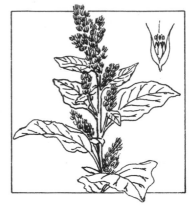

**APPLES** (*Malus communis*)
The chlorogenic and caffeic acids found abundantly in apples block formation of cancers and help prevent recurrences in women dancing with cancer. Raw and cooked apples, fresh-pressed apple cider, and unpasteurized apple cider vinegar are particularly good ways to get the anti-cancer benefits of apples.

**APRICOTS/APRICOT PITS** (*Armeniaca vulgaris*)
Apricots, especially when dried, are an exceptional source of anti-cancer carotenes. Bitter apricot pits (and peach pits) contain the famous anti-cancer compound laetrile, also known as amygdalin or vitamin $B_{17}$. Because laetrile breaks down into hydrogen

cyanide (and glucose and benzaldehyde) it is considered poisonous by the FDA. Nonetheless, apricots pits are available in many
Asian markets and by mail (*see* Resources). The standard daily
dose is one apricot or peach pit for every ten pounds/4.5 kilo-
grams of body weight. One source says a dose is "a little less than
what makes you queasy." Some people bake the pits for 20 minutes at 300° F in a well-ventilated kitchen and drive off the cyanide
gas (benzaldehyde is not affected by heat), but this may be counterproductive (*see* page 156).

**BARLEY/BARLEY GRASS** (*Hordeum vulgare*)
   Like all seeds (grains and beans are seeds), barley is a good source
of protease inhibitors and lignans. Barley grass, often sold in tablets, is rich in carotenes and chlorophyll. *See* cereal grasses.

**BEANS** (*Phaseolus vulgaris*)
   Dried (not green) beans are a superb ally for women concerned
about breast cancer. Dried beans offer cancer-inhibiting enzymes
that prevent the initiation and recurrence of breast cancer. They
contain or stimulate production of genistein, protease inhibitors,
lignans, phytosterols, and fatty acids. One cup/250 ml of cooked
or canned beans daily is ideal. To reduce gas, soak beans overnight and discard the soaking water before cooking them. *See* soybeans.

**BEETS/BEETROOT** (*Beta rubra*)
   Extract of beet root kills cancer cells in the laboratory. Grated
raw beets nourish the liver and strengthen immunity. *See* greens.

**BOK CHOY** (*Brassica chinensis*) *See* cabbage family.

**BROCCOLI** (*Brassica oleracea*)
   Not only an exceptional source of anti-cancer chlorophyll, carotenes, protease inhibitors, lutein, indoles, sulforaphane,
glucosinolates, and dithiolthiones, broccoli is also extraordinarily
good at blocking cancer initiation and a powerful ally for women
choosing radiation therapy. *See* cabbage family.

**BRUSSELS SPROUTS** (*Brassica oleracea*) (Yes, the same botanical name as broccoli, cabbage, collards, cauliflower, and kale.)
   These miniature cabbages are an exceptionally good source of
protease inhibitors, glucosinolates, and lutein. *See* cabbage family.

### BURDOCK ROOT (*Arctium lappa*)

Whether used as an anti-cancer food or an anti-cancer herb, burdock excels. Rich in benzaldehyde, phytosterols, glycosides, mokko lactone, and arctic acid, burdock root prevents cancers initiated by chemicals and radiation (whether environmental or as chosen treatments), thwarts *in situ* cancers of the breast and cervix, and helps block recurrences. Sold in Oriental markets as "gobo," burdock root is an exotic vegetable in most American kitchens, but its sweet, rich taste is wonderful in any cooked dish where you'd use carrot. *See* Materia Medica.

### CABBAGE (*Brassica oleracea*)

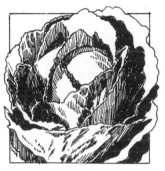

A garden mainstay and a prized medicine for over 4,000 years, cabbage shares the honors with broccoli and Brussels sprouts as the best anti-cancer food, but surpasses them in its ability to adapt to dozens of delicious recipes. (*See* page 307.) Cabbage is most medicinal and easiest to digest when fermented (sauerkraut) or cooked (but not overcooked). Cabbage contains chlorophyll, dithiolthiones, flavonoids, indoles, isothiocyanates, polyphenols, caffeic acid, ferulic acid, folic acid, antioxidants, carotenes, and lutein. Cabbage is also a superb ally used externally; *see* page 115.

### CABBAGE FAMILY (*Brassica* species)

(E.g.: arugala, broccoli, bok choy, Brussels sprouts, cabbage, cauliflower, collards, daikon, horseradish, kale, mustard greens, radishes, rutabaga, shepherd's purse, and turnips.)

Cabbage family plants contain more anti-cancer compounds than any other foods. One or more servings daily from this tasty group is a mainstay of any anti-cancer diet. Their ability to strengthen the immune system and block the initiation and growth of cancers is due to a variety of constituents. (*See* above, under "Cabbage.")

The more cabbage family plants you eat and the more frequently you eat them, the less your risk of developing cancer. Frequent small doses are more protective than occasional large doses. For the greatest benefit, eat some cabbage family plants raw, some fermented, and some cooked. Raw cabbage family plants slightly suppress thyroid activity; cooked or fermented ones have little effect on the thyroid.

**CARROTS** (*Daucus carota*)

Carrots are on everybody's list of foods that prevent and cure cancer. They are especially effective against cancers of the breasts and lungs, and are one of the best sources of antioxidant carotenes, carotenoids, and chlorogenic acids. (The word *carotene* is derived from carrot, in fact.) Carrots also contain asparagin, a kidney-active alkaloid found in asparagus and poke root. Eating carrots helps tissues resist radiation damage. Grated raw carrot poultices soothe inflamed breast tissues and are a folk remedy against tumors and abscesses of the breasts. Carrot broth can help relieve mouth sores caused by chemotherapy.

**CAULIFLOWER** (*Brassica oleracea*)   *See* cabbage family.

**CELERY/CELERY SEEDS** (*Apium graveolens*)

Celery, eaten in quantity, raw or cooked, is mildly anti-cancer. It is an excellent food for women with breast cancer, especially those choosing chemotherapy, because it is rich in antioxidants, folic acid, and mineral salts, as well as constitutents that strengthen liver functioning, improve production of hydrochloric acid in the stomach, protect the lungs from infection, improve cellular metabolism, build red blood cells quickly, and strengthen the adrenals. Celery seeds are richer in anti-cancer phytochemicals, especially polyacetylenes and phthalides.

**CEREAL GRASSES**

The grasses of most cereals (grains)—such as wheat, rye, barley, and rice—are edible, highly nutritious, and cancer preventive.[12] Ann Wigmore made a career of promoting wheat grass (sprouted for 7–10 days and freshly juiced) for health; but mature cereal grasses—like oatstraw—are actually more effective. Anti-cancer compounds such as chlorophyll, folic acid, antioxidants, carotenes, minerals, and essential amino acids peak in grasses just before they begin to joint, about 200 days from seed. If you don't grow your own (but do consider it if you have a garden or yard; it's really quite easy), oatstraw is sold in the herb section (and compressed cereal grass in the supplement section) of your health food store. *See also* barley, oats, and wheat.

**CHICKPEAS** (*Cicer arietinum*)

Also known as garbanzo beans, chickpeas contain asparagin and are one of the richest known sources of protease inhibitors.

**COLLARDS** (*Brassica oleracea*)  *See* cabbage family; *see* greens.

**CORN** (*Zea mays*)
A worldwide study found a very strong correlation between low death rates from breast cancer and high consumption of fresh or dried corn (or beans or rice). Corn reduces breast cancer risk by influencing the output of thyroid hormones and by providing protease inhibitors. *See* oil.

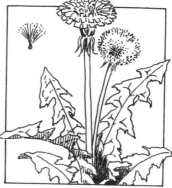

**CUCUMBERS** (*Cucumis melon*)
Garden cucumbers contain an anti-tumor compound called cucurbitacin as well as protease inhibitors. The roots of wild cucumber (*Echinocystis lobata*) are said to be strongly cytotoxic.

**DANDELION** (*Taraxacum officinale*)
*See* greens *and* Materica Medica.

**FASTING**
I do not fast. I believe that it is critically important to health to eat as hunger dictates. Snacking on fruits, vegetables, yogurt, and whole grain chips helps prevent cancer; fasting does not. Max Gerson, M.D., author of many books on natural treatment of cancer, felt that fasting caused those with cancer to "go downhill terribly."[13] Helmut Keller, M.D., who also specializes in natural treatments for cancer, concurs: Most fasting programs lead to malnutrition, and malnutrition leads nowhere but to an increase in tumors.

**FIGS** (*Ficus carica*)
Figs, mentioned in the Bible as a cancer cure, contain the anti-cancer phytochemical benzaldehyde. In Japanese hospitals, poultices and injections of fig distillate are used against human cancers.

**FLAX SEED** (*Linum usitatissimum*)
Flax seeds and flax seed meal are delicious additions to breads, pancakes, and muffiins. They are exceptional sources of anti-cancer lignans and acids such as gallic acid, ferulic acid, chlorogenic acid, and coumaric acid. They appear to be anti-estrogenic and quite specific against breast cancer.[14] *See* oil.

## FRESH FOOD

Fresh food–food which has not been stored, shipped, frozen, dried, precooked, or preserved–is the best source of anti-cancer, antioxidant vitamin C. Vitamin C is easily dissipated by exposure to light, moisture, air, heat, water, or freezing, thus, the fresher the food, the more vitamin C it contains.[15]

Inadequate vitamin C intake is well-documented as an independent risk factor for ductal carcinoma *in situ,* lobular carcinoma *in situ,* and cervical dysplasia.

Eating just two weed leaves a day, especially if they're eaten within seconds of being picked, will give you lots of real vitamin C, strengthen your immune sytem, and help you prevent cancer. Synthetic ascorbic acid, whether added to foods or sold as vitamin C, can disturb normal vitamin C metabolism. *See* vitamins.

## GARLIC *(Allium sativum)*

Garlic, the queen of cancer-preventive and cancer-inhibiting foods, counters the initiation, promotion, and recurrence of many kinds of cancer.[17] Unusually rich in anti-tumor elements selenium and germanium, garlic also contains an abundance of antioxidants, isoflavones, and allyl sulfides.

Garlic has been clinically proven to inhibit the growth of breast cancer cells. The National Cancer Institute recognizes it as a preventive against cancer. In Russia, doctors use fresh garlic extracts to treat human cancer. In the laboratory, garlic cured breast can cers in mice. Garlic prevents cancer best when consumed at the same time as carcinogens. Its effectiveness is dose-dependent.

Garlic is a superb complementary medicine for women choosing chemotherapy. Clinical studies show that it protects the liver, the heart, and the blood vessels better than capsules of vitamin E.

Raw garlic is far more effective than cooked or encapsulated garlic; the active principle is linked with the smell. As little as half a clove of raw garlic a day strengthens immunity and increases the number and power of natural killer cells. Eating an entire bulb daily makes these cells 140-160 percent more effective at killing cancer than usual. Hard to envision eating raw garlic? Try " Garlic Toast Country Style," page 310.

*"In Corsica there are villages where cancer is unheard of. There the people live chiefly on garlic, home produce, and goat's cheese, and no chemical fertilizers are used."* Maurice Messegue, herbalist [16]

### GINGER (*Zingiber officinale*)

Ginger, used consistently, even in small doses, is remarkably effective at preventing the initiation of breast cancer. Ginger contains many anti-cancer phytochemicals, including antioxidants and carotenes. *See* Seasoning Herbs; *see* Materia Medica.

### GRAPES/RAISINS (*Vinis vinifera*)

The grape cure has always fascinated me, as I crave grapes with an overwhelming passion whenever I'm ill. Consuming nothing but grapes for several weeks is said to put primary tumors into remission and prevent recurrences. Grapes supply an abundance of anti-cancer trace minerals, selenium, antioxidants, and acids such as ellagic acid. Dried grapes (raisins) are rich in tannins and caffeic acid. They're antimutagenic and particularly good at preventing breast cancers that arise with age.

### GREENS

Dark leafy greens (e.g., collards, mustard, dandelion, nettles, kale, amaranth, and lamb's quarter) are rich in cancer-preventing carotenes, chlorophyll, antioxidants, folic acid, flavonoids, and—if fresh and lightly washed—vitamin C. It's a rare day that I don't eat a cup or more of greens, cooked or raw, seasoned with a big spoonful of my homemade, calcium-rich herbal vinegars. Greens are excellent complementary medicine for those choosing radiation therapies. I do limit my consumption of cooked swiss chard, spinach, and beet greens as they interfere with calcium metabolism.

### HERBS *See* Greens; *see* Nourishing Herbal Infusions; *see* Seasoning Herbs. *See also* "Plants That May Induce Cancer," page 290.

### HORSERADISH (*Amoracia rusticana*)

This cabbage-family plant with a pungent root offers many anti-cancer acids, such as carbonic acid, silicic acid, phosphatic acid, sulfuric acid, and hydrochloric acid. *See* cabbage family.

### JUICING

There is an immense literature on the supposed benefits of juicing raw fruits and vegetables. Although not detrimental to health, raw juice is no more nourishing than a milk shake from organic ingredients. Few of the claims made for juices are factual. Juices are not as easily digested as cooked foods. The mechanical action of the juicer does not break open a significant number of cell walls.

(Max Gerson, M.D., who advocated using fresh juices as part of cancer treatment, complained that no juicer did a good job and used a shredder and a press instead.) Fresh juice is not predigested; the enzymes in the raw juice are not a significant aid in digestion. It's more difficult—not less—to assimilate anti-cancer nutrients and phytochemicals from juices. The fiber in fruits and vegetables—which improves uptake by slowing transit time—is thrown away, allowing the juice to move through the gut too quickly to be absorbed. For optimal health, I eat some foods raw (more in hot weather) but most food cooked. And have a glass of carrot juice only every now and then, as a treat.

## KALE (*Brassica oleracea*)

Kale is an excellent source of chlorophyll, indoles, and carotenes, especially the ultra anti-cancer carotene, lutein. Kale is a top-of-the-list cancer preventive vegetable. *See* cabbage family; *see* greens.

## LAMB'S QUARTER (*Chenopodium album, C. quinoa*)

Like amaranth, lamb's quarter is both a cultivated grain crop and a common garden weed. Consumption of the leaves (rich in carotenes, folic acid, and antioxidants) and/or the seeds (rich in protease inhibitors) can help prevent cancer initiation. During the summer I eat the greens raw and cooked, and freeze extras. In the fall I harvest and dry the whole plant, seeds and leaves. I replace up to 20 percent of the flour in any recipe (brownies, cornbread, pancakes) with lamb's quarter seeds and leaves ground in a blender. I add them whole to soups, bean dishes, and tomato sauces.

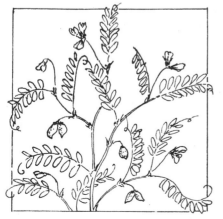

## LENTILS (*Lens culinaris*)

Lentils are one of the oldest of all cultivated crops. Extraordinarily rich in protease inhibitors, genistein, and lignans, all kinds of lentils have proven themselves capable of reversing cancerous cellular changes and helping cells repair damaged DNA.[6] Highly recommended for women at high risk of breast cancer and those wanting to prevent recurrence.

**MILLET** (*Panicum milliaceum*)
This tasty seed is the staple grain crop for many Africans, and is a good source of protease inhibitors, lignans, laetrile, and carotenes.

## NOURISHING HERBAL INFUSIONS
My daily cup of nourishing herbal infusion is my safeguard against cancer, my longevity tonic, and my beauty treatment—all in one cup. Herbal teas are pleasant, but they don't extract the anti-cancer compounds and mineral richness that is available from nourishing herbal infusions. (Instructions for making an infusion are on page 294.) I use one nourishing herb at a time, rather than mixing them, so I can savor their individual flavors and their unique effects on me. Nourishing herbal infusions that are renowned for helping prevent—perhaps even cure—cancer include comfrey leaf, stinging nettle leaf, violet leaf, burdock root, red clover blossoms/tops, and oatstraw. They also help prevent side effects from chemotherapy and radiation. Nourishing herbal infusions contain antioxidants, phytosterols, chlorophyll, carotenes, and acids. *See* Materia Medica for individual herbs.

## NUTS & SEEDS
Organically grown nuts (especially almonds, walnuts, black walnuts, and pecans) and seeds (such as sunflower, sesame, flax, and amaranth seeds) were excellent cancer preventives in clinical studies. All nuts and seeds are good sources of anti-cancer protease inhibitors, essential fatty acids, and antioxidants. Rancid nuts (e.g., pre-roasted nuts, and nuts sold shelled and broken) can be carcinogenic. *See* almonds; *see* flax; *see* oil; *see* sunflower.

## OATS/OATSTRAW (*Avena sativa*)
Oats, being seeds, are a good source of protease inhibitors. Oatstraw, the grass of oats, is rich in carotenes and folic acid. Both are good sources of antioxidants and chlorogenic acids. Oat cereal and oatstraw infusion are important parts of an anti-stress, anti-cancer diet. Oats eaten regularly can increase libido, balance hormones, protect the adrenal glands, balance the thyroid, and improve the

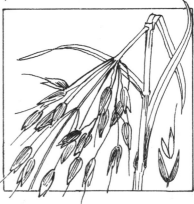

strength of the veins. Everyone loves a cup of mellow oatstraw infusion, especially women worried about a breast lump, women choosing chemotherapy, and women in the midst of sudden menopause.

## OIL

Have you heard that breast cancer is connected to fat intake? Do you eat less oil because of that?[18] I don't. While I do agree that there is a connection between breast cancer and dietary fat, it's not the one we usually hear about. **The kind of fat you eat is more important than the amount.** Rancid fats and hydrogenated fats, even in small amounts, increase the risk of cancer.

I use olive oil. Fresh, organic olive oil is an anti-cancer food, even when consumed lavishly.[19] Women of Crete get 45-60 percent of their calories from fat—mostly fresh olive oil—yet are the least likely of any women in the world to die of breast cancer.

Studies show the strongest link between fat and breast cancer when the diet is high in linoleic acid, the major fatty acid in safflower, corn, soy, and sunflower oils. These oils, although promoted as healthy, are unstable and go rancid shortly after being extracted. **Rancid oil is carcinogenic.** Olive oil resists rancidity.

Oil-bearing seeds (including grains, beans, and nuts) are protected from rancidity by antioxidant vitamin E. Once they are broken open, they (and their oils) lose vitamin E to oxygen, heat, and light. When the available vitamin E is gone—usually within 36 hours—the oil starts oxidizing, that is, it becomes rancid.

Oils sold in clear glass bottles are rancid. (Buy oil in cans or dark bottles.) Oils used for repeated frying are very rancid. Oils in roasted nuts are rancid (unless they're eaten immediately after being roasted). The vast majority of fats eaten in industrialized countries are rancid or hydrogenated, or both, and thus carcinogenic.

Anti-cancer oils include:

• **CANOLA OIL** (*Brassica napus*) is my choice if olive oil is unavailable. Canola oil, made from the seeds of a cabbage family plant, is usually fresh and rarely expensive, even when organically grown.

• **FLAX SEED OIL** (*Linum usitatissimum*) is a rich source of essential fatty acids and antioxidants. It adversely affects both the initiation and growth stages of breast cancer[20] and has been shown to be anti-tumor, antimiotic, and antiviral (so long as it is not heated). I buy only absolutely fresh flax seed oil (in a dated bottle) and keep it frozen or refrigerated. Rancid flax seed oil can cause vomiting and purging. The price of this oil restricts its use.

• **OLIVE OIL** (*Olea europaea*) of good quality (extra virgin, virgin, or regular) is an important part of my personal anti-cancer diet, and I use it freely. Exceptionally rich in antioxidants, olive oil has a special ability to help cells protect themselves from free radical damage, and it's the oil most likely to make it to your table with its antioxidants intact. Women dancing with breast cancer may want to use olive oil exclusively since recent studies find no statistically significant difference between breast cancer metastasis in women on a low-fat diet versus women on a high-fat olive oil diet.

• **SESAME OIL** (*Sesamum indicum*), fresh tahini, and sesame seeds are rich in antioxidants, lignans, and phenols which inhibit the formation of cancer.

## ONION (*Allium cepa*)

Like her sister garlic, onion can prevent as well as reverse cellular changes that initiate cancer. Onions are rich in selenium and allyl sulfides. In laboratory tests, onion extracts inhibited proliferation of some cancer cells and killed others.

## ORANGE PEEL (*Citrus* species)

All citrus fruits (e.g., oranges, lemons, grapefruits, limes, bitter oranges, and tangerines) are rich sources of antioxidants, flavonoids, coumarins, triterpenoids, and limonene. The part usually thrown away—the rind—is the most medicinal, *but only from organic fruits.* Bitter orange peel has a long and powerful reputation as a cancer preventive and a cancer cure. *See* Materia Medica.

## ORGANIC FOOD

Several studies done in the past five years have found organically grown foods to be both richer in minerals (up to 400 percent more selenium ) and lower in heavy metals and carcinogenic compounds than non-organic foods.[20A] For a free copy of one of these studies, write to Doctor's Data. (*See* "Resources," page 54.)

Every renowned specialist working with non-orthodox cancer therapies—from the early 1950s (when the first non-organic foods came to market) until the present day—has emphasized the use of organically grown foods. Rene Caisse, who popularized the anti-cancer herbal formula, Essiac, said: "Patronize [those] who are growing foods in soil not contaminated with chemicals." And the man behind the Gerson anti-cancer diet, noted simply: "Organic food seems to be the answer to the cancer problem."

Choosing organically grown food keeps both us and the Earth

healthy. Organic farmers don't use organochlorine-based petrochemicals which promote breast cancer.[21] They work to enrich the
soil, insuring that succeeding generations will inherit fertile land and
the chance to reap rich crops of vital, healthy food.

## PARSLEY (*Petroselinum crispum*)

Ordinary parsley in your salad can help prevent the formation
and growth of cancer cells in your breasts. And it's easy to grow,
even on a windowsill. Parsley is incredibly high in carotenes, folic
acid, chlorophyll, and vitamin C. It also contains antiseptic, anti-
cancer, and antioxidant essential oils including terpenes and
pinenes. In addition, parsley contains phytosterols which specifically hinder recurrence of breast cancer. Parsley poultices soothe
breasts sore from mammograms, surgery, infections, or swelling.
Drinking fresh parsley juice is harsh on the kidneys; I avoid it.

## PINEAPPLE (*Ananas comosus*)

Fresh, canned, or dried pineapple is a good source of protease
inhibitors, and acids (including citric, folic, malic, and chlorogenic
acids). The digestive enzyme bromelain, concentrated in the un-
ripe fruit, has been found to disrupt the glyco-protein shield that
tumors use to protect themselves, and to reduce metastatic recurrence. Bromelain also reduces prostaglandin production. *See* essential fatty acids for more on prostaglandins.

## POTATOES (*Solanum tuberosum*)

Delicious, inexpensive potatoes are a very rich source of antioxidants and protease inhibitors. Potato protease inhibitors can stop
cancer-causing viruses even better than soybean protease inhibitors—formerly the fiercest antiviral agents known. Eating potatoes
strengthens the immune system. Potatoes are also a good source
of chlorogenic acid, a polyphenol that prevents cancer initiation.

Virtually every member of the potato family has been regarded
as a cure for cancer, even poisonous ones such as *Belladonna atropa*.
(*See* page 291.) *Organic Gardening* magazine reports that soaking
potatoes in cold water before cooking them increases their vitamin C content substantially.

## PURSLANE (*Portulaca oleracea*)

This common garden weed is a superb source of antioxidants,
folic acid, carotenes, omega-3 fatty acids, and glutathione. I enjoy
it in salads in the summer and preserve it in vinegar for winter use.

**RADISHES/DAIKON** (*Raphanus sativus*)
Radishes are exceptional anti-cancer foods. They are rich sources of vitamins C and D, protease inhibitors, and other cabbage family phytochemicals. Daikon is used to increase the lifespan of the terminally ill in Chinese hospitals. *See* cabbage family.

**RHUBARB** (*Rheum rhaponticum*)
The stalks of garden rhubarb are as effective at inhibiting cancer as the more famed roots, far tastier to consume, and safer as well. Cooked rhubarb stalks contain carotenes, flavones, antioxidants, and rhein and emodin—two phytochemicals shown to reduce the growth and spread of tumors. To improve on a good thing, and avoid white sugar, sweeten rhubarb with organic raisins, black mission figs, and a little maple syrup.

**RICE** (*Oryza sativa*)
Like all grains, rice is a good source of protease inhibitors. Women who eat the most rice have the lowest rates of breast cancer. Brown rice is the staple anti-cancer food of the macrobiotic approach, and rice in many forms—wild, basmati, short grain, and long grain—is one of the most important grains in my anti-cancer lifestyle diet.

**RUTABAGA/SWEDE** (*Brassica napus*)  *See* cabbage family.

**RYE** (*Secale cereale*)
Another grain; another source of anti-cancer protease inhibitors.

**SEASONING HERBS**
Even the herbs used to season your food can help prevent cancer. All members of the mint family, including **rosemary**, **thyme**, **basil**, **oregano**, **lavender**, and **sage**, are excellent sources of anti-cancer antioxidants, acids, polyphenols, phenolic diterpenes, flavonoids, and phytosterols. **Turmeric** contains the potent flavonoid curcumin, as well as carotenes, antioxidants, and phytosterols. Many other widely used seasoning herbs such as **nutmeg**, **cloves**, **caraway**, **cayenne**, **cumin**,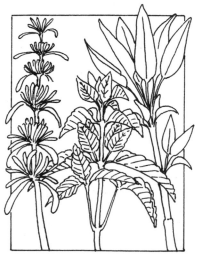

**celery seed**, **coriander**, and the Asian culinary herbs, **lemon grass**, **galanga**, and **betel nuts,** are strong anti-cancer agents. They emulsify cancer-initiating chemicals, whether from the environment or "in-vironment," and transport them out of the body.

Seasoning herbs like **ginger** act as tonics when used in small amounts frequently. Japanese scientists found ginger remarkably effective at blocking mutational changes that initiate cancer. Ginger roots contain antioxidants, gingerol, and carotenes. Ginger enhances production of glutathione-S-transferease, thus improving the body's ability to remove and resist carcinogens.

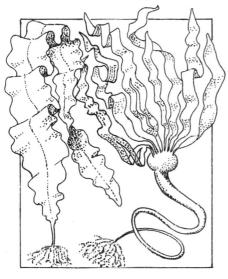

**SEAWEED** (*Alaria, Lamanaria, Nereocystis*)

Brown seaweeds such as **wakame**, **kelp**, and **kombu** provide a treasure chest of cancer preventive constituents: antioxidants, carotenes, selenium, and the star: alginic acid, which absorbs heavy metals, radioactive isotopes, and some chemicals, escorting them harmlessly out of the body. (Laboratory rats who ate seaweed before being exposed to cancer-causing chemicals had 30 percent less breast cancer.[22]) Seaweed in the daily diet protects the thyroid, strengthens the lymphatic and immune systems, and prevents the initiation of cancer. Those dancing with cancer use seaweed for its active anti-tumor effect and its ability to prevent recurrence. (In the study mentioned above, continued ingestion of kelp acted on the rats who did develop cancer "as a chemotherapeutic agent," slowing the cancer's progression in 95 percent of them.)

Seaweed is a vital part of my anti-cancer lifestyle and is an important complementary medicine for the woman choosing chemotherapy or radiation. A therapeutic dose is 2 ounces/60 grams dried seaweed daily during treatment or after a mammogram.

Cookbooks with seaweed recipes are listed on page 222; for mail order sources of seaweeds, *see* page 54. (I avoid buying powdered kelp unless I know the person who has harvested and powdered it, as it is often lacking the beneficial alginic acids.)

## SOYBEANS (*Soja hispida*)

Soybeans and soy products—especially fermented ones (e.g., **tamari, miso, tempeh**, and **natto**)—are exceptionally rich in phytochemicals which prevent the initiation, promotion, and recurrence of breast cancer: phytates, phytosterols, phenolic acids, lecithin, essential fatty acids, antioxidants, protease inhibitors, saponins, isoflavones, and anticoagulants.[23] Daily ingestion of a half-cup of tofu, tempeh, or miso, or a cup of soymilk, may reduce risk of breast cancer in women.[23a] Soy also protects cells from the cancer-promoting effects of radiation and chemicals (both environmental and medical). After exposure to x-rays, soy-fed rats developed breast cancer only half as frequently as rats not eating soy. Tamari added to the diet of mice reduced their actual incidence of cancer in a dose-dependent fashion. *See* beans.

## SPINACH (*Spinacea oleracea*)

Spinach offers anti-cancer protease inhibitors, chlorophyll, folic acid, unusually high levels of lutein, and three times more carotenes than an equal amount of carrots. Those who eat the most spinach have the lowest rates of cervical and endometrial cancers.

## SPROUTS

You may be surprised that I don't eat sprouts. I prefer plants grown in the earth; they're more grounded in their energy and much richer in such nutrients as minerals. But more importantly, I want to avoid the staggering array of carcinogenic natural chemicals produced by sprouting plants trying to protect themselves.

## SQUASH *see* Winter Squash

## STINGING NETTLE (*Urtica dioica*)

Stinging nettle is one of my favorite anti-cancer foods. Nettle is the world's richest source of carotenes and chlorophyll, as well as an excellent source of folic acid and selenium. Nettle is a powerful ally for women choosing chemotherapy, as it protects the blood itself from the mutagenic changes (which can lead to leukemia) caused by the chemotherapeutic drugs. *See* nourishing herbal infusions.

## STRAWBERRIES (*Fragaria vesca*)

Of 1,271 elderly Americans, those who ate the most strawberries were least likely to develop cancer. In fact, lessened cancer risk was more accurately gauged by looking at strawberry consumption than any other food. Strawberries are rich in antioxidants, chlorogenic acids, folic acid, ellagic acid, and polyphenols.

### SUNFLOWER SEEDS (*Helianthus annuus*)

Sunflower seeds can inhibit the formation and recurrence of breast cancers. Instead of a vitamin E supplement, I eat nutty sunflower seeds loaded with anti-cancer antioxidants and genistein. *See* nuts.

### SWEET POTATOES (*Ipomoea batatas*)

Sweet potatoes (unrelated to potatoes) are a superior source of anti-cancer carotenes, carotenoids, and phytosterols. They have a powerful reputation for lowering cancer risk, and are especially good allies for women exposed to environmental organochlorines and for those wishing to avoid breast cancer recurrence.

### TEA (*Camillia sinensis*)

Tea, ordinary black or green tea, drunk in ordinary amounts, checks the initiation, promotion, and growth of breast cancer (and eight other cancers including lung and liver).[24] Every cup of tea contains antimutagenic, anti-cancer tannins (green tea has twice the tannins of black) and antioxidant, anti-cancer polyphenols (especially epigallocatechin gallate). Green tea is the strongest

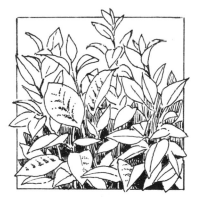

antimutagen of any plant yet tested, completely suppressing solid tumor formation in mice at risk and protecting habitual drinkers in Japan from many cancers. Russian, Indian, and Japanese studies validate tea's reputation for providing protection against radiation, but only if drunk daily for at least a week before exposure. Be aware that tea does contain caffeine, and caffeine can aggravate breast tenderness and lumpiness in some women.

### TOMATOES (*Lycopersicon esculentum*)

Like potatoes, tomatoes are members of a plant family long considered more related to sorcery than medicine. However they do it, tomatoes are an excellent anti-cancer food, rich in antioxidants, chlorogenic acids, flavonoids, coumarins, carotenes, lycopene, and carotenoids. High consumption of tomatoes correlates strongly with lessened risk of cancer. Women over the age of 65 who ate tomatoes infrequently were twice as likely to have breast (and other) cancers as those who ate tomatoes regularly. Tomatoes are exceptionally effective at preventing the initiation of cancer.

**TURNIPS** (*Brassica rapa*)
Both the roots and the greens of the turnip are edible, so there's a double dose of anti-cancer compounds. Actually, it's more like a quadruple dose, because turnips have twice as much glucosinolates as Brussels sprouts or watercress. *See* cabbage family.

**WATERCRESS** (*Nasturtium officinale*)
Watercress is an excellent source of anti-cancer compounds such as chlorophyll, antioxidants, gallic acid, folic acid, and glucosinolates. Regular consumption stimulates hair growth, builds blood, improves appetite, and strengthens the immune system, making it a healing food for those using chemotherapy or radiation. In animal studies, injections of watercress extract stopped cancer.

**WHEAT/WHEAT GRASS** (*Triticum vulgare*)
Freshly milled whole grain wheat flour (not white flour or its products) is a good source of anti-cancer lignans, diferulic acid, and protease inhibitors. Wheat grass is an excellent source of chlorophyll, folic acid, and antioxidants. *See* cereal grasses; *see* oil.

**WILD & EXOTIC MUSHROOMS**
Exotic and wild mushrooms such as **puffballs** (*Calvatia* species), **reishii** (*Ganoderma lucidum*), **oyster mushrooms** (*Pleurotus ostreatus*), **shiitake** (*Lentinus edodes*), **straw mushrooms** (*Volvariella volvacea*), **maitake** (*Grifolia frondosa*), **Zhu ling** (*Polyporus umbellatus*), **polyporacea** (*Poria cocos*), **chaga** (*Inonotus obliquus*), **enokidake** (*Flammulina velutipes*), and **tree ears** (*Tremellae fructiformis*) have been shown to enhance immune functioning, deactivate viruses, prevent the promotion and initiation of many cancers, slow tumor growth, and increase lifespan. [25, 26]
Wild and exotic mushrooms are rich in selenium, antioxidants, lignans, and adaptogenic compounds. For cancer prevention, I eat them once a month. Those dancing with cancer can partake more freely and frequently. Mushrooms foraging is risky. Mushrooms that smell good and taste great can kill you. For safety's sake, buy mushrooms at a store, or check your find with an expert or three

field guides. Even after 30 years, I still do. *See* pages 86–87 for more details on preparation and use of wild mushrooms.

## WINTER SQUASH (*Cucurbita maxima*)

Pumpkin, butternut, Hubbard, acorn, delicata, and turban squashes are sweet-tasting, orange-fleshed, hard-rinded and exceptionally rich in cancer-preventing carotenes and antioxidants.

## YOGURT

A quart of yogurt a week not only helps me prevent cancer, it strengthens my immune system, and promises me a healthy long life. Fermented milk—known variously as yogurt, leben, youghurt, kafir, koumiss, and yakult—is the daily drink of the world's healthiest citizens, no matter where they live. Milk from goats and cows (and sheep and yaks) who graze on weeds and grasses free of pesticides and herbicides is one of the very best foods available. And when that milk is cultured with beneficial bacteria, its health-promoting and cancer-inhibiting qualities are more than doubled. (And the amount of available calcium is increased by half.)

Helpful prostaglandins and fatty acids found in yogurt and milk inactivate the kinds of prostaglandins that initiate cancer. Special antibodies found in yogurt mitigate the cancer-promoting effects of viral and bacterial infections. Yogurt is especially recommended for those at high risk of cancer, as it is superb at blocking cellular changes that initiate the cancer cascade. Several studies have shown that the more yogurt a woman eats, the lower her risk of breast cancer.[27] Eating a quart of yogurt a week also protects the vagina and bladder from infections, and improves digestion.

Those who claim milk is unhealthy are throwing the baby out with the bath water. Hormones, antibiotics, and organochlorines in milk are unhealthy and to be avoided, not milk. Nor is milk fat a problem, except when that fat is the carrier of unwanted hormones and organochlorines. In fact, conjugated linoleic acid, a fat found only in animal products (including milk and cheese), decreases lifetime risk of breast cancer by 50 percent if consumed in sufficient quantity before puberty. Most women experience health benefits when they seek out optimal sources of organic milk and milk products and use them in moderation.

If you are lactose-intolerant or suffer stomach distress after drinking milk, you'll be happy to know that fellow sufferers attest to the fact that home-made yogurt, cultured for 24 hours before being refrigerated, is lactose-free.

# Anti-Cancer Phytochemicals

The hundreds of thousands of different substances in plants, including nutrients, are known collectively as phytochemicals. Although I describe them one by one, phytochemicals work synergistically, not individually. Supplementation with individual phytochemicals can actually increase cancer risk.

It is possible to get mega-doses of nutrients without taking pills. For example, 8 oz/250 ml of nettle infusion contains 1,000 mg calcium and 5,000 IU of carotenes. A cup of violet infusion supplies 6,000 IU carotenes. A serving (100 grams) of dandelion leaves contains 60,000 IU carotenes.

The following phytochemicals and nutrients can prevent and reverse the initiation, promotion, and growth of breast cancer.[28, 32]

**Acids** (e.g., **alginic acid** in seaweed, **arctic acid** in burdock, **diferulic acid** in whole wheat, and **gallic, caffeic, ferulic, chlorogenic**, and **ellagic acids** in fruits) prevent the initiation of cancer by protecting DNA from damage. They also discourage the formation of carcinogenic metabolic by-products during digestive action in the intestines and emulsify some carcinogenic chemicals, making them more soluble in water and thus easier to eliminate. *See* phytic acid.

**Allyl sulfides** (e.g., S-allylcysteine, dialkyl sulfides) increase the production of glutathione S-transferase, which increases the excretion of carcinogens and slows the reproduction of tumor cells. Allyl sulfides are damaged by heat. *Best Sources:* Garlic, onions, leeks.

**Anticoagulants** thin the blood and are known to reduce the risk of stroke. Circumstantial evidence suggests that frequent ingestion of anticoagulants helps prevent the initiation and recurrence of cancerous tumors. *Best Sources:* Soy products, willow bark (*Salix* species), red clover blossoms, woodruff leaves (*Asperula odorata*), May wine, and cleavers herb. (Aspirin and warfarin are anticoagulants.)

**Antioxidants** quench free radicals, thus preventing the initiation phase of cancer. Capsaicin (the hot in peppers) is a particularly potent antioxidant, as are selenium, germanium, vitamins A, C, and E, carotenes, and the **diterpenoids** in mints such as rosemary. *Best Sources*: Fresh, whole foods, minimally processed.

**Benzaldehyde**, in a gluconated form, has been used by traditional healers in Japan and naturopathic doctors in North America to slow the growth of cancerous tumors.[35] You can buy it at the supermarket in the form of almond extract (containing about 700 milligrams of benzaldehyde per ounce). The dose used in Japan is the equivalent of three-quarters of an ounce of almond extract. It is diluted in a glass of juice which is divided into fourths, one fourth taken every six hours. Benzaldehyde is "GRAS" (generally regarded as safe by the FDA) but can be toxic if more than 50 ounces are consumed at once. Benzaldehyde is a form of laetrile. *Best Sources*: Almonds, apricot pits, peach pits, figs, burdock root.

**Carotenes** and **carotenoids** are a large group of antioxidant phytochemicals. Over 800 different carotenes have been found, including **lycopene**, **lutein**, **zeaxanthin**, and the familiar **beta carotene**. Carotenes block the initiation and promotion of cancer by binding free radicals, protecting the DNA from radiation and chemicals, and nourishing the production of anti-cancer enzymes in the digestive tract. Carotenes enhance production of interleukins, lymphocytes, and many kinds of T-cells (e.g., helper cells and natural killer cells); they also enhance intracellular communication.

   Those who eat carotene-rich foods (even as little as half a cup/125 ml of cooked carrots daily) are seven times less likely to develop cancer than those who don't. In one study of people over 65 years old, those who ate the least carotenes had a 300 percent greater risk of dying of cancer than those who ate the most. In another, blood samples taken from women 10-15 years before they developed breast cancer showed significantly lower levels of carotenes and vitamin E than blood from women who remained cancer-free. *Best Sources*: Dandelion leaves, violet leaves, nettles, dark leafy greens, carrots, sweet potatoes, winter squash, pumpkin, cantaloupe, watermelon, pink grapefruit, papaya, and apricots.

   **Important:** When foods rich in carotenes are cooked, they are up to five times more active at inhibiting cancer than if eaten juiced or raw.

**Catechins** are antioxidant tannins; they help prevent the initiation of cancers. *Best Sources*: Green tea, berries.

**Chlorophyll**, the green color in plants, is a concentrated source of carotenes. Clinical studies show chlorophyll-rich diets capable of preventing cancer initiation (especially from environmental chemicals) and of stopping the growth and spread of most cancers. *Best Sources*: Dark leafy greens, nourishing herbal infusions, cereal grasses.

**Coumarins** are anticoagulant phenols which enhance production of anti-cancer enzymes. *Best Sources*: Tomatoes, citrus.

**Dithiolthiones** prevent cancer initiation by activating the production of specific anti-cancer enzymes which stop damage to cellular DNA. *Best Sources*: Broccoli, cabbage family.

**Essential fatty acids** (EFAs) (e.g., **omega-3** and **omega-6**), are not made by our bodies. Most fatty acids are formed in the intestines from a diet rich in lignans, but essential fatty acids cannot be made, they must be consumed. Blood rich in essential fatty acids contains low levels of prostaglandins. Blood lacking essential fatty acids becomes overwhelmed with troublesome prostaglandins which can promote tumor growth. Several studies found low levels of prostaglandins linked to low rates of breast cancer. High levels of specific prostaglandins are typically found in the blood and tumors of those with breast cancer.[33] Clinical studies of herbal seed oils containing EFAs show them able to prevent breast cancer and adversely to affect its progress once established. I do not use essential fatty acids in capsules as they are likely to be rancid and to do as much harm as good. *Best Sources*: Purslane, flax seeds, walnuts, and wild fish of cold waters (e.g., herring, sardines, mackerel, halibut, tuna, and salmon. Farmed fish—such as virtually all catfish, trout, and salmon sold in restaurants—contain little or no fatty acids). The seeds and seed oils from borage (*Borago officinalis*), evening primrose (*Oenothera biennis*), and hemp (*Cannabis indica* or *sativa*) are also excellent sources of essential fatty acids.

**Flavonoids** (e.g., catechin, coumarin, quercetin, morin, rutin, kaempferol, and silymarin), or **bioflavonoids**, are a very large group (4000 and still counting) of antioxidants which prevent cancer-promoting hormones from attaching themselves to cells. They also inhibit the production of enzymes needed for cancer cell metastasis. Flavonoids are anti-cancer, anti-inflammatory, antimicrobial, and immunosupportive. They protect the liver and the heart. *Best Sources*: Citrus, berries, yams, soy, dark leafy greens, seasoning herbs, milk thistle seeds, broccoli, cabbage, squash, carrots.

**Folic acid** is critical to the breakdown of proteins, and the growth and reproduction of all cells. When blood levels are low, onco-genes are more easily activated; when blood levels are high, can-cer cells have difficulty reproducing. *Best Sources*: Leafy greens, whole grains.

**Germanium,** an antioxidant, is a biological-response modifier that helps the body change its response to cancer. Germanium strengthens the immune system, promotes production of inter-feron and natural killer cells, and inhibits many kinds of cancer. *Best Sources*: Ginseng, garlic, comfrey leaf, wild mushrooms, aloe.

**Genistein** inhibits the initiation of estrogen-sensitive cancers of the breasts, ovaries, and cervix. It also stops metastasis from es-tablished tumors by blocking their ability to form new capillaries. *Best Sources*: Lentils, seeds, beans, peas. *See* isoflavones.

**Glutathione**, an antioxidant enzyme, is a key anti-cancer agent. *Best Sources*: Purslane, raw spinach, parsley.

**Glycosides** (e.g., saponins, phytosterols, and isoflavonoids) are carbohydrates which split into a sugar and a non-sugar when di-gested. Glycosides are immune-enhancing, cancer-preventive, and adaptogenic. *Best Sources*: Roots, including burdock, dandelion, Siberian ginseng, sweet potatoes, yams.

**Indoles** (e.g., indole-3-carbinol) nourish the production of enzymes that inactivate cancer-promoting estrogens and estrogen-mimics. Indoles lowered breast cancer rates 450 percent when given to laboratory mice. *Best Sources*: Cabbage family plants.

**Isoflavones**, or **isoflavonoids** (e.g., genistein), are phytosterols which are superb cancer inhibitors. Their anti-cancer, anti-estro-gen effects help prevent cancer in all reproductive areas: breasts, ovaries, cervix, uterus, prostate, and testes. Isoflavones inhibit the replication of oncogenes by destroying a critical enzyme and have been clinically shown to cause initiated cancer cells to convert to normal cells.[34] Women whose diet (and urine) is high in isoflavones have the lowest breast cancer rates: Japanese women's excretion is 117 times greater than American women's. *Best Sources:* Dried beans, soy products, red clover, sage, garlic, fennel, licorice root.

**Isothiocyanates** are especially active in breast tissues, where they promote the production of specific enzymes that protect DNA from damage and inactivate a range of carcinogens. *Best Sources:* Kale, radishes, horseradish, daikon, Brussels sprouts; cabbage family.

**Lecithin** makes fat-soluble chemicals, such as organochlorines, water-soluble and speeds their excretion, thus helping to prevent both the initiation and promotion stages of cancer. *Best Sources:* Flax seeds, egg yolks, unclarified soy oil. (I do not use powdered lecithin; it is extracted with the use of petrochemical solvents.)

**Lignans** have antioxidant, anti-cancer, antibacterial, antifungal, antiviral, and insecticidal actions.[36] They stop all phases of the cancer cascade. Lignans block the action of cancer-promoting prostaglandins, plus they are converted by colon bacteria into anti-estrogenic substances that reduce age-related breast cancer risk and inhibit recurrence. Postmenopausal women with breast cancer have consistently low levels of lignans in their urine. *Best Sources:* Seeds, grains, walnuts, and beans. Flax seeds have 800 mcg lignans per gram, rye has 6 mcg/gram; buckwheat, millet, soy, and oats all have 2 mcg/gram; barley, corn, and wheat have 1 mcg/gram.

**Limonene, D-limonene,** and **limonoids** are oils that nourish the production of digestive enzymes which break down carcinogens (and perhaps even cancer cells) and escort them out of the body. *Best Sources:* Peels of organic oranges and lemons.

**Lycopene** is an antioxidant carotenoid especially effective in preventing the initiation of cancer. *Best Sources:* Tomatoes, pink grapefruit, watermelon.

**Monoterpenes** are mild antioxidants needed for the production and utilization of anti-cancer enzymes. *Best Sources:* Fruits, vegetables, mints, basil, seasoning herbs.

**Phytic acid**, or **phytate**, is a plant-based phosphorus which prevents the formation of cancer-promoting free radicals in the intestines and inhibits tumor growth in a wide range of cancers. *Best Sources:* Wheat, whole grains, fruits, vegetables, and beans.

**Phytosterols** are plant hormones which are frequently (usually mistakenly) compared to human hormones. I've seen several articles and a book or two that postulate that women with breast cancer or those at high risk should avoid plant hormones. I disagree. Phytosterols block the cancer-promoting effects of our own hormones by binding to the receptor sites first. They prevent the initiation and the recurrence of cancer. Phytosterols also nourish and strengthen the immune system, and act as precursors to the production of anti-cancer vitamin D. *Best Sources:* Beans, whole grains, edible and medicinal roots (e.g., dandelion, burdock, yams, carrots, parsnips, parsley), red clover blossoms, and sage.

**Polyphenols** such as **polyacetylenes** are found in virtually all plants; they are highly colored and strongly flavored antioxidants. Polyphenols are antiviral, antibacterial, and anti-cancer. They act in conjunction with flavonoids. Some, such as **phenolic acid**, protect DNA against damage. *Best Sources:* Fresh food, soy products, red wine, green and black tea, carrots, parsley, celery.

**Protease inhibitors** block the action of cancer-promoting enzymes called proteases, thus preventing the activation and expression of oncogenes, and the promotion and growth of breast cancers. Protease inhibitors shield cells from the effects of radiation and prevent the formation of free radicals. Protease inhibitors are even capable of reversing cancerous changes in the DNA and healing cellular damage caused by radiation. Best of all, the effects continue even if you forget to eat protease inhibitors regularly, since they stay active in the body for months. High heat damages protease inhibitors. *Best Sources:* Dried beans, especially soybean products, unless cooked at temperatures above boiling (like in a pressure cooker), nuts, raw corn, green tomatoes.

**Quinones** inhibit the action of carcinogens and co-carcinogens. *Best Sources:* Rosemary.

**Saponins** are antioxidants that are especially effective at preventing cellular mutations that would lead to cancer. They inhibit cancer-promoting enzymes, break down dioxin, and stop reproduction of cancer cells. *Best Sources:* Chickweed, beans, soy products.

**Selenium** is the anti-cancer mineral. Cancer rates drop as selenium is added to the diet. Selenium stops all phases of the cancer cascade. Selenium stops initiation by increasing adaptability at the cellular and humoral levels, protecting the DNA from disruption by chemical carcinogens, and by stopping viral oncogenesis. Selenium disrupts cancer promotion by working as an antioxidant, an enzyme nourisher, and an immune system strengthener. In addition, selenium has been shown to depress the growth rate of established tumors. Organically grown foods have much more selenium than foods raised with chemical fertilizers. *Best Sources*: Garlic, onions, greens, grains, mushrooms, brazil nuts.

**Sulforaphane** extracted from broccoli created "quite dramatic results" when fed to rats bred to develop breast cancer: Fewer animals developed tumors, and when they did, it was much later than usual, and the cancers were fewer and smaller than usual. *Best Sources*: Broccoli and other cabbage family plants.

**Tannins** (e.g., catechin) are common plant compounds that cause cellular contraction, making them useful in tanning leather, healing burns, and preventing cancer. Tannins are antimutagenic and antagonistic to cancer growth in all stages. *Best Sources*: Green and black tea, nourishing herbal infusions, oak leaves and acorns. **Caution**: Excessive amounts of tannins in the diet (e.g., 30 cups of black tea daily for years) can initiate cancer.

**Triterpenoids** and **terpenes** inhibit hormones that promote breast cancers. *Best Sources*: Citrus, licorice root.

*"Cancer development is a multistage, longtime event, and interfering with it anywhere along the line can retard or halt its deadly march."*
Jean Carper, *Food Pharmacy*, 1988

# Vitamin and Mineral Sources

**Boron:** Organic greens, nettles, dandelion, yellow dock.
**Calcium:** Yogurt, leafy greens, seaweed, dried beans, nettles, mint, sage, yellow dock, red clover, oatstraw, plantain leaf, dandelion.
**Chromium:** Mushrooms, nuts, liver, beets, whole wheat, oatstraw, nettles, red clover, seaweed, echinacea.
**Copper:** Seafood, leafy greens, bittersweet chocolate, whole grains, dried beans, nuts, skullcap, sage, horsetail, chickweed.
**Folic acid** (a B vitamin): *See* page 49.
**Iodine:** Seaweed, seafood, mushrooms, beets, parsley, celery.
**Iron:** Molasses, leafy greens, liver, bittersweet chocolate, mushrooms, whole grains, potatoes, seaweed, burdock, milk thistle seed, dandelion, yellow dock, echinacea, plantain, nettles, licorice, mint.
**Laetrile** (vitamin $B_{17}$ or amygdalin): Fruit pits, almonds, millet, grasses, roots. *See* benzaldehyde, page 47.
**Magnesium:** Seaweed, leafy greens, yogurt, whole grains, nuts, oatstraw, licorice, nettles, burdock, sage, red clover, yellow dock, dandelion, parsley, potato skins.
**Manganese:** Seaweed, leafy greens, milk thistle seed, yellow dock, ginseng, echinacea, nettle, dandelion.
**Potassium:** Fruits, vegetables, sage, seaweed, mint, red clover, nettle, plantain leaf or seeds.
**Selenium:** Seaweed, organic garlic, mushrooms, liver, seafood, milk thistle seeds, ginseng, echinacea, yellow dock.
**Sulfur:** Eggs, yogurt, garlic, cabbage family, nettles, plantain.
**Zinc:** Pumpkin seeds, sage, echinacea, nettle, seaweed, milk thistle.
**Vitamin A:** Produced from carotenes, *see* page 47.
**Vitamin B complex:** Whole grains, greens, dried beans, seafood, red clover, parsley.
**Vitamin $B_6$:** Potato skins, broccoli, dried beans, lentils, meat, fish.
**Vitamin C:** All fresh fruits and vegetables, pine needles, dandelion greens, red clover, parsley, plantain leaf, paprika.
**Vitamin D:** Sunlight, butter, egg yolks, fatty fish, liver.
**Vitamin E:** Cold-pressed food oils, freshly ground whole grains, nettles, seaweed, dandelion, nuts, greens, sunflower seeds.
**Vitamin K:** Nettles, alfalfa, kelp, green tea.

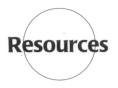

# Resources

## Seaweed
These seaweed harvesters are conscientious, ecologically aware, and willing to be listed. There are many other sources of seaweed. I encourage you to support local harvesters or to spend one weekend a year at the ocean harvesting your own. Good quality dried seaweed smells and tastes like a fresh ocean breeze.

• Ryan Drum, Superior Seaweed, Waldron Island, WA 98297

• Lewallen Sea Vegetables
  PO Box 1265, Mendocino, CA 95460; 707-937-2050

## Organic Food
• Free report on nutrients in organic food from Doctor's Data, PO Box 111, West Chicago, IL 60185-9986

• Walnut Acres, Penns Creek, PA 17862; 1-800-433-3998

• Mt. Ark Trader, Fayetteville, AR 72702-3170; 1-800-643-8909

• National Organic Directory, PO Box 464, Davis, CA 95617; 916-756-8518

• Apricot pits: Choice Metabolics, 1-800-227-4473

## Further Reading:
• *Beating Cancer With Nutrition*, P. Quillin, Nutrition Times, 1994
• *Healing With Food*, Melvin Werbach, M.D., Harper, 1993
• *Cancer Free*, S. J. Winawer, M.D., and M. Shike, M.D., Simon & Schuster, 1994
• *Diet, Nutrition & Cancer Prevention: A Guide to Food Choices*, available free from 1-800-4-CANCER.

# Ancient Breasts

"Deep within you, whether you are aware of it or not, is your primal need for breast. It is part of you; it was born with you. It has been with you for millions of years.

"When you emerged into the world of air, hunger came with you. And linked to hunger was the remedy for hunger, already known to you. You had, at birth, the skill to guide yourself to it by touch, by smell, by warmth, by sweetness. You had, and still have, internal, ancient coding to find the breast and suck.

" 'Find the breast and suck.' This message sings in you, in every one of us, from birth to death. It says: 'Find the breast, source of nourishment, source of contentment.' It urges: 'Find the breast, where hunger ceases, where you are one with the mother, one with the pulsing heart of the Mother, at one with Breast/Heart/Mother/All.'

"The breast is bliss. The breast is enlightenment. The breast is the emblem of our most sacred aspirations. The Madonna holds the infant to her breast. Ka'aba (Hajar-e-aswad), the holy rock of Mecca, is known as the Mother's Bountiful Breast.

"Breast is nourishment is life is sun is round and warm and full. A simple drawing of a breast is the symbol for Sun, nourisher of all life. And life is sacred, so breasts are sacred, so women are sacred, holy, whole. Always and everywhere women's breasts have been honored.

"Has anyone ever told you that your breasts are holy and sacred and moving with the energy of life? Has anyone ever told you that your breasts are a source of power? Has anyone ever given you permission to love your breasts, touch your breasts, adore your breasts? Has anyone encouraged you to honor your breasts and all women's breasts as life, as the support of life?

"Were you allowed to suckle at your mother's breast? Have you ever received, ever given, nourishment from your breasts? Have you drunk from the breast of Mother Earth? Have you drunk from the wild springs of the Earth? Taken bites of plants still rooted? Spilled warm, raw milk into your mouth? Have you put your mouth upon the source and received fulfillment, ecstasy?

"Do your breasts have a story? If you ask, they will tell you. Do you remember when your breasts emerged? What were you feeling about them then? Excited? Eager? Awkward? Embarrassed? Angry? Tender?

"Do you remember the first time you felt your breasts move as you ran? The first time you felt your breasts float as you swam? The first time you stood in the shower and watched the water arch out over your breasts and waterfall off your nipples?

"We are the Ancient GrandMothers and our breasts are ancient. Perhaps you find them ugly. See how they drift yearningly toward the Earth, lower with every passing year. We smile knowingly; we know our breasts contain a power that is resilient, flexible, supple, easy, and impossible to restrain. Whether the whim of fashion says our breasts are to be large or small, pointed or flattened, with cleavage or without, padded or bound, accented or obscured, it matters not to us. Our breasts fall free, untouched by current notions. The power of our breasts is the power of life.

"The power of our breasts is the power of every woman's breasts. As our breasts are life, so every woman's breasts are life. And this is true of you, too, GrandDaughter: The power of your breasts is the power of life. Your breasts are sacred."

# 3.
# Taking Our Breasts Into Our Own Hands
# Breast Self-Massage

Breast self-massage is simple.
Breast self-massage is pleasurable.
Breast self-massage helps prevent cancer as well as detect it.
Breast self-massage helps keep breast skin supple.
Breast self-massage adds resiliency to breast tissue.
Breast self-massage is a way to be intimate with your breasts.
Breast self-massage is a piece of women's wisdom.
Breast self-massage is safe.
Breast self-massage is free.

Many of the women I've talked with say they don't do breast self-exams, though most think they ought to. No one wants to look for (or, heaven forbid, find!) cancer. We've been trained to avoid danger, and looking for cancer sounds like looking for trouble. Our bodies are influenced by what we think, so how can it be safe to spend time every month doing a breast self-exam, worrying if we're about to find a lump? But we feel guilty when we don't.

   And what are we supposed to feel when we touch our breasts anyway? They feel full of lumps! Most of us aren't sure how to touch or examine our breasts or what we'd do if we did feel something truly suspicious. Our guilt and confusion make it all even more complex.

   Breast self-massage offers a way to let go of this tension and get in touch with yourself. This soothing, nurturing self-massage is a pleasurable and relaxing way to get to know your breasts. It avoids the worry of checking for cancer, while providing an excellent early-warning system should cancer arise. Regular, loving touching of our breasts allows us to recognize normal breast changes without fear, and gives us time to respond thoughtfully to abnormal changes. Breast self-massage is also a quiet, focused time that allows the Wise Healer Within (*see* page 83) to alert us to any changes that require our attention.

57

Infused (not essential) herbal oils are an important element of breast self-massage. When herbs are infused into oil, active plant components are liberated and can be massaged into breast tissue—where they help reverse abnormal cellular changes such as hyperplasia, atypia, precancers, and *in situ* cancers. It's fast and fun to make your own infused oils (*see* page 297), or you can buy them (*see* page 75). But if you don't have any, plain olive oil works fine.

If you already know breast self-exam techniques, let them inform your fingertips during your breast self-massage. If this is all new to you, take a few months to learn about your breasts with self-massage before doing breast self-exam. They complement each other: Let the pleasure of the massage infuse the exam, and let the effectiveness of the exam inform the massage.

### When should I do my breast self-massage?

Now. Anytime. All the time. Sure, your breasts are less lumpy at some times of the month. But you can do breast self-massage whenever you want, even if you're lumpy. If the best time for you to pay attention to yourself is when you bleed, because that's when you take time to be alone, then that's the time to do breast self-massage. You could do it every week and get to know how your breasts change with your cycle and with the moon, but most likely you'll do it every month. I like to do my breast self-massage when the moon is new.

## Breast structures change.

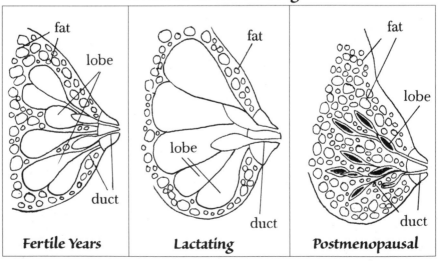

Fertile Years          Lactating          Postmenopausal

**How do I do breast self-massage?**

First, make or buy some infused herbal oils or ointments. You'll want several, as each offers unique benefits.

Then, create a comfortable, private place where you can lean back: in a warm bath or propped up with cushions in bed. (Protect linens and clothing from oil stains.) Arrange yourself there, bare-breasted, with your infused herbal oils close at hand.

Let your eyelids fall. Put your hands over your heart and hum. Cup your breasts with your hands and hum. Imagine or visualize energy streaming out of your nipples. Allow your breasts and heart to open and flow as you hum.

Open your eyes. Transfer some herbal oil or ointment to your palms. Rub your hands together briskly until they feel warm. Place them on either side of one breast and hum.

Cup your fingers alongside or under your breast, thumbs touching and up as high on the chest as possible. (If your breasts are very large, rest the right breast in the right palm and massage with the left thumb, starting in the armpit and moving toward the center of the chest.) Press in and slide your thumbs down toward the nipple, pressing the breast tissue into your fingers and palms. Stretch your thumbs up toward the collarbone again, but slightly farther apart, press in and slide down.

Continue until your thumbs are as far apart as possible (the middle of your chest and your armpit). Repeat, gradually increasing pressure, but only as long as it feels good.

**Caution:** There is a slight possibility of spreading breast cancer through vigorous massage, rough handling, or very deep pressure.

Transfer more oil or ointment to your palms and rub your hands together. Cup your breast as before, thumbs up and touching. Hum. Repeat the previous pattern, but break up the stroke: Instead of a long, slow, smooth stroke, use your thumbs to make a lot of overlapping short strokes, gradually moving down the chest. Try various degrees of pressure.

Raise the arm of the breast you're massaging, and put your hand behind you or on your head. If your breast leans to the outside, prop a pillow under that shoulder or lean over. Cover your breast with your free hand and hum.

Dip your fingers into your oil or ointment and, starting in your armpit, press the fingerpads of your first two or three fingers down with enough pressure to hold the skin, and make a small circle. Don't let your fingers slide over the skin. Keep making

little circles (with enough pressure to feel the underlying structures) as you trace an imaginary spiral from your armpit around
and around your breast, growing ever smaller until you reach
your nipple. (If it is difficult or impossible for you to use your
fingerpads, use your palm.) Cover your breast with your hand
and hum.

Curl your fingers into your armpit and gently grasp the
ridge of lymph-rich tissues and muscles that extend from the shoulder down into the breast. Move up and down this ridge several
times, using small squeezes or long glides or little spirals or your
own strokes.

As you touch your breasts, imagine or visualize your fingertips emitting healing pink sparkles that embrace and nourish
your breasts. Let your fingerpads sink deeply into your breasts.
Allow any held distress to be soothed by the balm of the infused
herbal oil/ointment. Let overactive energy be calmed by the
rhythm of your fingers circling, circling, spiraling, spiraling.

Apply more oil or ointment with your fingerpads, making
large gliding circles from midchest to under your breast, up toward the armpit and over and around, again, and again, with a
steady rhythm.

When you're done massaging your breast, close your eyes
and relax. Hum. Call to your Wise Healer Within as you hum.

Massage your other breast, starting from the beginning:
Put your hands over your heart. Hum. Cup your breasts. Hum.
(Is there a difference between the breast that has already been massaged and the one that hasn't yet?) Rub your oily hands briskly
together; hold either side of your breast and hum. Extend your
thumbs and massage as before, including all of the previous strokes
and ending with your eyes closed, relaxing deeply and allowing
yourself to contact and listen to your Wise Healer Within.

### Afterwards . . .

After your breast self-massage, take a moment to record
your experience. This will help you learn more quickly what's
normal for you. You can draw a map of your breasts to help you
remember what you've felt. Try using colors. Write down any
messages offered to you by your breasts or your Wise Healer
Within. If you like, make up a little song to hum during your massage. The keynote in breast self-massage is **pleasure**.

# A Slippery Assortment of Herbal Oils

Using infused herbal oils is an easy and pleasurable way to keep your breasts healthy, prevent and reverse cysts, dissolve troublesome lumps, and repair abnormal cells. Breast skin is thin and absorbent, and breast tissue contains a great deal of fat, which readily absorbs infused herbal oils. The healing and cancer-preventing actions of herbs easily migrate into olive oil–creating a simple, effective product for maintaining breast health.

Add beeswax to any herbal oil and you have an ointment. The antiseptic, softening, moisturizing, and healing properties of beeswax intensify the healing actions of the herbs and carry them deeper into the breast tissues.

Whether you want to maintain breast health–or have had a diagnosis of cancer–infused herbal oils and ointments are soothing, safe, and effective allies. (Learn how to make your own, beginning on page 297. Mail order suppliers are listed on page 75.)

**Burdock seed oil** (*Arctium lappa*)

One of the world's most valued allies for nourishing the scalp, thickening the hair, and restoring hair growth is burdock seed oil. It won't make more hair grow on your breasts, but it will do a wonderful job of keeping your breast tissues healthy. Burdock seed oil strengthens cells and quickly relieves bruises caused by fine needle aspirations, biopsies, breast surgery, injections of chemotherapeutic drugs, and other medical procedures. If your breast skin breaks out in a rash (from surgical tapes or drains or nervousness), burdock seed oil offers quick relief.

**Calendula blossom oil** (*Calendula officinalis*)

Calendula blossom oil is a reknowned old wives' remedy against breast cancer, yet it's gentle enough for regular use. Older books call it pot marigold, causing some people to confuse it with the unrelated modern garden marigold. In addition to keeping breast tissues healthy, calendula excels at preventing–and, with patience, removing–adhesions and scar tissue, even keloid scars.

*Keloid scars* are elevated, hard scars, usually with irregular edges. They can be painful, especially when they occur as a result

of breast surgery. Keloid scars are caused by an overgrowth of
scar tissue at the site of an injury or incision and are more frequent
in dark-skinned women than light-skinned women. *Adhesions* are
bands of scar tissue that bind together internal body surfaces that
ought to be free to slide by each other. Adhesions are common
after abdominal surgery but can form after breast surgery.

For maximum effectiveness, infuse slightly dried calendula
blossoms in lard (organic if possible). The animal fat is taken deeper
into the tissues than vegetable oils and rapidly dissolves lumps.

Golden calendula oil brings new life to dull skin and is
highly recommended for breast self-massage.

### Cancerweed root oil (*Salvia lyrata*)

This uncommon plant contains ursolic acid, and is a folk
remedy for cancer. The roots of the more common ground ivy
(*Glechoma hederacea*) are similiar in action. Oil/ointment of either
plant, used several times a day, is said to eliminate cysts and abnormal breast cells including indeterminate lesions and hyperplasia.

### Castor oil (*Ricinus communis*)

The commercially extracted
(not infused) oil of the seeds of this
poisonous plant was the remedy
most frequently recommended by
the psychic healer Edgar Cayce for
resolving lumps and growths. (The
poison isn't in the oil, but–if taken
internally–castor oil is a strong laxative.) The classic application is a hot
castor oil compress made by baking a flannel cloth saturated in castor oil in the oven until it is thor-
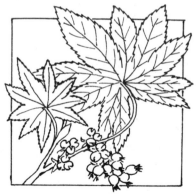
oughly heated. This hot compress is applied, covered with plastic
and/or layers of towels to hold in the heat, and kept on as long as
possible. In extreme cases, compresses are applied continuously,
day and night. For small lumps, room temperature castor oil is
applied morning and night ( before bed), and covered completely
with a regular adhesive strip (or two).

### Comfrey root oil (*Symphytum officinale*)

Comfrey root oil/ointment is a specific remedy for those
with sore breasts. It is especially wonderful for breast self-massage.

Infused oil of comfrey root (best) or leaves is one of the most amazing healing agents I've ever used. Comfrey oil/ointment both strengthens tissues and helps them become more resilient and flexible. As a pre- and post-surgical ally, it has no peer. Time after time, I've seen deep wounds, old wounds, stubborn wounds, and persistent ulcers heal fast, with little or no scarring, when dressed with comfrey.

If you've heard scare stories about comfrey—or read elsewhere, even in this book, to use only comfrey leaves—this remedy may alarm you. Substantial, lengthy *internal* use of comfrey root can cause liver damage (not cancer) in rare instances. But *external* use of comfrey root, even for extended periods, has never been connected to liver damage, nor any other harm.

### Dandelion oils (*Taraxacum officinale*)

Dandelion has a special affinity for breasts. Regular use of **dandelion flower oil** promotes deep relaxation of the breast tissues, facilitating the release of held emotions. Applied regularly to the entire breast area, glowing golden dandelion flower oil can strengthen your sense of self worth as well as your immune system. Easily made, this oil is a superb ally for regular breast self-massage, and highly praised by those doing therapeutic breast massage.

**Dandelion root oil,** used alone or in conjunction with the flower oil, can help clear minor infections, relieve impacted milk glands, and reduce cysts in the breasts.

### Essential oils

Essential oils are concentrated oils obtained from aromatic plants by steam distillation or with chemical solvents. They are capable of killing normal as well as abnormal cells, and severely disrupting liver and kidney functioning. Essential oils are quite different from infused oils (which are made by steeping fresh plants in an edible oil). Essential oils can cause poisoning; infused oils cannot. Essential oils can't be made at home; infused oils can. Essential oils can be costly (up to $300 per ounce); infused oils are reasonably priced (generally under $10 per ounce). Essential oils can irritate tender skin; infused oils rarely do. Essential oils are used in small amounts; infused oils are used lavishly.

**Caution:** Test your sensitivity before using essential oils. Put a drop of the oil on the sensitive skin inside your elbow. If your skin gets red or mottled, itches or burns in the next 12 hours,

be very cautious with essential oils and certainly don't use them
on your breasts. My cat's neck fur fell out after I anointed her chin
with three drops of essential oil to (successfully) rid her of fleas!
    Essentail oils of **citrus, rosemary, lavender, marjoram,
juniper**, or **clary sage**–ten drops diluted in one ounce/30 ml of
olive oil–have been used to increase circulation to the breasts,
warm them, activate the immune system, and offer the healing
benefits of their aromas as well.

### Evergreen oils

    Wonderfully fragrant infused oils can be made from all kinds
of evergreen needles. (*See* page 298.) Evergreen oils are superb for
regular breast self-massage, especially for those troubled with painful
or lumpy breasts. Evergreens, including the renowned yew, contain compounds clinically proven to kill cancer cells. The most
powerful in this respect are arbor vitae (*Thuja occidentalis*) and cedar (*Juniperus virginia*). But all evergreens contain antiseptic, antifungal, antiviral, and anti-tumor oils. I make my infused evergreen
oil from white pine (*Pinus strobus*), the most common evergreen in
my area; friends use spruce, cedar, and hemlock.
    Infused evergreen oils are generally non-irritating (a few
women report sensitivity to spruce needle oil), but essential oils of
evergreens can cause a rash. Essential oil of the evergreen **tea tree**
(*Melaleuca* species) has been poured into cancers that have ulcerated, causing some to go into remission. This is dangerous and
may be painful; I strongly advise you to seek counsel before you
use tea tree, or any essential oil, in this way.

**Ground Ivy** (*Glechoma hederacea*). *See* cancerweed.

### Olive oil (*Olea europea*)

    The oil pressed from the fruits (olives) and seeds (pits) of
these magnificent, long-lived trees is neither an infused oil nor an
essential oil. It is my favorite oil for eating, cooking, and using as
a base for infusing herbs. Virgin or extra virgin oils are great for
eating, but have a rich smell which is overpowering in an infused
oil or ointment. As a base for infused oils, I use the less expensive
(and less aromatic) pomace oil–made by pressing the ground pits
after the olives have been squeezed dry. No matter what type you
use, fancy or plain, olive oil will no doubt uphold its ancient and
venerable reputation for healing and nourishing skin and scalp.

**Plantain leaf oil** (*Plantago lancelota, P. majus*)
With its brilliant color and its solid reputation as a breast cancer preventive, plantain oil/ointment is another favorite for breast self-massage. Frequent applications of the jewel-green oil– as many as ten times a day–have been used successfully by women to reverse *in situ* cancer cells in the breasts. Plantain oil is very easy to make at home. (The aroma of the finished oil reminds me of salami.) Plantain ointment is the *first* first aid I reach for when I itch, when I get a sting, when I need to heal torn muscles, when I want to draw out thorns, splinters, or infection, and when I need to relieve pain and swelling.

**Poke root oil** (*Phytolacca americana*)
That strange-looking weed with the drooping black berries that towers over gardens and roadsides throughout much of eastern North America is pokeweed–an old favorite of wise women dealing with breast lumps and breast cancer. If I felt a suspicious lump, I'd reach for poke root oil. It reduces congestion, relieves swelling, and literally dissolves growths in the breasts.
Jethro Kloss, author of the classic herbal *Back to Eden*, used freshly grated raw poke root poultices to burn away breast cancer. **Caution**: Fresh poke placed directly on the skin is strong enough to damage healthy tissues as well as cancerous ones.
The infused oil is also effective and far safer. A generous amount is gently applied to the lump, covered with a flannel cloth and then with a hot water bottle (no heating pads), and left on for as long as you're comfortable. This is repeated at least twice a day.
Poke root oil is too powerful for regular preventive care. **Caution**: Poke oil can cause a rash on sensitive skin. Ingestion of poke oil can cause severe intestinal distress.
**Poke root tincture** can be used instead of poke root oil. The properties are quite similar, though the oil is absorbed better and may be considerably more effective.

**Red Clover blossom oil** (*Trifolium pratense*)
The infused oil of red clover blossoms is a remarkable skin softener. It melts away lumps, counters cancer, and helps the lymph system reabsorb unneeded cells. Combine it with internal use of red clover blossom infusion for an even better chance of eliminating abnormal cells and preventing breast cancer recurrence. It's gentle enough for regular use in breast self-massage.

### St. Joan's Wort blossom oil (*Hypericum perforatum*)

The vermillion red oil of the flowers or flowering tops of St. Joan's (St. John's) wort is mild enough to be used regularly to promote breast health, yet powerful enough to seem positively miraculous as it repairs damage to the skin and nerves of the breasts. I consider it an indispensable ally for all women. In addition to using it for breast massage, I favor it for assistance in healing the armpit and breast area after surgery, reducing skin damage from radiation, and relieving nerve and muscle pain. Its antiviral powers pass through the skin and into nerve endings, preventing and checking a wide variety of skin problems, including virulent hospital-bred infections such as shingles.

I find St. Joan's wort oil an exceptionally useful ally for women dealing with nerve damage caused by removal of axillary lymph nodes. Frequent applications restore sensation, promote good lymphatic circulation, help prevent lymphedema, and offer prompt and long-lasting relief from pain.

Women who apply St. Joan's wort oil before and after radiation treatments report that their skin stays healthy and flexible even after dozens of treatments. In addition to preventing radiation burns, this oil prevents sunburn, too. It's the only sunscreen I use to protect my skin, which gets plently of sun. And it's a superior healer of sunburn, as well.

St. Joan's wort oil is an invaluable ally for those with sciatica pain, leg and foot cramps, back pain, neckaches, arthritis pain, bursitis, or any other ache. I use it externally (along with 25 drops of the tincture internally) as often as every 10 to 15 minutes when dealing with the acute phase of a cramped, spasmed muscle. For long-term pain, I use oil and tincture as frequently as needed, sometimes as often as ten times a day.

St. Joan's wort oil is also the best remedy I've found to relieve the pain and promote rapid healing of nerves and skin troubled by shingles, cold sores, mouth and anal fissures, genital herpes, and chicken pox. Hourly applications of oil, plus 25 drops of tincture taken internally at the same time, is not excessive in the initial, acute stages of these problems. As symptoms abate, I use fewer applications. In chronic conditions, I use the oil and tincture four times a day.

Used as a scalp oil during chemotherapy, St. Joan's wort encourages rapid regrowth of healthy hair.

*See* Materia Medica for further information on this wonderful green ally.

**Yarrow flower oil** (*Achillea millefolium*)

Yarrow flowers and leaves infused in oil make a sparkling green oil that promotes fluid flow in the breasts and inhibits bacterial growth. Women have noted that consistent use of yarrow oil seems to prevent the growth of new blood vessels that cancerous tumors need for growth. Yarrow is also a wonderful ally for relieving swollen, tender breasts and nipples. As it may irritate the skin slightly, I use yarrow only as needed.

Yarrow is a plant imbued with a reputation for psychic powers and energy healing. The aroma of the oil is said to give power to the heart and strength to the vulnerable. Sleep with yarrow, and you'll have a dream of the future.

**Yellow Dock root oil** (*Rumex crispus, R. obtusifolia*)

This dark yellow, orange, or burnt-sienna-colored oil is a classic remedy against all hard swellings, tumors, growths, and scabby eruptions. It softens tissues and helps the body reabsorb lumps. The ointment excels as an ally for those dealing with skin ulcers (bed sores), burns from radiation, or mouth sores from chemotherapy. Yellow dock has been known to resolve worrisome nipple discharges. Yellow dock oil does not recommend itself for regular use; I reserve it for occasional intense use.

# Poke Oil Plus
## by Donny Yance, CNMH
*makes 2 ounces/60 ml*

1 ounce/30 ml poke root oil (*Phytolacca americana*)
2 teaspoons/10 ml arnica blossom oil (*Arnica montana*)
2 teaspoons/10 ml tincture of mistletoe (*Viscum album*)
1 teaspoon/5 ml vitamin E oil
1 teaspoon/5 ml St. Joan's wort oil (*Hypericum perforatum*)

This blend is used externally to inhibit free radical damage, cell mutation and local breast cancer recurrence. Its trauma healing ability is useful after a lumpectomy or other breast surgery. Application is twice a day, followed–three days of the week–by a poultice of ground: flax seeds, marshmallow root, slippery elm, and fenugreek mixed with water to make a paste.

# Breast Self-Exam Questions

• Are my breasts the same size and shape as last month? *Yes.*

• Are the curves of my breasts distorted from their norm? *No.*

• Is one different from the other in an unusual way? *No.*

• Is one unusually higher or lower than the other? *No.*

• Any new bulges, indentations, dimples, or puckers? *No.*

• Do my nipples look the same as each other? *Yes.*

• Are my nipples suddenly inverted, retracted, or bulging? *No.*

• Has the slant or tilt of my nipple changed? *No.*

• Any cracks, sores, secretions, or flaky skin on my nipples? *No.*

• Any evidence of nipple discharge in my clothing or bra? *No.*

• Is my breast skin the usual texture and color? *Yes.*

• Are the pores enlarged, the skin stretched or shiny? *No.*

• Are my breasts redder, hotter, more veined than usual? *No.*

• Do I feel areas of unusual tightness, thickening, or tension? *No.*

• Does either breast feel heavy, dense, or strange? *No.*

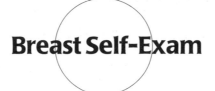

# Breast Self-Exam

One self-help technique available to any woman concerned about breast cancer is monthly breast self-exam (BSE). You can add this exam to your established breast self-massage routine. Or you can learn it first and then add breast self-massage. The two techniques work wonderfully together, as well as alone, because both encourage us to focus our attention on our breasts.

Breast cancer causes distinct changes in the breast tissue. When we observe our breasts as closely as we do our faces, and touch them as often, these changes are more obvious. Combined with journeys to the Wise Healer Within (who can alert you to microscopic cellular changes before they can be seen or felt), breast self-exam can provide extremely early detection of cancer, giving you time to take appropriate action to reverse those changes with non-invasive natural remedies.

Women doing breast self-exam with attention and consistency can find cancers as small as one-eighth of an inch and locate masses that may be undetectable otherwise. As many as one-third of all breast cancers found by women couldn't be imaged by a mammogram. This is especially true of younger women whose denser breast tissues obscure small lumps to the x-ray "eyes"—but not to the touch. Whether you choose to have regular screening mammograms or not, an important aspect of breast health is touching your breasts regularly. Mammograms can't take the place of knowing your own breasts, whether through breast self-massage, breast self-exam, or a combination of the two.

Before we can notice changes, we have to know what our breasts look and feel like; and that's what BSE is about. It gives us a format for knowing our breasts intimately; it helps us gauge what's personally normal and what needs attention. It's more accurate, and much more affirming, to think of breast self-exam as being about getting to know your breasts, not about trying to find cancer.

# Positions for Breast Self-Exam
*Affirmations by Clove*

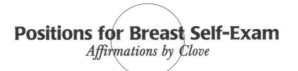

In positions 1–6 you are looking at your breasts in a mirror, first standing still, then turning slowly from side to side. The best light is from the side rather than overhead. Refer to the checklist of BSE questions on page 68 as you assume these positions.

**Position 1.** Look
Stand in front of a mirror with your arms at your sides.
*I see myself, a beautiful goddess.*

**Position 2.** Look
Stretch both arms over your head.
*I welcome the healing rays of the heavens.*

**Position 3.** Look
Clasp your hands and bring them down behind your head; push your elbows back hard.
*I open my heart and my lungs.*

**Position 4.** Look
Push your palms together hard in front of your forehead.
*My body is strong and healthy.*

**Position 5.** Look
Bend from the hips until your nipples point down. You can rest your hands on your knees or a wall.
*My breasts receive the healing rays of the Great Mother, the Earth.*

**Position 6.** Look
Put your hands on your hips (fingers pointing down) and push down hard.
*I am woman, the source of life, creating my own life.*

**Position 7.** Touch
Sit in a bath or on a bed and lean back, or stand in the shower. Raise your right arm and put your hand behind your head. Use a

spiral, clock, or row pattern and three levels of touch (see page 73) to explore your right breast thoroughly with your left hand. Change sides; touch your left breast with your right fingerpads.

**Position 8a.**   Touch
Lie down and relax. Place a pillow under your right shoulder. Bring your right arm up and tuck it under your head. Bend your knees and roll slightly to the left until your right nipple points up. Using an orange segment or row pattern, touch the outer half of your right breast. Continue with 8b before switching sides.

**Position 8b.**   Keeping your hand firmly in place, roll onto your back and examine the inner half of your breast, using the same pattern. Repeat 8a and 8b on your left breast.

## Breast Self-Exam Patterns

A good breast self-exam covers every portion of both breasts. These patterns help us scan thoroughly from collarbone to under breast, from midchest to armpit.

- **Spiral pattern**
  Begin at your nipple; spiral out using small circles.

- **Clock Circles pattern**
  Envision a clock with your nipple at the center. Begin at noon, high on your chest. Using at least six small overlapping circles, move to 3 o'clock (in your armpit), then six o'clock (under your breast), then nine o'clock (the middle of your chest). After completing one clock, do smaller ones inside it, until you do one last clock around your nipple.

- **Row pattern**
  Envision even rows, like knit fabric, an orchard, or rows and rows of braids or beads. Make small circles along these rows, going up and down, or back and forth.

- **Orange Segment pattern**
  Make small circles along 12 or more lines (as many as you need to cover your breast completely) which radiate out from your nipple.

### Do I need to do all those positions and that muscle flexing?

In breast self-exam, the ideal is to look at and touch as much breast tissue as possible, not just what we usually think of as our breasts. Breast tissue extends from collarbone to just below the fold of skin under the breast, and from midchest to mid-side and armpit. By assuming different positions and tightening the various muscles of the chest, we can highlight different areas of the breast.

### What's the best time to do breast self-exam?

Any time you can do it is the best time. You may find your breasts less tender and less lumpy about a week after your menstrual flow begins, but you can do BSE any time of the month. Postmenopausal women may wish to examine their breasts at the new moon. Doing BSE at a regular time helps jog your memory, but doing it as the mood moves you will help you get to know your breast tissues with all their changes. Since breast structures change monthly and throughout our lives (*see* illustration page 58), it is beneficial to touch our breasts at a variety of times.

### I keep forgetting to examine my breasts. Help!

Do it every day. Like brushing your hair, doing a quick breast check only takes a minute in the morning, and it's easier to remember if you do a little every day. Check a different quarter of your breast each day. Once a week do a more thorough check: BSE position 7 in the shower, BSE positions 1–6 after drying off. Several times a year do breast self-massage and go on a journey to visit your Wise Healer Within. If you do all that, you can forget monthly checks.

### What's the least amount of BSE I can do and still take care of myself?

The average doctor spends less than two minutes—and only once a year—examining your breasts. If you only check your breasts once a year, but spend 20 minutes on it, you'll receive 1000% better care than if you rely on "professional" attention.

If you're at high risk for breast cancer, 15 minutes per month will cover all positions every month. If you're at normal risk for breast cancer, you can cut this to ten minutes by omitting position 7 one month and 8 the next. If you're at low risk for breast cancer, five minutes once a month (positions 1 through 7) plus a yearly massage could be enough.

## Is there a special way to touch my breasts in BSE?

Like this: Hold the first two or three fingers of one hand close together. Place the pads (not the tips) of those fingers on the opposite breast. (Left hand examines right breast; then right hand examines left breast.) Press gently toward the ribcage and make a small circle, moving the skin with your fingers.

Then press a little more deeply, and make another small circle. Then press very firmly (but don't hurt yourself) and make a third circle.

Move your fingers a finger's width away, in your chosen pattern, and make another three circles at varying pressures. Move another finger's breadth and continue your pattern (*see* page 71), circling with light, moderate, and firm pressures.

## Can't I just slide my fingers around on my breasts?

Breast lumps are moveable, like lumps in pudding. If you slide your fingers across your skin, lumps can slide out of the way and you won't feel them. To feel a lump, you have to trap it. You can trap it between your chest wall and your finger pads. Or trap it between your two hands if your breasts are large: Put your breast on your palm and press down with your other hand with a gentle, firm pressure.

No grabbing. No squeezing. Circle, circle, circle; circle, circle, circle; circle, circle, circle. Soapy is fine; oil, lotion, powder is fine; but keep your fingers pressed firmly to skin when making circles—no slipping and sliding.

## What am I feeling in there?

If it's **soft** or **spongy**, it's **fat**. The older you are, the more fat you'll feel. Fat is a normal part of breast tissue.

If it's like **lumpy cream of wheat** or **large curd cottage cheese**, it's **lumpy glandular tissue**. The older you are, the less of it there will be. Lumpy glandular tissue is a normal part of breast tissue, as is non-lumpy glandular tissue.

If it's **ridgy, corrugated, fibrous, bony, and big**, it's **your ribs** (and the connective tissues and muscles around and between your ribs). The thinner you are, the more of this you'll feel. Ridgy, corrugated, fibrous, bony ribs are normal.

If it's thick, **gel-like**, or **softly firm**, it's a **thickening**. Thickenings are a normal part of breast tissue. Thickenings are commonly found in a semicircle under the breast (like a built-in bra) and perched in the upper, outer chest near the armpits.

If it's like a **regularly shaped pea**, pebble, or marble, it's most likely a **cyst**. A slippery lump that suddenly appears in the breast is more likely a cyst than a cancer, but it needs to be watched closely. If it shrinks (or swells and shrinks) over time, or if it stays the same, it's probably a harmless cyst, especially if you're under 50 years old. If it only gets bigger, or if you have a sense that it's cancer, seek assistance. (And read Chapter 6, "There's a Lump in My Breast.")

If it's hard and dense, like a **dried grain of rice**, like an **uncooked lentil**, like a **dried bit of cheese**, it could be **cancer**. Is there a mirror-image in the other breast? If so, it's probably normal for you. If not, seek help. This kind of lump may or may not be normal breast tissue.

If it's a **tender, rounded lump in your armpit**, it's probably a **swollen lymph node**. Lymph nodes are normal tissue, but swollen lymph nodes indicate injury, infection, or possibly cancer, in the adjacent arm, lung, or breast. I assist my immune system when my glands are swollen by taking 10 drops of cleavers tincture once or twice a day for up to a month. If my lymph nodes are swollen *and* tender, I use 1–4 drops of poke root tincture daily for a week or more instead. (More information on these herbs can be found in the Materia Medica.) If your lymph nodes remain swollen or tender for more than a month, seek help.

### I feel clumsy and don't know what I'm doing.

Take a break from BSE. Learn breast self-massage. Come back to breast self-exam in a few months. It takes time to get to know your breasts. Give yourself that time. Touch yourself without judging it. Touch because you want to be intimate with your breasts, with their power. Love your breasts. Hum.

*"Ninety percernt of lumps—and I am talking about lumps that ultimately turn out to be cancer—are detected by women [themselves]. . . ."*
Pat Kelley, breast cancer activist, 1993

# Breast Massage Oils by Mail

Burdock seed oil: 3, 5, 9
Calendula oil: 1, 2, 4, 5, 7
Castor oil: 1, 6
Dandelion flower oil: 1, 2, 3, 9
Evergreen oils: 4, 9
Poke root oil: 1, 3, 4, 9
St. Joan's wort oil: 1, 2, 3, 4, 5, 7, 9
Special breast massage blends: 1, 8, 9

1 • **Avena Botanicals/Deb Soule**
219 Mill St. Rockport, ME 04856; 207-594-0694

2 • **Blessed Maine Herbs/Gail Edwards**
PO Box 4074, West Athens, ME 04912; 207-654-3994

3 • **Catskill Mt. Herbs/Whitefeather**
PO Box 1426, Olivebridge, NY 12461; 914-657-2943

4 • **Hygieia/Deborah Maia**
PO Box 893, Great Barrington, MA 01230; 413-528-6085

5 • **Green Terrestrial**
1449 Warm Brook Rd, Arlington VT 05250; 802-375-8087

6 • **Heritage Products**
PO Box 444, Virginia Beach, VA 23458

7 • **Mountain Rose Herbs**
PO Box 2000, Redway, CA 95560; 1-800-879-3337

8 • **NaturaSacredplay/Elaine Geouge**
PO Box 32, Buckhorn, NM 88025; 505-535-2255

9 • **Red Moon Herbs/Corinna Wood** and **Jessica Godino**
1039 Camp Elliot rd, Black Mt, NC 28711; 828-669-1310

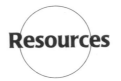

# Resources

- "Breast Cancer Protection Program," free; Strang Cancer Prevention Center, 428 E. 72nd St., NY, NY 10021; 212-794-0077

- Breast self-examination card, free; National Breast Cancer Foundation, PO Box 5939, Abilene, TX 79608

- Breast self-exam card, free; First Response, PO Box 562, Gibbstown, NJ 08027

- "Breast Self-Examination, A New Approach," free booklet from American Cancer Society, 1599 Clifton Rd., NE, Atlanta, GA, 30329; 1-800-ACS-2345. This excellent resource is a favorite of mine and was highly recommended by several women. ACS will give you the names of women who offer hands-on training in BSE at no charge.

☆ These small images can add to the pleasure of taking your breasts into your own hands. (Catalogs are free.)

- **Life-Sustaining Goddess** (2000 B.C.E.) from
Grand Adventure, RD 6, Box 6198A, Stroudsburg, PA 18360;
717-992-6393

- **Inanna** (2500 B.C.E., *see* front cover) from Star River,
PO Box 510642, Melbourne Beach, FL 32951; 407-953-8167

- **Breast Goddess Box** and **Offering Goddess** from
Mission Studio, 1937 Crestview, Ashland, OR 97520;
503-488-2451

# Weaving the Web of Immunity

"Dear GrandDaughter, we hear your desire for health: Your desire makes us audible, your need makes us visible. We are the Ancient Ones, old beyond your reckoning, and wise in the ways of health and healing. Though you may think of us as guardian angels or guides, the form you give us doesn't matter. We call ourselves the GrandMothers. We are the wisdom that exists in rock and water, air and fire, and within you. We hear you and we respond:

"You want a powerful immune system, one strong enough to weather the storms and stresses of your life, to keep you free from cancer, vital and resilient. To strengthen your immunity, it is wise to know it well. And to know it, we must enter its realm. We will take you there, dear one, but first we must warn you: Powerful immunity is deep, dark and cutting; severe, certain and decisive. Are you willing to enter the darkness? To encounter the edge?

"Few are. Most prefer the light and the smooth, fearing the dark and shunning edges. But the dark is as much a source of strength as the light. Some aspects of immunity are birthed only in darkness. And though it may seem safer to avoid jagged edges, your immunity must be sharp as broken glass. We invite you to honor the dark, nourish your uneven edges, embrace what is crude and unrefined, what is primal and wild. This supports immunity in ways that smoothness and slickness cannot.

"We see that you are willing. Enter with us now the deep underground of your own being. Meet the symbolic queen of the web, the virtual center of your immunity. She is threaded through with impulses from every nerve, every emotion, every vibration of life beating within you. Like a spider, she is aware of the sound of every insect, alert to the special hum of the flies you call cancer cells. She listens, she acts. She sends her messages to the living threads of your immune system. Like a spider catching a fly, the strands snare cancerous cells and wrap them for later feasting.

"The cancer-fly awaits its fate, the fate of all life, to be the nourishment for more life. When all is well with you, special cells are created every time a cancer-fly is captured. Guided by the fly's hum and the immune web, these cells find the captured cancer-fly and consume it with great appetites.

"But these bundled feasts, these caught cancer-flies, can, like zombies from your nightmares, awaken if not consumed in time. They can awaken like the living dead to breed and feed as maggots upon the parts of yourself you have failed to nourish, the parts that are rotting within you.

"You asked for enhanced immunity and we, your Ancient GrandMothers, offer you this: carrion birds, the vultures who nourish themselves as they pick clean your rotting flesh, leaving nothing for the maggots.

"We offer you the ancient image of Mah, Mother Destroyer, She Who Holds the Knife. Mah who nourishes and supports all that is you by ordering death for all that is not you. How can you support her work? Honor the vultures within you. Follow the spider's sacred spiral from your center to your edges. Cut through and nourish the abandoned parts of yourself. Together, dearest GrandDaughter, we will build powerful immunity."

# 4.
# Building Powerful Immunity

Can a powerful immune system prevent cancer? Can a strong immune system put cancer into remission? Can it prevent the recurrence of cancer that has been treated? Stop a cancer from metastasizing?

Orthodox medicine rarely focuses on the immune system as a means of preventing or curing cancer. In fact, orthodox medicine urges women to detect and treat cancer with techniques known to suppress the immune system.

But building powerful immunity can help us remain cancer-free. Building powerful immunity is also an important part of treatment, whether alone or as complementary medicine. Immune system strengthening is especially useful against cancers initiated by viruses. (Epstein-Barr virus is associated with breast cancer.[1]) Building powerful immunity provides long-lasting benefits for relatively little effort.

To prevent cancer, I use immune-strengthening techniques from Steps 0, 2, and 3 on a regular basis. Women dealing with grey areas of cancer diagnosis (such as *in situ* cancers, ambiguous findings, greatly differing pathology reports, indeterminate microcalcifications, and moderately differentiated cells) would include Step 4 as well. I consider Steps 4, 5, and 6 most appropriate for women dancing with cancer, dealing with an acute infection, or healing chronic immune problems.


**Step 0.** *Do Nothing*

• Meditate on the great void; think nothing, see nothing.

• Eliminate time for at least one day (two weeks is ever so much better). How? Remove your watch. Hide or unplug all clocks. Turn off the radio and TV. Go to bed when you want to. Eat when you're hungry. Wake up when you feel like it.

**Step 1.** *Collect Information*

★ Look at *The Body Victorious* by Lennart Nilsson, especially pages 94-109 and 127-130, which bring you eye-to-eye with cancer-eating macrophages, T-lymphocytes, and monocytes.[2]

• The immune system is said to consist of large basic parts (tonsils, adenoids, thymus, spleen, lymphatic vessels, and lymph nodes) plus specialized cells that those parts make (white blood cells, mast cells, and serum factors such as interferon).

★ But Candace Pert (discoverer of pleasure receptors in the brain, and visiting professor of neuroscience at Rutgers University) has proven that every cell of the body participates in the immune system through a "psychosomatic communication network."[3] The immune system is a complex, integrated network of chemical, electrical, and hormonal signals. It is a vibrational network that is as affected by emotions as by bacteria, as impacted by thoughts as by drugs, which resonates with the vibrations that surround it.

**Step 2.** *Engage the Energy*

• The immune system is particularly sensitive to energy messages whether the obvious ones of **fragrances, colors, music, rhythms, movement, symbols**, and **prayers**, or the more subtle ones such as **breath, intention,** and **environment**. Classic vibrational healing techniques–**such as shamanic journeys**, religious **pageants**, healing **ceremonies**, sand paintings, and personal **rituals**–activate multiple vibrational messages, vastly increasing their effectiveness.

• Visit your immune system with the Wise Healer Within (page 82).

★ **Laugh! Sing! Cry! Rage!** Really, these do strengthen your immune system. The ancient Greek healing temple complexes always included clowns and theater. Laugh 'til you cry. Sing 'til everybody else does. Have a tantrum. Long-standing low-level depression, smouldering anger that is rarely or never expressed, bitterness and vengeance harbored for decades, and frozen silences that endure long past the hurt, all depress immune functioning. Expressing these feelings in some safe way is a powerful means of strengthening the immune system and countering the cancer cascade.

• Flower essences, homeopathic remedies, crystal elixirs, chakra meditations, and other unorthodox techniques for strengthening the immune system are not so strange as they sound. Explore their scientific basis in *Vibrational Medicine* by Richard Gerber, M.D.[4]

★ To strengthen my immune system, I use the color orange. I visualize **orange,** I eat orange foods, I even imagine that the air is tinged a peachy orange and breathe it in. I gather orange energy into my belly chakra. I concentrate the orange into my navel: the mark of my separation from my mother, from the Goddess, from the bliss of being one with All. The navel is the symbolic center of my immune system (the system that keeps me embodied and separate from the All until it's time to merge again with the All at my death). From my belly button, I circulate the orange of immune vitality throughout my body, bringing it into my breasts and any other areas where I feel it is needed. I imagine every cell of my immune system vibrating with orange. When I am filled with orange, I breathe out with a great sigh. For more on chakra healing, see *Pranic Healing* by Choa Kok Sui.[5]

• Both **light and dark** are necessary for a strong immune system. Melatonin, a hormone that helps protect us against cancer, is produced only in the dark, while full spectrum sunlight is needed to trigger the production of other important immune system components. To build powerful immunity, sleep in a totally dark room at night and spend at least 15 minutes a day outside without glasses or contacts.

★ **Listen** to what you say—out loud and to yourself; your body and your immune system do.[6, 7] Affirmation, positive thinking, prayer, or mantra, no matter what you call it, talking lovingly to yourself is a daily practice that builds powerful immunity. One of the fiercest old women I know, and a valued mentor, healer Margo Geiger, taught me to not only think good thoughts but also to unthink immune system stressing phrases like: "This is killing me," or "I'm dying to . . ." ("Let's live for it!" she'd say.)

• The smell of a drop of pure **essential oil of rosemary, lavender, tea tree**, or **rose geranium** is said to strengthen the immune system.[8] (No synthetics, please, they depress the immune system.)

## Journey to the Wise Healer Within

*Have someone read this to you, or read it into a tape recorder and play it back for yourself.*

*Find a place and time to be alone for half an hour, away from the demands of family, work, telephone. Loosen constricting clothing; unhook your bra (better yet, take it off); remove your shoes, and eyeglasses or contact lenses. Lie comfortably on your back with a pillow under your knees. Close your eyes and breathe out.*

Breathe out and relax. Breathe out until you're empty. Breathe out any thoughts. Breathe out any tension. Breathe slowly and evenly, like you're swinging or rocking, like you're flapping large wings or moving in a little boat on calm water. Let go to the easy rhythm of this movement. Let this gentle sighing out and inhaling in hold you. Give in to the sensation of being moved effortlessly by your own breath, by a rhythm and a power much larger than you.

As you breathe and surrender to your own rhythm, bring your attention to your heart. Was there a time when your heart yearned for something? Feel it again, that yearning, wanting, aching, opening, needing. This time your yearning is heard. This time there is an answer to your desire. This time the Wise Healer Within answers you.

*You may perceive the Wise Healer Within in any number of guises: female, male, animal, plant, rock, alien, insect, the cosmos. You may just "know" that the Wise Healer Within is present and communicating with you; or you may see or hear something.*

Introduce yourself to your Wise Healer Within and offer a small gift, perhaps something you have in your pocket, perhaps your smile, or a hug. You can ask the Wise Healer Within questions: What's your name? What gift would you like next time I visit? Do I pay enough attention to you? Do you have any complaints or compliments about our relationship? Any comments about how I treat myself?

Ask your Wise Healer Within to take you on a tour of your breasts and the nearby lymph nodes. You'll need to make yourself small enough to fit into the ducts and lobules of the breast tissue and to glide through the lymphatic vessels. First go to healthy breast tissue. Note carefully what you sense, see, hear, or feel. Let your inner healer know that optimal health is what you want for every part of your body and every aspect of your life.

Ask your Wise Healer Within to point out any pre-cancerous or cancerous cells in your breasts or anywhere in your body. Ask your inner healer to keep a sharp lookout for atypical cells and to notify you immediately if any begin to proliferate. How can your Wise Healer Within alert you? Decide together on a way to communicate.

If your Wise Healer Within does show you cancerous or pre-cancerous cells, ask for help in changing them. You can go into those cells and, with the help of your inner healer, make a plan of action. What needs to change? How? Do you need other help? Who or what? What do you need to do to initiate those changes? To sustain the changes? How can you be sure that the abnormal cells have returned to normal? How frequently do you need to monitor those cells?

Ask your Wise Healer Within to take you to the healthiest, happiest cells in your body. Bask in their life force. If you want, ask to go to the area of your body that would most benefit from your attention, and ask for help in giving those parts of yourself exactly what they need.

*Spend as long as you like with your Wise Healer Within. You'll know when it's time to go.*

Now feel yourself walking away from your Wise Healer Within, knowing that you can return whenever you wish. Feel your entire body walking away, the right side and the left side, walking away. Feel your arms and legs moving rhythmically, walking away, yet staying connected. Your feet pressing the ground, walking away. Let the rhythm of your walking gradually bring you back to full size and take you to the very place where you are right now. Open your eyes, stretch, and sit up, feeling energized and at ease.

*Take the time to record your journey in pictures or words.*

**Step 3.** *Nourish and Tonify*

• Much of the immune system is created on demand. Specialized cells which eliminate cancer cells, bacteria, and viruses are made as needed. When the immune system is richly supplied with nutrients, it creates plentiful amounts of these specialized cells: interferon, macrophages, tumor-suppressor cells, natural killer cells, and T-cells. When nutrients are lacking, the immune system falters, leaving one susceptible to many diseases, including cancer.

 The nutrients most critical for building powerful immunity are **selenium**, **germanium**, **trace minerals**, and the **antioxidant vitamins A, C,** and **E. Caution:** Supplemental forms of these nutrients may initiate or promote cancer. *See* "Vitamin and Mineral Sources," page 53, for safe sources.

• How do **nutritional deficiencies** hinder immune functioning? The number of tumor-suppressor and helper T-cells diminishes, the activity level and number of tumor-eating T-cells falls, interferon production slows, there are fewer immunoglobulin cells, and deficiencies of healthy red and white blood cells develop.[9]

★ **Beets, carrots, garlic, green tea, wild mushrooms, seaweed,** and **dark leafy greens** are the best foods to nourish and strengthen the immune system. For rapid results, try miso soup with seaweed, garlic, leafy greens, and wild mushrooms for lunch, and "Immune A Go Go Soup" (page 309) or "Good Enough To Live (Not Die) For Stir-Fry" (page 308) for dinner for several weeks.

★ My favorite herbs for nourishing the immune system are **stinging nettle, astragalus, American ginseng, Siberian ginseng,** and **wild mushrooms**.

• **Stinging nettle**—infusion of dried leaves, or broth from cooking the fresh tender tops—is one way I strengthen my immune system, increase my energy, and regenerate and protect my adrenal glands. Those who've used nettle during severe illness (including cancer and AIDS), second my rave reviews of her life-enhancing, life-extending benefits. *See* Materia Medica.

• **Astragalus** root is said to be one of the safest herbs for building powerful immunity, and it is often taken daily for extended periods. In addition to general immune strengthening, astragalus offers powerful help when immunity is severely challenged. Clinical studies show astragalus infusion highly effective at improving and restoring T-cell functioning, improving bone marrow activity, and augmenting interferon response. Chinese hospitals give astragalus to strengthen the immune systems of those with cancer, and to protect them from the detrimental effects of chemotherapy and radiation treatments.[10] *See* Materia Medica.

★ One of the most studied of all herbs, **ginseng** root (*Panax quinquefolius* or *Panax ginseng*) is an exceptional ally for the im-

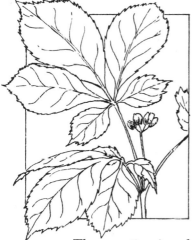

mune system under stress.[11, 12] Ginseng nourishes production of interferon, phagocytes, antibodies, and killer T-cells.[13] Ginseng increases energy and raises antioxidant levels. It shrinks and eliminates tumors, protects the adrenal cortex, and is strongly anticarcinogenic in the presence of radiation and chemicals, making it superb complementary medicine for those choosing aggressive orthodox treatments. I use ginseng to mitigate the effects of physical stresses such as lack of sleep, travel, and temperature extremes

The question is, which of the bewildering variety of types and preparations of ginseng to buy? I prefer American ginseng. I generally use a tincture made from fresh ten-year old roots (taking 25–100 drops daily), but whole dried roots of good quality can also be used (the dose is 1–9 grams cooked for 4 hours in 1–2 cups/250–500 ml water). Powders, capsules, and teas of ginseng are generally of such poor quality that they have little or no effect. So long as you need ginseng, there's no overdose; if you take it when you don't need it however, ginseng may produce an unpleasant, jittery, speedy sensation.

★ **Siberian ginseng** (*Eleutherococcus*) is widely considered the single most effective immune tonic and adaptogen (herb that mitigates the effects of stress) in the herbal realm. Safe and inexpensive, it helps the immune system respond to cellular damage caused by radiation, air and water pollution, and stresses such as constant noise, overwork, and grief.[14] Siberian ginseng grows like a weed, and is much less expensive than *Panax. See* Materia Medica.

★ **Wild mushrooms** were my first love. Long before I became enamored with green plants, I was stalking mushrooms—on my belly in the Catskill mountains. Mushrooms are the great regenerators, unlocking centuries of stored mineral wealth from dead trees. We feed our immune systems these concentrated minerals, as well as a host of other anti-cancer compounds, when we eat wild and exotic mushrooms. I eat wild mushrooms frequently when they're in season, drying and freezing any surplus. Those with cancer may benefit from daily use. **Play it safe**; don't taste unknown mushrooms; triple check before eating any wild mushroom. You can buy exotic mushrooms in capsules or fresh in some markets. Here's what laboratory and clinical studies have discovered about their adaptogenic and immune enhancing effects:

• **Maitake** (*Grifolia frondosa*), the dancing mushroom—whether fresh, tinctured, or in tablets—is more effective than any other tested mushroom, including shiitake, at inhibiting tumor growth in laboratory animals. More importantly, it is highly effective when taken orally. (Shiitake is most effective intravenously.) When you buy maitake, take care to get the fruiting body. The mycelium, which is frequently sold (read the label), is much less effective.

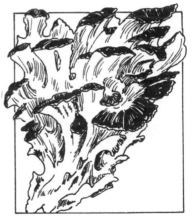

• **Reishii** (*Ganoderma lucidum*) are one of the most respected immune tonics in Oriental medicine. All *Ganoderma* are adaptogenic, revitalizing, and regenerative—especially to the liver. Daily use during radiation treatments reduces damage to normal cells. Even occasional use builds powerful immunity and reduces risk of cancer. In clinical studies, reishii increased T-cell and alpha interferon production, shrank and eliminated tumors, and improved the quality of life for those with terminal disease. Reishii are said to work exceptionally well with shiitake, the effects of one enhancing the effects of the other.

*Eating Reishii*: Reishii are more frequently sold as tablets or tinctures than fresh or whole. After boiling one for six hours with little result, I understand why. This is one tough mushroom. Reishii contain so little water that they weigh the same fresh or dried. The classical method of preparation is to simmer 1 ounce (30 grams) of *Ganoderma* in a pint of water in a tightly covered pan for 24 hours. The resulting liquid is sipped for the next 24 hours. Slow cooking of *Ganoderma* is easier nowadays; a crock pot avoids the risk of scorching. The usual dose of the tincture (whole mushrooms in alcohol) is 20–40 drops, 3 times a day.

• **Shiitake** (*Lentinus edodes*) builds powerful immunity and directly suppresses chemical and viral oncogenesis. Regular use of shiitake improves vitamin D production and utilization (important in preventing cancer), and increases production of cancer-fighting alpha interferon. Shiitake are also anti-inflammatory. In Japan, shiitake extract given intravenously enhances and prolongs life for those with advanced breast cancer. Side effects, even from large doses, are rare.

*Eating Shiitake*: I buy fresh shiitake, slice the caps, sear them in a little olive oil, add slices of garlic and a handful of water, cover, and steam about 15 minutes. Dried shiitake are wonderful in soups. The stems are tough and rubbery, and don't soften when cooked, but don't discard them. Try this: Fill a little jar with shiitake stems, add apple cider vinegar to the top, screw on a tight plastic lid, and wait 6-8 weeks. Heaven smells and tastes like shiitake vinegar, I'm sure. It adds a sensational flavor to salads, is very high in minerals, and is anti-cancer as well. To maintain powerful immunity, I use shiitake once or twice a month. To help prevent side effects of chemotherapy, a tablespoon/30 ml of vinegar daily or a side dish of the caps several times a week wouldn't be too much. Use **enokidake** the same way.

• **Zhu ling** (*Polyporus umbellatus*), prized for thousands of years as an aid to longevity and vitality, produces edible mushrooms above ground and a tuber-like mass underground which is used medicinally. *In vitro* (in a test tube), zhu ling only increased alpha-interferon, but *in vivo* (in real life), when ingested by Chinese people with cancer, zhu ling was strikingly helpful. Use like reishii.

• **Chaga** (*Inonotus obliquus*) grows on white birch trees. In Russia it has been used extensively as an immune nourisher, cancer preventive, and aid to those dancing with cancer, especially melanomas. (The most common mushroom on birches in my woods is *Ganoderma applamatum*.) Prepare and use chaga like reishii.

• **Puffballs** (*Calvatia* species) are common wild mushroom with powerful anti-cancer properties.

## Building Powerful Immunity with Herbs

• **White blood cells** are produced in the thymus gland and the bone marrow. They come in many different forms (such as helper T-cells, killer T-cells, and B cells), but all destroy cancer cells and viruses.

    These herbs enhance white blood cell production: **astragalus, echinacea, Siberian ginseng, ginseng, reishii, wild mushrooms, licorice,** and **goldenseal**.

• **Macrophages** live in the lymph nodes, the liver, and the spleen, where they eat bacteria and cellular debris, and prevent damage to the immune system.

    These herbs enhance macrophage activity: **echinacea, Siberian ginseng, ginseng,** and **licorice**.

• **Interferon** binds to cell surfaces and initiates the creation of viral-inhibiting proteins.

    These herbs enhance production and use of interferon: **astragalus, echinacea, licorice,** and **boneset** (*Eupatorium perfoliatum*), and **reishii, shiitake** and **zhu ling** mushrooms.

• **Echinacea** is the all-American immune system tonic and anti-cancer herb. It activates production of white blood cells, interferon, leukocytes, T-cells, and B-lymphocytes. It also directly inhibits the growth of most bacteria and viruses. Echinacea is my first choice for countering infection anywhere. Unlike prescription antibiotics or herbal antibacterials (such as goldenseal) which counter infection but weaken immune functioning, echinacea strengthens and nourishes the immune system. *See* Materia Medica.

★ **Usnea**, a common lichen, is especially rich in a powerful antibiotic and anti-tumor bitter called usnic acid (also usinic acid), and in immune-strengthening minerals, too. *Usnea barbata* is the one I use, but other lichens show similar immune-enhancing and tonifying properties. There are no side effects reported from use of usnea tincture. I'm quite impressed with its ability to rally the immune system. Here's a marvelous healing stories that stars usnea: The hip replacement went awry; infection set in and raged, sneering at the antibiotics. Should they operate again, or wait and risk losing the leg? Thirty drops of usnea tincture every two hours turned the infection around in less than a day (just as it did for me when I was smitten with a vertigo-producing, teeth-clenchingly painful sinus infection). I've found usnea on the branches of fruit trees and conifers in the Pacific Northwest, the Canadian North, and all over New Zealand. I tincture it—fresh or dried, it makes no difference—in 100-proof vodka in a brown glass bottle until it turns orange (the color of immune strength). Herbalist Cascade Anderson-Geller intensifies the strengthening and tonifying properties of usnea by boiling it briefly in water before tincturing it.

★ **Exercise** is an excellent way to tonify the immune sytem. A number of clinical trials have shown regular exercise to be strongly linked to heightened immunity and resistance to cancer. The emphasis is on *regular*. It is better to walk one mile four times a week for a month than to jog 16 miles once a month.

## Step 4. *Stimulate/Sedate*

★ **Poke** root kicks the immune system into high gear, especially the lymphatic drainage of the breast tissue. Poke is a specific for women with breast infections, painful underarm lymph glands, breast cancer, or lung problems. *See* Materica Medica.

Women living with persistent, painful breast lumps report good results from use of 5–10 drops of poke root tincture daily for no more than three months. Those dancing with cancer sometimes use as much as 30 drops a day for up to a year. Dose is one drop a day, increasing by a drop every 2–3 days, until it takes effect.

**Caution**: You can feel spacey and out of your body when taking poke, especially at higher doses. The first few times, take it after dinner and stay home so you can judge your reaction. Large doses used for more than three months can stress the kidneys.

• Clinical studies show that grief and stress lower the number and activity level of T-cells and natural killer cells, slowing immune response, and increasing cancer risk.[15] Counter with ginseng or motherwort tinctures (10–20 drops of either) and a support group.

★ Vibration strengthens the thymus and the immune system. One simple way to vibrate the thymus is to tap on the chest (between the breasts) 300 beats a day. Playing the harp, drumming, and dancing are other ways.

★ **Licorice** root (*Glycyrrhiza glabra*) is one of the world's safest and most widely used immune system stimulants. It is especially effective at inhibiting herpes viruses and preventing virally-induced cancers from growing or spreading. Licorice tincture (25–75 drops a day) or tea (not infusion) supports plentiful antibody production, is anti-inflammatory, and protects the adrenal cortex. **Caution**: Large doses of licorice used for extended periods raise the blood pressure and disrupt electrolyte balance.

• **Intense heat** stimulates the immune system. Getting really hot 4-6 times a year is an excellent way to build powerful immunity. How? A sauna, a steam room, an epsom salt bath (as hot as possible, while drinking yarrow or sage infusion), or a Native American sweat lodge (as hot as possible, while burning yarrow and sage). **Intense cold** (don't overdo it) stimulates the immune system, too.

• **Chronic infection** is a severe strain on the immune system. Take action when infections linger: For the gums, try a rinse of 1–5 drops of myrrh (*Commiphora myrrha*) tincture in a little water; for the vagina and uterus, use condoms and other latex barriers to prevent infections, echinacea to treat them; and for chronic sinus infections, try a salt water nasal douche (*see* page 236).

**Step 5a.** *Use Supplements*

• **Selenium** builds a healthy immune system as well as blocking the initiation and proliferation of cancer cells. Those dancing with cancer use up to 1000 mcg (1 mg) of selenomethionine or 1–5 mg a day of sodium selenite daily (extremely high amounts) to stimulate immune functioning. **Caution**: Overdoses can occur. *See* page 157. Herbal sources of selenium: organic garlic, astragalus.

• **Zinc** is another important immune system nutrient. Without it, white blood cells have less energy, T-cells dwindle, and thymus activity falls. But, like any good thing, it can be overdone. Supplemental zinc in excess of actual need will suppress the immune system. Herbal sources of zinc: echinacea, nettles, seaweed.

• The B-vitamin complex, especially **B₆** (pyridoxine), is critical to immune system health. Lack of $B_6$ causes a diminishment of thymus function. The usual supplemental dose is 100 mg daily. Foods rich in pyridoxine include broccoli, prunes, and lentils.

★ **Carotenes,** or pro-vitamin A, strengthen and activate the immune system. Daily doses begin at 20,000 IU (the amount in a serving of dandelion greens or two large carrots) but ten times that much can be consumed without causing side effects. Carotenes nourish and support the production of interferon, tumor-suppressor cells, killer T-cells, and helper T-cells (sometimes increasing them by 30 percent within a week). Carotenes are especially important for the health of the thymus—master gland of the immune system. And they are used in large amounts when the immune system communicates with itself. Warning: Large doses of vitamin A can cause dry lips, dry nails, falling hair, and liver problems.

### Step 5b. *Use Drugs*

• Virtually all drugs depress the immune system, at least temporarily. This includes caffeine and nicotine, as well as steroids, most prescribed drugs, chemotherapeutic agents, sedatives, and stimulants.

• Antibiotics are life savers when it comes to countering some infections, but overuse (and overconsumption, through animal products) leads to a weakened immune system.

• The drug Nuprogin, used to boost white blood cell count, severely weakens the immune system.

### Step 6. *Break & Enter*

• Surgery, and the attendant anesthesia, suppresses the immune system for 7–10 days.

• Radiation therapies suppress the immune system, sometimes for months after treatment has ceased.

• One extraordinary means of strengthening the immune system is to break habitual mind-body patterns with **mind-altering plants**, allowing new beliefs and functional patterns to be entered through carefully planned ceremony. Because the immune system is highly

interactive with brain chemicals, it is powerfully affected by psychoactive plants. Ingesting these "power plants" (e.g. psilocybin
mushrooms, peyote cactus, ayahuasca, marijuana) under the
skilled guidance of a shaman or a wise woman can initiate powerful changes in immune system functioning which more than offset
the potential for immune system depression from their use.[16-19]

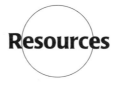

# Resources

## Engaging the Energy

• *Humor and Healing,* Bernie Siegel, M.D., audiotape from Sounds
  True, 735 Walnut St., Boulder, CO 80302; 303-449-6229.

• *Meditations for Enhancing Your Immune System,* Bernie Siegel, M.D.,
  audiotape from Hay House, PO Box 6204, Carson, CA 90749;
  1-800-654-5126.

• *Sacred Verses, Healing Sounds,* Deepak Chopra, audiotape from
  New World Library, 58 Paul Dr., San Rafael, CA 94903.

## Immune-Enhancing Mushrooms

• Gourmet mushrooms, including shiitake, wood ear, and orange
  chanterelles from Spices, Etc.; 1-800-827-6373

• Organic shiitake from Mt. Ark; 1-800-643-8909

> *"Human immunity is ecology in action."*
> David Hoffman, herbalist (1993)

# 5.
# Mammograms–Who Needs Them?

Perhaps no aspect of breast cancer is more widely publicized than screening mammography. Ads on television, in magazines, and in the daily paper urge women to deal with fear about breast cancer by having a yearly mammogram. We're even told that doing this is a way to "really care for yourself."

But screening mammograms don't prevent breast cancer. A mammogram is an x-ray and x-rays cause cancer. The ads promoting regular screening mammography are paid for by those who stand to profit from their widespread acceptance and use–the manufacturers of the equipment and x-ray film. Whose health does this technology really benefit? Women's health? Or corporate health?

Should you have a screening mammogram? At what age? How frequently? Science hasn't agreed on answers to these questions.[1] I believe that my anti-cancer lifestyle (see page xv) will decrease my risk of dying from breast cancer in a way that regular mammograms won't. I care for my breasts with infused herbal oils, regular loving touch, organic foods, and healthy exercise–and forgo regular screening mammograms. Of course, you can do it all in the Wise Woman Tradition. The point is to *pay attention to your breasts.*

### All mammograms are x-rays.

A mammogram uses radioactive rays to "see" breast tissues. X-rays are known to cause DNA damage in breast cells.

A *diagnostic mammogram* is used when a woman or her practitioner feels a lump and wants to see it. (Sonograms–a non-radioactive test–can be used instead.) Most diagnostic mammograms are not one x-ray, but a series of x-rays.

A *screening mammogram* is done on a healthy woman to determine if there are unsuspected signs of cancer, such as a shadow or micro-calcifications. A screening mammogram is not one x-ray, but a series of x-rays, usually two per breast, four in all.

### Mammograms are inaccurate.

Low-radiation mammograms are safer mammograms, but less radiation means a fuzzier picture. Standard x-rays—rarely used any more for breasts—create an easy-to-interpret high-radiation image. Xerograms use half that radiation, but are twice as hard to read. Film-screen mammography, the latest very-low-radiation exam, gives an image that's even more difficult to interpret. More than 10 percent of all screening mammograms done at one large center in 1992 couldn't be read and had to be redone.[2]

A 1994 study showed wide variation in the accuracy with which mammograms are interpreted. Understandably, those who read screening mammograms regularly are more accurate than those who rarely do; in some hospitals, however, work loads are so heavy that accuracy suffers from lack of time, not inexperience.

Roughly 8 out of 10 "positive" mammographic reports are "false positive," that is, a subsequent biopsy does not confirm the presence of cancer. And as many as half (10–15 percent at an excellent facility) of all "negative" mammographic reports are "false negative."[3]

According to current data, if all American women 40–50 years old were screened yearly by mammogram, 40 out of every 100 breast cancers would be missed.[4] If all women over 50 were screened, 13 out of every 100 breast cancers would be missed. Half of all breast cancers in women under 45 are invisible on a mammogram.[5] Screening mammograms often miss the deadliest breast cancers: fast-growing tumors in premenopausal women.

### Mammograms can't tell if there's cancer.

Neither diagnostic nor screening mammograms detect cancer. Mammograms can reveal areas of dense tissue in the breasts. These areas may be cancer, or may be associated with cancer, or may be normal tissue, but a mammogram can't tell.[6] The only medically accepted way to tell is to do a biopsy. Over 80 percent of the biopsies done to follow up on a suspicious screening mammogram find no cancer.

### Mammograms don't replace breast self-exams.

Women find their own breast cancers most of the time. (Ninety percent of the time according to one English study.[7])

Monthly breast self-exam (or breast self-massage) provides early detection at lower cost, with no danger—and more pleasure—

than yearly screening mammograms.

Most breast cancers (80 percent) are slow growing, taking between 42 and 300 days to double in size. A yearly mammogram could find these cancers 8-16 months before they could be felt, but this "early detection" does little to improve the already excellent longevity of women with slow-growing, non-metastasized breast cancers.

The 20 percent of breast cancers that are fast growing are the trouble-makers. They can double in size in 21 days. Monthly breast self-exams are much more likely to find these aggressive cancers than are yearly mammograms. (A 21-day doubling cancer will be visible on a mammogram only 6 weeks before it can be felt.) If you massage or examine your breasts even six times a year, you can take action on fast-growing lumps. If you rely on mammograms exclusively, the cancer could grow undetected for months.

In a recent look at 60,000 breast cancer diagnoses in the United States, 67 percent were found by the woman or her doctor —and over half of these were not visible on a mammogram—while 33 percent were discovered by mammogram. (This may seem like a substantial number of cancers found by mammography, but the majority of them were *in situ* cancers, a controversial type of cancer that may—but often does not—progress to invasive cancer.)

## Mammographic screening increases risk of breast cancer mortality in premenopausal women.

A Canadian study of 90,000 women (published in *Lancet,* November 1992) showed a 36–52 percent increase in mortality from breast cancer in women 40–49 who had annual mammograms. [8, 9] The Swedish Malmo Screening Trial (as reported in *The British Medical Journal,* 1988) which also included tens of thousands of women, showed 29 percent greater mortality from breast cancer in women under 55 who were regularly screened with mammograms. (Studies of women 50–59 showed no difference in breast cancer mortality between women who did and women who didn't have regular screening mammograms.)

Critics of these studies claim that newer mammographic equipment uses less radiation. This belies the point that mammograms are inherently dangerous. Orthodox medicine tells me again and again to overlook the harm that it has done to women and promises a future where the machines will be better calibrated and safer. But what of the harm that's been, and is now, done?

Mammographic screening is not and never will be a safe way to find breast cancer. Although safer after menopause than before, mammography is never without risk entirely.

**Why I haven't had a baseline mammogram.**

The idea behind having a baseline mammogram—that there will be a norm to refer back to—is erroneous. Breast tissues are constantly changing as menstrual, ovulatory, pregnancy, lactational, and menopausal hormones change. Science, the constant straight line, meets woman, the ever-changing spiral. And younger breast tissue is especially sensitive to radiation. According to J. W. Gofman (M.D., Ph.D., authority on dangers of radiation exposure), a 35-year-old woman whose normal risk of developing breast cancer is 1 in 1500 increases it to 1 in 660 by exposing herself to the radiation of a baseline mammogram. The National Women's Health Network says baseline mammograms should be abolished.[10]

If you've already had a baseline mammogram and now feel worried, make yourself a soup of lentils (to restore damaged DNA to normalcy), seaweed (to remove radioactive isotopes), and

---

**Excerpt from a report by Rosalie Bertell, Ph.D. on the Ontario [Canada] Mammography Program**

*This program, proposed May 1989, and since enacted, calls for the use of low-dose film-screen mammograms to screen 300,000 women aged 50–64 every other year until they reach the age of 70.*

"To recoup my estimates: The mammography program will cause 15 to 40 breast cancers of which 7 to 18 will be fatal. Most of these will be diagnosed after the age of 70 years when . . . [the women] are no longer in the program. About 163 women will have unnecessary breast surgery due to the program, and roughly 10,000 will have retests because of false positive mammograms.

"Roughly 8 or 9 women will be significantly benefitted by the program because of early detection. . . . About 300 women may benefit indirectly because of the educational and consciousness-raising aspect of the screening program." [23]

carrots (to support your immune system). Season with miso and tamari (to stop the promotion of cancer cells), and thyme, rosemary, and garlic (to further strengthen the immune system). Breathe in, relax, don't worry.

## Mammograms aren't safe.

Professor Anthony Miller, Toronto National Cancer Institute, says cancer cells may be squeezed into the bloodstream under the pressure of the mammographic plates.[11] Screening mammograms are unsafe other ways, too: they expose sensitive breast tissues to radiation, and they increase your chances of having a biopsy and being overtreated for carcinoma *in situ.*

### Radiation Dangers

Scientists agree that there is no safe dose of radiation. Cellular DNA in the breast is more easily damaged by very small doses of radiation than thyroid tissue or bone marrow; in fact, breast cells are second only to fetal tissues in sensitivity to radiation. And the younger the breast cells, the more easily their DNA is damaged by radiation. As an added risk, one percent of American women carry a hard-to-detect oncogene which is triggered by radiation; a single mammogram increases their risk of breast cancer by a factor of 4–6 times.[12]

The usual dose of radiation during a mammographic x-ray is from 0.25 to 1 rad with the very best equipment; that's 1–4 rads per screening mammogram (two views each of two breasts). And, according to Samuel Epstein, M.D., of the University of Chicago's School of Public Health, the dose can be ten times more than that. Sister Rosalie Bertell—one of the world's most respected authorities on the dangers of radiation—says one rad increases breast cancer risk one percent and is the equivalent of one year's natural aging.[13]

If a woman has yearly mammograms from age 55 to age 75, she will receive a minimum of 20 rads of radiation. For comparison, women who survived the atomic bomb blasts in Hiroshima or Nagasaki absorbed 35 rads. Though one large dose of radiation can be more harmful than many small doses, it is important to remember that *damage from radiation is cumulative.* Many women born in the 1930s and '40s—who are now considering the benefits of postmenopausal mammographic screening—have already absorbed quite a bit of radioactivity into their breast tissues from fallout from the atomic bomb tests of the 1950s. (*See* page 18.)

The American Cancer Society claims that the radiation danger from a screening mammogram is no more than that caused by natural radiation in the environment. Not so. The amount of radiation from even one breast x-ray is 11.9 times the yearly dose absorbed by the entire body, according to Diana Hunt, former saleswoman for an x-ray manufacturing company, UCLA Medical Center graduate, and senior staff x-ray technologist for 20 years.[14] (See page 18 for a list of rads absorbed while skiing in Denver, flying in an airplane, and other activities often cited as comparable to mammographic screening.)

A study published in the October 20, 1993 issue of *Journal of the National Cancer Institute* found a statistically significant increase in the incidence of breast cancer following radiation treatment of various benign breast diseases even among women older than 40 at the time of the first treatment.

*Treatment Dangers*

You increase your risk of being overtreated for breast cancer whenever you have a screening mammogram. Eight out of ten masses detected by screening mammogram are false alarms, but if something is seen in your mammogram you'll be urged to undergo a biopsy.

### Screening mammograms lead to overtreatment.

Many of the "cancers" found by mammographic examination are carcinoma *in situ*. At least 75 percent of these will remain non-invasive and can be removed surgically, if desired, at any time, or simply left alone. Of the 25 percent of *in situ* cancers that do become invasive, the number that metastasize is quite small (and unmetastasized breast cancer rarely kills).

Early detection of tiny *in situ* tumors often leads to orthodox treatments which do not prolong life and which can cause immune system suppression, severe drug reactions, even death. Of course, early detection can also lead to life-enhancing wholistic treatments.

### Screening mammograms don't increase your chances of being cured . . . or of surviving longer.

Early diagnosis of breast cancer by mammographic screening produces higher rates of cure and longer survival times without actually increasing the number of women cured nor lengthening their lives. How can that be? It's sleight of hand with numbers.

Survival, when it comes to breast cancer statistics, is defined as being alive five years after the diagnosis of cancer. Cure is defined as being disease-free five years after diagnosis. A women who dies of breast cancer more than five years after her diagnosis can still be included in statistics as a "cure."

A woman with a slow-growing metastasizing breast cancer will live, on the average, 15 years after the cancer's inception.[15] A mammogram can detect a slow-growing breast cancer when it is about eight years old. (15 – 8 = 7 more years to live.) If this woman dies seven years after her diagnosis, she will be counted as "cured" because she lived for more than 5 years.

The same slow-growing metastasizing breast cancer will be 11 or 12 years from its inception when noticed by a woman who neither touches her breasts regularly nor has mammograms. (Women who do regular breast self-exam or breast self-massage usually notice a slow-growing cancer nine years after its inception, just one doubling bigger than visible to a mammogram.[16]) This woman will live as long as the woman whose cancer was discovered by screening mammogram, but won't be "cured" because she didn't live for five more years. (15 – 11 = 4 years).

The cure is only a statistic. There is no difference in the number of years lived after the inception of the cancer, no difference in the length of life, only a difference in number of years lived after diagnosis.

### Mammograms don't find cancer before it metastasizes.

Breast cancers generally don't begin to metastasize until they contain at least one million cells. It takes an ordinary breast cancer—one that doubles every 100 days—about six years to grow that large.[17] (Some very slow breast cancers take 20 years to accumulate a million cells. A very fast breast cancer can get there in a year.) But a million cells is still only as big as the dot at the end of this sentence. And that's undetectable by either touch or mammogram. (But not by intuition. I've met several women who "felt" their cancers at this tiny size but couldn't convince anyone they had cancer because the medical diagnostic equipment, though technologically advanced, wasn't as perceptive as their inner wisdom.)

By the time a cancer is big enough to be seen on a mammogram, it's usually 8 years old, has 500 million cells, and is approximately one-quarter inch (half a centimeter) long.[18] It has been large enough to metastasize, if it is going to, for a year or more. (Some breast cancers never metastasize, no matter how large they get.)

> ### Statement from the Friends of Elenore Pred
> #### (1934-1991)
> #### co-founder of Breast Cancer Action
>
> "Because Elenore lived for ten years after her initial
> breast cancer diagnosis, she is in the record book as hav-
> ing been cured. Elenore wants all of us to stop clinging to
> this false hope about early detection equaling a cure. A
> five-year survival rate is just that and nothing more, cer-
> tainly not a cure. Stop the misleading information now.
> For you, Elenore, we will stay in their faces."

### Aren't mammograms life saving for women over 55?

In several studies, yearly mammograms of women aged
55 and older reduced breast cancer mortality by one-third. But
this doesn't mean any one woman's risk is reduced by one-third
according to Dr. Peter Skrabenek, a critic of mass screening. Furthermore, the women enrolled in these very successful mammographic studies received regular physical examination of their
breasts, which–by itself, without risk–reduces breast cancer mortality. The vast majority of breast cancers found in older women
are slow-growing, non-metastasizing, and not life-threatening, no
matter when they're found.

### Yearly screening mammograms aren't cost effective to so-
### ciety nor are they safe environmentally.

The *Southern Medical Journal* reports that the cost effectiveness (defined as the number of dollars spent so one person can live
one year longer) of mammograms for women under 55 is
$82,000.[19] A recent analysis found that it cost $195,000 to detect
one breast cancer using screening mammograms.

Dr. Charles Wright of Vancouver General Hospital estimates that the cost of saving one life by mass screening is $1.25
million (Canadian).

The mammography industry could gross $1 billion per
year if every woman aged 40–49 was screened yearly. Less than
10 percent of all breast cancers occur in women that age.

Choosing screening mammograms means I choose to contribute to the stream of low-level radioactive waste leaving hospi-

tals. Will my mammogram increase my daughter's risk of developing breast cancer by increasing the amount of radioactivity in her environment? What is the real cost of this choice?

### Is there a less risky way to participate in screening mammography?

The American College of Obstetricians and Gynecologists, as well as the national health plans of England, Holland, Italy, and Sweden, recommend screening mammography no more than every two years and only after menopause. Several studies show no advantage to yearly mammograms. Once every two or three years confers the same decrease in five-year mortality, with less radiation hazard to individuals and society, and at far less cost.

### Mammograms distract us from the need for societal commitment to true prevention.

Many of the cancers found by mammographic screening are *in situ* cancers. Women with *in situ* cancers rarely die from them. With or without early detection and treatment, 93 percent survive more than five years. When *in situ* breast cancers are found by mammogram, treated, and added to the statistical base, breast cancer cure rates and longevity statistics improve. No wonder mammography is praised. It has done what decades of research into cures for breast cancer have failed to do: make it appear that there is some progress in stemming the tide of breast cancer. But finding and treating an ever-increasing number of breast cancers isn't real progress; commiting to reducing chemical and radioactive pollution is.

### Are there other ways to find early-stage breast cancers?

In addition to physical examination and breast self-massage, thermography and ultrasound are safe tests available to women who wish to avoid mammograms. Thermography gives a picture of the heat patterns in the breasts (cancers are hotter than the surrounding tissues). Ultrasound bounces sound waves off the breast tissues to measure their density (cancer is denser than the surrounding tissues). Other techniques used to image breast tissues, such as digital mammography and scintimammography rely on radioactivity and are inherently unsafe.[20-22]

### Mammograms don't promote breast health.

Breast self-massage, breast self-exam, and lifestyle changes do.

## If You Decide to Have a Mammogram

• Get the best, even if it means a long journey.
• Go where they specialize, preferably where they do at least 20 mammograms a day.
• Be sure the facility is accredited by the American College of Radiology.
• Insist on personnel who specialize in mammograms. (Taking and reading mammograms are skills that require intensive training and a lot of practice.)
• Ask how old the equipment is. Newer equipment exposes the breasts to less radiation. A dedicated unit (one specifically for mammograms) is best.
• Ask how they ensure quality control. When was their unit calibrated?
• Load your blood with carotenes for a week before the mammogram to prevent radiation damage to your DNA.
• Expect to be cold and uncomfortable during the mammogram, but do say something if you're being hurt.
• The more compressed the breast tissue, the clearer the mammogram. (But pressure may spread cancer cells if they're present.)
• If your breasts are tender, reschedule. During your fertile years, schedule mammograms for 7–10 days after your menstrual flow begins.
• Don't wear antiperspirant containing aluminum; it can interfere with the imaging process. (Those clear stones do contain aluminum, as do most commercial antiperspirants.)
• If you want another opinion, you'll need the original mammographic films, not copies. (X-ray facilities only keep films for 7 years.)
• Get your doctor to agree, in writing, *before* the procedure, to give you a copy of your mammogram. The U.S. Public Health Service advises women to ask for written results from a mammogram.
• Given the high percentage of "false normal" mammograms, if you think you have cancer, trust your intuition.
• Remove radioactive isotopes from your body with burdock root, seaweed, or miso.

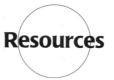

# Resources

- "Mammography Screening: A Decision-Making Guide," $6 from the Center for Medical Consumers, 237 Thompson St., New York, NY 10012

- Comprehensive statement on the risks and benefits of screening mammography from National Women's Health Network, 514 Tenth Street, N.W., Suite 400, Washington, DC 20004

- Information on mammograms from the Women's Cancer Resource Center, 3023 Shattuck Ave, Berkeley, CA 94705

- For information on accredited mammography facilities: Call 1-800-4-CANCER, the National Cancer Institute's information line.

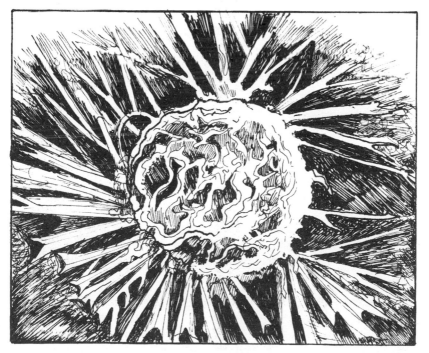

*A Breast Cancer Cell*

# Breast Lump Option Circuit

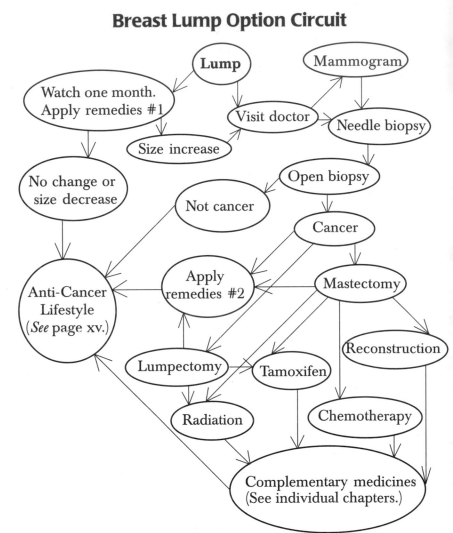

**Remedies group #1•** Anti-cancer Lifestyle plus
• Violet, red clover, burdock root, or nettle infusion daily
• Ginger, cabbage, or potato compress 2-15 times a week
• Cleavers, Siberian ginseng, or echinacea tincture daily
• Anoint with infused herbal oils daily

**Remedies group #2** • Do all of group #1 plus:
• Increase frequency of poultices and amount of tinctures
• Add poke, sundew, mistletoe, or pau d'arco
• Be sure to consult with experienced healers

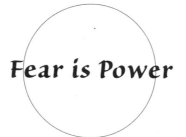

# Fear is Power

*There's a lump in my breast and I'm afraid. I'm afraid it may be cancer. I'm afraid I'll lose my breast. I'm afraid I'll die. I'm afraid of being cut, of the way other people will treat me if they think I have cancer, of cold doctors and harsh treatments and pain. I don't know what to do. Maybe I should just ignore it. Maybe I'm making it up. But I can't ignore it; I think about it all the time. I find myself touching it all the time, too. I'm afraid.*

"We sense your fear, GrandDaughter. Fear can immobilize you, like a wild animal in sudden light, making you unsure of which way to move. Fear can make you close your eyes, hoping that nothing bad will ever happen. Fear can torture you, deflecting your attention from caring for your breasts, loving your body.

"Fear can also motivate you. Fear can empower you, move you, stir you. Do not try to repress or deny, sublimate or eliminate your fear. Use your fear. It is powerful. Use your fear as energy for the journey you now begin. Use your fear as your ally for awareness. Use your fear to feed you rather than freeze you.

"Let the energy of fear slowly emerge, without judgment. Savor your fear; do not let it consume you. Let the vitality of your fear feed your immunity. Allow it to temper you to a more flexible strength.

"Use fear as a messenger, as a window to your soul. Let fear motivate you to care for yourself, to reach out for support, to research your options. Let it challenge you to frame your own definition of health and define your own healing paradigm. Embrace your fear and you will embrace your health/wholeness/holiness.

"Look into our eyes, GrandDaughter. You are part of our lineage. You are not alone with your lump and your fear. We are here within you, the ancient, earthy women's wisdom. See us within yourself so you can find us outside. We are here, as real as you allow, holding you – now and forever – in loving hands of healing."

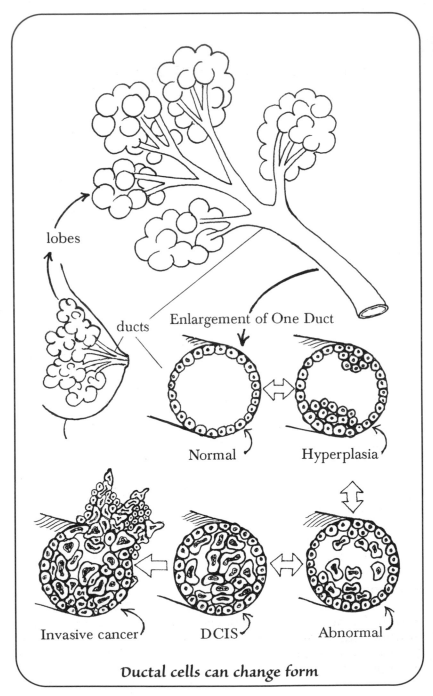

lobes

ducts

Enlargement of One Duct

Normal

Hyperplasia

Invasive cancer

DCIS

Abnormal

*Ductal cells can change form*

# 6.
# There's A Lump in My Breast

Few events in a woman's life are as troubling as finding a suspicious lump in her breast. Even if she's reasonably sure it's benign, there's a worm of worry until some expert has been consulted, or the lump has been lived with for sufficient time to become part of herself, or labeled "not me" and urged to leave. Until it is named and known, addressed and attended to, the lump is a lurking companion, disrupting dreams and edging the days.

For many of us, finding a lump compels us to go to the doctor as soon as possible. But most M.D.s have been trained to assume that a breast lump is malignant until proven otherwise, and will urge you (often with fear-inspiring language) to agree to invasive x-rays and biopsies, none of which will be regarded as sufficient to rule out cancer definitely.

Since test results that are negative for cancer are suspect, both negative and positive test results can draw you deeper into the orthodox maze—on to the next and the next (more and more invasive) procedure. (Of course, there are also stories of M.D.s who say, "It's nothing. Don't worry." And–after you have tried not to worry for too long–it turns out to be cancer.)

Although that lump in your breast (or shadow in your mammogram) is probably benign, you need to start envisioning *now* what you'll do if it is cancer. Some of the suggestions in this chapter may seem too deep or too intense for women who only have a lump, but–unfortunately–it is quite easy to go from worry about a lump to major breast surgery with alarming speed. Use the "Breast Lump Option Circuit" (page 104) to envision your path through the maze of choices you'll face in your desire to learn about and treat your lump.

Taking care of yourself does not necessarily mean going to an M.D. the moment you find a lump. You can take some time to work with Steps 0, 1, 2, and 3. This will improve your health no matter what kind of lump it turns out to be. (And, if it is cancer, the sooner these steps are used, the more effective they are.)

# What Is This Lump in My Breast?

• **Fibroadenoma** (fibroma, adenoma, or adenofibroma): *Benign*. Generally regular in shape, round or oval. Rubbery, firm texture. Rarely painful. Moves freely. More common in younger women than in postmenopausal women.

• **Cyst** (macrocyst, microcyst, fibrocyst): *Benign*. Can hide a cancer (rare). Generally regular in shape, round or oval. Squishy to quite firm in texture. Often painful. Moves freely. May appear overnight (literally) and change size quickly—shrinking and expanding with changes in your menstrual cycle, emotions, and diet. Very common in premenopausal women; uncommon after menopause, except in women using hormone replacement. Cysts do not increase risk of breast cancer. Some studies find that women with lumpy, fibrocystic breasts are slightly less likely than average to have breast cancer during their reproductive years.[1]

• **Lipoma** (fat necrosis): *Benign.*Usually irregularly shaped. Soft or firm textured. Usually painless. Fixed, not movable. Initiated by an injury to the breast, lipomata may take years to become apparent. Lipomata occur in women of all ages.

• **Calcifications** and **micro-calcifications**: *Benign, but may signal cancer.*(*See* page 110.) Calcifications can be felt; micro-calcifications are detected by mammogram. Occurring in women of all ages, these deposits cluster around dead and abnormal cells. Benign breast changes in older women, such as sclerosing adenosis, also cause calcifications.

• **Cancerous mass** (cancerous tumor or lesion): *Malignant*. Almost always irregular in shape. Texture quite firm: like a grain of uncooked rice, like a bit of wire. Cancerous lumps rarely cause pain, but they can. Fixed, they move only with the underlying tissue. A cancerous mass may grow quickly or slowly, but rarely shrinks on its own. Breast cancer is more common and less invasive among postmenopausal women.

**Step 0.** *Do Nothing*

• Remember that "do nothing" does *not* mean "ignore that lump." It means **find the still point within yourself before you act.** Sit in silence and beingness. With a solid centering point you won't be buffeted this way and that by your fear and, even more unnerving, by everyone else's fear. (Many women felt others were more fearful of their lumps than they were.)

• Health/wholeness/holiness is more visible in the dark, louder in the silence, more graspable with open hands. The Great Void may reveal your own truth, your own path, your next step.

★ Do nothing for others for a while. Stop nurturing others. Stop saying "yes" to others, and **say "yes" to yourself.**

• **Float** or lie on your back, in the dark, in silence, in enough warm water to cover your breasts, allowing them to be weightless and free. Breathe.

**Step 1.** *Collect Information*

• **Most breast lumps are harmless.**[2]

• The majority of women develop one or more benign lumps in their breasts sometime during their fertile years.

• Is your lump **freely moving or fixed**? Put your finger on your eyelid and move it around on your eyeball; it is freely moving. Put your finger on the very tip of your nose and try to move the skin; it is fixed. Freely moving lumps are almost always benign; fixed ones, most often cancerous.

• If someone tells you (or told you) that you have **fibrocystic breast disease**, tell them to think again. There is no such disease according to some M.D.s and most wise women.[3, 4] Insurance payments for treating breast cancer can be denied due to a "previous condition" if this appears on your health records, even though it has been shown that women with fibrocystic breasts are not at increased risk of developing breast cancer.

• If your lumps and cysts are benign but painful, many of the remedies in Steps 0, 1, 2, 3, and 4 can help you.

# There's Something in My Mammogram

A mammogram can locate and reveal "suspicious" shadows and calcifications in the breasts, but cannot diagnose cancer. Orthodox medicine diagnoses cancer only by means of a biopsy. Nine out of ten biopsies done for calcifications will find no cancer; in the other 10 percent, the cancer found is almost always Stage 0, *in situ.*

**Shadows**—*Dense tissues cast shadows on x-ray films.*
• If the shadow is round, with smooth, regular edges—a cyst or fibroadenoma is the most likely cause.
• If the shadow is star-shaped, jagged, or radiating—cancer, fat necrosis, or radial scarring (the last two are benign) are the most likely causes.

**Calcifications** and **micro-calcifications**—*Tiny deposits of calcium (some as fine as dust) are visible in x-rays.*
• Abnormal and dead cells, including scar tissue and dead cancer cells, attract calcium.
• Calcifications that are large, few in number, widely dispersed, and round imply benign causes.
• Calcifications in both breasts that are small and numerous imply benign causes.
• Calcifications that are small, numerous, clustered, asymmetrically shaped (stellate, branched, teardrop-like) and found in only one breast imply cancer.
• Indeterminate calcifications (none of the above) may be examined with a magnification view, a biopsy, or another mammogram in 2–6 months to see if the calcifications are the same (probably benign) or have changed (more likely to be cancer). Depending on the skill of the person reading your mammogram, indeterminate means cancer 1–20 percent of the time.

• For more information on calcifications, contact the **Women's Cancer Resource Center**, 3023 Shattuck Ave., Berkeley, CA 94705; 510-548-9272.

• Most M.D.s are more frightened of cancer than you are, and frightened of malpractice suits as well.[5] "Check every breast lump for cancer, no matter how many biopsies and mammograms it takes," is standard. But remember, these are invasive procedures that carry an inherent risk of injury, even death.

You don't have to agree to anything while in the doctor's office. You can go home and research, emotionally and intellectually, any treatment. But be forewarned, I've heard many awful stories of women threatened with imminent death by physicians intent on doing the biopsy, right then, right there. On the other hand, an M.D. told me that the hospital she is associated with won't let her order a breast sonogram unless she also orders a mammogram. When she pushed the issue, she was threatened with suspension.

Take a friend along when you ask an orthodox medical professional for an opinion on your lump. Take a tape recorder, too (not instead). A confrontational friend who's willing to be pushy is invaluable. This may seem extreme for dealing with a lump that's likely benign, but many women told me they were bullied into procedures they didn't want for lack of a friend to stand up with them. And a few had to be assertive to get tests they wanted.

One way to handle a bulldozing doctor is to make an appointment a week or two in the future for the invasive procedure suggested, leaving yourself enough time to consider (and reconsider) your options. And to cancel if you wish.

★ For an overview of your options, *see* page 104.

★ The quest to find out what's inside has led us to develop x-rays, C-T scans, MRIs, and other technological eyes. We've come to believe that machines are impartial (and therefore to be trusted) and that people aren't. But machines don't make the diagnosis. It's a person who reads the mammogram; it's a person who interprets the biopsy sections. Because I believe cancer is a message from the wild side of ourselves, I think it is important to solicit the help of someone who gives a diagnosis from (what looks to most Westerners as) the wild side. **Get an opinion from someone highly experienced in non-Western diagnosis**, such as a shaman, a psychic, or someone skilled in Chinese diagnostic techniques. (Practitioners of Chinese pulse diagnosis claim to be able to tell whether a mass is cancerous or not, and whether or not it has metastasized.)

• Do you need a biopsy? How soon? No evidence indicates that you will decrease the length of your life if you wait two months before getting a lump biopsied, even if it is cancerous, unless it is a rare fast-growing tumor.[6] If the lump grows steadily, or if you sense that time is of the essence, make that appointment now. If not, use remedies from Steps 2 and 3, and watch for one or two months. If the lump changes with your menstrual cycle, you can stop worrying after two months, but stay in touch with your breasts.[7]

★ The **anti-malignin antigen in serum assay** (AMAS blood test) is a way to investigate a lump or a suspicious mammographic finding without a biopsy. This test measures the amount of anti-malignin (antibodies against an antigen called malignin which is produced when cells undergo malignant transformations). Those without cancer produce very little anti-malignin. Those with cancer show a marked elevation. Sensitivity rate is 95 percent. (Available to health-care professionals from Oncolab, 36 The Fenway, Boston, MA 02215, 1-800-922-8378.)

• Another noninvasive way to distinguish between malignant and non-malignant breast changes is the **breast biophysical exam**. This test can detect very tiny electrical differences between normal regions and abnormal regions. According to the *Medical Tribune*, biophysical exams identified 178 of 182 cancers (98 percent sensitivity), with an 86 percent specificity.[8]

★ Two excellent references: *The Informed Woman's Guide to Breast Health: Breast Changes That Are NOT Cancer,*[9] and *The Breast Cancer Handbook: Taking Control After You've Found a Lump.*[10]

**Step 2.** *Engage the Energy*

★ **Take off your bra**. It's not just feminist folklore: Wearing a bra more than 12 hours a day, or wearing a bra that leaves red marks on your skin, increases the number of lumps in your breasts and the possibility that they'll be malignant. Many women confirmed that cutting down on wearing a bra cut down on their breast lumps.

• An important means of engaging the energy when you have a lump in your breast is to **talk about it**. Talk to other women, talk to your beloved, talk to yourself, talk to the lump, talk. Silence is not golden in this instance.

## Breast Meditation

Sit comfortably in front of a large mirror in a warm, private space. Bare your breasts. Look in the mirror. Tell your breasts something like: "I love you. You are just the way you are supposed to be. I see your perfection. I know your beauty. I honor your power." Use your own words. Repeat as many times as you like. When you are done, close your eyes. Slowly bring your hands up and cup them under your breasts. Say: "My breasts are healthy. My breasts are powerful." Open your eyes and look at yourself in the mirror, saying, "My breasts are my strength. My strength nourishes me and others." Close your eyes and let your hands return to your lap. Sit quietly and breathe as you visualize glowing pink clouds within your breasts spiraling in toward your nipples for a minute. Continuing to breathe, let this sparkling pink energy spiral out for a minute. As you breathe, imagine the energy doing figure-eights from breast to breast for a minute. Finally, imagine that you are plunging your hands into vibrant pink energy. Feel it flowing up your arms, through your armpits and out of your nipples. Open your eyes, smile at yourself in the mirror, and come out of the meditation.

★ A visit with your Wise Healer Within (page 82), and a quiet time doing the Breast Meditation (above), are inner journeys that help you decide what you, and your lump, need for health.

• **If your breasts could speak, what would they say?** Are they angry? Sad? Embarrassed? Confused? Afraid? Do they receive enough attention and care? Do they feel put down? Do your breasts like you? Do you like them? Do you feel comfortable with your breasts? Write it down.

• Breasts are symbols of love, sex, nurturance, and primal survival needs. **What does the lump in your breast symbolize?** A thwarted desire to love or be loved? A pulled-back area of sexual expression? A blocked-off wish to nurture (yourself or others)? A knot of fear about survival?

• **Homeopathic remedies** for shrinking and resolving breast lumps include *Phytolacca, Conium,* and *Hypericum* (not all at once). The cell salt *Silica* is also suggested.

★ **Pay attention to your intuition**. Not only are most breast lumps found by women themselves – "My hand went to it as I was showering without any conscious thought." "I was in bed reading when I realized my fingers were rubbing a lump in my breast." "I wasn't looking for anything, my hand was just suddenly touching this hard little lump."– but most women have a very strong sense of whether or not the lump (or calcification in a mammogram) is benign or malignant.

    Your fear of cancer isn't to be trusted; your sense of cancer is. Some women *know* they have cancer, but face medical denial. Other women fear cancer and allow themselves to be overtreated by doctors who fear cancer even more. If you *know* you have breast cancer, please demand what you need, without delay, no matter what the tests or experts say.[9] Finding someone who will listen to you, believe you, and address your concerns is one of the most important aspects of healing. Remember, you're as likely to be right as a test. And please stand up for yourself if you feel secure taking your time or using non-orthodox methods.

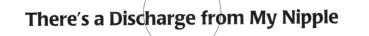

## There's a Discharge from My Nipple

• Fluid coming from your nipple, either by itself or when you supply gentle pressure, may be a sign of cancer if:
    The discharge is tinged with blood.
    The area around your nipple is scaly and itchy.
    *If you have either of these signs of cancer, seek help.*

• A nipple discharge is not a sign of cancer if: the discharge is clear or straw-colored or milky *and* you are breast-feeding or pregnant or in the midst of menopause or taking hormones or drinking more than four cups of coffee a day.

If you *know* you have breast cancer, you may want to rush immediately into Steps 5 and 6. Don't rush. Take it easy; take the time to choose and activate remedies from Steps 0, 2, 3, and 4 first. Use the global approach, too; *see* page xviii.

**Step 3.** *Nourish and Tonify*
Combine external and internal remedies for best effect.

Step 3: *External Remedies to Nourish and Tonify*

★ **Poultices** are messy and time-intensive, but provide a deeply penetrating power that can dissolve benign lumps and calcifications, and check the promotion and growth of malignant lumps. **Cabbage, comfrey, dandelion, poke,** and **violet** poultices are favorites. Learn to make them on page 299. *See* Materia Medica for cautions and applications.

    **Cabbage poultices** are an old wives' remedy for painful, lumpy breasts.[11] Apply a hot leaf (boil it or iron it) to the breast and lie down for 15 minutes or go to sleep. Keep the leaf in place with a tight T-shirt. If you like, apply castor oil before the cabbage leaf.

    **Violet leaf poultices** soothe and dissolve problem areas in the breasts. I consider them especially invaluable when dealing with *in situ* carcinomas. One way to do it: Make a quart of violet leaf infusion (page 294). Reheat half the infusion and leaves. Strain. Drink the liquid and apply the warm, wet leaves to your breast. Leave this soothing, dissolving poultice in place for many hours if possible. Another way to do it: Pick fresh violet leaves and chew them until they get sticky. Apply this sticky mass of leaves directly to your breast and allow it to dry.

• Poultice-like applications of cloths saturated wih infused herbal oils/ointments are classic remedies for dissolving lumps and cysts.

    Healers speak glowingly of castor oil's ability to dissolve worrisome lumps, nourish breast tissue, and soothe painful breasts. Many lumps shrink noticeably after the first two or three applications of **castor oil packs** (*see* page 62). Alternating with ginger compresses (*see* page 305) increases the effect.

    Herbalist Hildegard of Bingen (1098-1179) heated together the pressed juice of fresh **violets** with one-third part (by weight) olive oil and an equal part **billy goat fat** to make an ointment she used against cysts, lumps, precancerous growths, sore muscles, and headaches.[12]

**Pine-based salves** also have a long history of use in dissolving all manner of unwelcome growths in the breasts. Choices range from simple oils made at home from local pines such as **Evergreen Breast Massage Oil** (page 298), to complicated salves of pitch and turpentine such as **Yellow Salve** (page 302) and **Black Ointment** (page 304).

**Dandelion flower oil** and **poke root oil** are also highly praised for providing prompt relief from a variety of breast lumps. For more information on these oils, *see* pages 63 and 65.

• A lump-dissolving poultice can be made by soaking a cloth in an herbal tincture and applying the wet cloth to the area over the lump. A recipe for a such a tincture–**Lump Liniment**, used successfully against breast lumps a century ago–is on page 305.

• Here's an interesting way to shrink breast lumps, relieve breast soreness and congestion, and improve lymphatic circulation in the breasts: **Massage the tender area on the bottom of the foot where your toes attach** for 10 seconds per toe (longer is fine). Use firm pressure.

• **Yoga postures** can tonify the breasts and improve circulation to the breast area, especially if you focus your attention and energy toward them. Try the bow, the camel, or the cobra.

Step 3: *Internal Remedies to Nourish and Tonify*

★ My favorite breast-nourishing, lump-dissolving herbs are taken as infusions–up to a quart a day of any of these:

**Red clover:** Consistent use of infusion of the blossoms softens lumps, reverses pre-cancerous conditions, and has even been known to restore cancerous cells to health. Red clover, like soy, keeps breast cells from absorbing cancer-causing estrogens.

**Nettles:** Infusion of this "noxious" weed encourages and nourishes good flow of blood, lymph, and energy through the breasts, helps tissues lose excess fluids, and strengthens the immune system. Nettle helps calm feelings of panic and powerlessness, too.

**Violet:** The common flower of our gardens offers a leaf that brews into a slippery, soothing, lump-dissolving drink. And should the lump be a cancer, violet can slow or check its growth while further treatment is considered and selected.

• Herbs that tonify the lymphatic system—such as cleavers, calendula, and burdock—help dissolve lumps. They are usually used as tinctures. (To make your own, *see* pages 295-296.)

**Cleavers:** A dose of 20 drops a day is generally sufficient to shrink cysts and other benign lumps, sometimes within a few days, but I wouldn't hesitate to use it for longer. Large amounts of cleavers can thin the blood and may increase menstrual flow.

**Calendula:** These easily grown orange blossoms are praised by medical herbalist Amanda McQuade-Crawford and by Jeanine Parvati Baker, director of Hygeia College of Healing, as a particularly effective ally for women dealing with numerous fibrocystic lumps. The usual dose is 5-20 drops of tincture three times a day. For even better results, use infused calendula oil/ointment or fresh blossom poultices twice a day, too.

**Burdock:** Safe enough to use daily for years, burdock root has a reputation for improving lymphatic flow and reversing abnormal cellular changes. It is a powerful ally for women with indeterminate calcifications and *in situ* cancers. The dose is 30 drops of the fresh root tincture 3–8 times a day (or a cup or more of infusion daily).

★ When the breasts are lumpy, look to the liver. **Dandelion** root is the liver's best friend, and a specific remedy for women with cysts, lumps, growths, and abnormal cells in their breasts. Internally: 20–30 drops of fresh root tincture up to 4 times a day. Externally: freshly grated root, or 15–25 drops of the root tincture on a clean cloth, or the warmed oil of the blossoms on a cloth, applied twice a day.

★ **Seaweed** for dinner and seaweed for snacks. East and west agree that seaweed slides away lumps and stops initiated cancer cells in their tracks. With so many delicious varieties to choose from, eating it frequently isn't a problem.

• Older women—whose breast lumps are quite sensitive to hormones—and menopausal women—whose breast lumps may be due to erratic hormone levels—agree that hormone-moderating herbs such as **raspberry** (*Rubus idaeus*), **chaste tree** (*Vitex agnus-castus*), **motherwort**, and **licorice** are wonderfully helpful. A daily dose is a cup or more of dried raspberry leaf infusion, 60–90 drops of chaste tree berry tincture, 25–50 drops of motherwort tincture, or a cup of licorice root tea.

★ A very old (but up-to-date) remedy from China for women with cysts in their breasts (or their ovaries): Equal parts flowering tops of **chickweed** (*Stellaria media*), **motherwort** (*Leonurus cardiaca*), and **cronewort/mugwort** (*Artemisia vulgaris*). The dose is 10 drops of tincture of each plant, 3 times a day. This combination has been quite successful for many women, but it works slowly and may take 6–10 months to dissolve some cysts completely.

• Donny Yance, herbal specialist in breast cancer treatments, is particularly fond of **redroot** (*Ceanothus americanus*) as a tonic for women with breast lumps. He uses up to 80 drops of tincture daily or one cup of tea. Herbalist John Lust says redroot raises the spirit.

• It makes sense to nourish and tonify your immune system anytime, but especially if you're concerned about a lump in your breast. For help, read Chapter 4.

**Step 4.** *Stimulate/Sedate*
Combine external and internal remedies for best results.

Step 4: *External Remedies to Stimulate/Sedate*

★ Many women have had excellent results from massaging **poke** oil into their lumps morning and night for several weeks.
    Herbalist Rosemary Gladstar, founder of the California School of Herbal Studies, favors a poke root poultice made by putting 15 drops of the tincture on a cotton cloth. She places the wet area directly on the lump, wraps it up, and goes to sleep. She repeats this for five nights out of seven, and continues for 3 weeks, taking a week off before doing any more.

★ **Ginger compresses** are successfully used by many healers and women to reduce and eliminate breast lumps. (Instructions, page 305.) Women who've dealt with many kinds of breast lumps tell me that ginger compresses reduced benign masses quickly but sometimes irritated cancerous ones. (It doesn't mean you have cancer if your skin gets irritated.)

• Traditional healers in Polynesia and Japan follow the ginger compress with an **albi** (taro) poultice, made from freshly grated taro root or dried taro root powder mixed with water to the consistency of peanut butter. (European healers use ground **flax** seed—those of North America, grated **potato**—the same way.) One woman dissolved her postmenopausal breast lump in 3 months with the help of ginger, albi, and acupuncture. Before bedtime she applied ginger compresses for 15 minutes, then thoroughly covered the area over and around her lump with albi paste, wound a loose cloth around her breasts and torso, and went to sleep. She repeated the ginger compresses (same ginger) followed by albi (fresh albi) each morning, letting the albi remain on all day.

Fresh taro may be found in ethnic markets. Dried, powdered albi is available at some health food stores or by mail from Mt. Ark, 1-800-643-8909.

★ **Clay poultices** are a classic remedy for women with breast lumps. Pure powdered white or grey clay is often less expensive, and less irritating to the skin, than the fancy, colored clays. Bentonite clay is used by many healers. Ask around at pottery shops as well as health food stores and pharmacies to purchase clay. I don't buy wet clay; it can contain molds that may infect the skin.

I mix a handful of clay powder with enough water to make a paste as thick as mayonnaise which I apply thinly but generously. As the clay slowly dries, it falls off, or it can be brushed off.

Some women add a few drops of essential oil (see next page) or infused herbal oil (e.g., poke, calendula) to the clay.

Here's a dramatic experience I had using clay poultices: One of my goats was due to give birth in a week when she came into her milk with a very swollen and lumpy udder. When I milked her, I discovered an udder filled with three quarts of pus and blood. In the house, I put some cabbage leaves up to steam and filled a dropper bottle with poke and echinacea root tinctures (10 drops of poke for every 50 of echinacea). Back in the barn, I gave her 100 drops (4 ml) of the tinctures (repeated every other hour for the next two days) and poulticed her udder with the hot cabbage leaves (four times a day).

After a month of gradually decreasing treatment and attention (we were down to one poultice and 50 drops of tincture mix once a day), I proclaimed her cured. Within the week, the infection was back, worse than ever: Four lumps ulcerated right through her udder. Over the next seven days I put every ointment from my cupboard on her udder, but none of them seemed to really counter the infection and congestion. Even Bag Balm, an old standby yellow salve, didn't work its magic.

A visiting healer insisted on poulticing her udder with clay. Within the first few days (doing three poultices a day and giving her tincture every three hours) the lumps changed character and began to shrink, the ulcers healed, and she was definitely on the mend. We continued this successful treatment for three more weeks, gradually easing off while making sure she got plenty of kelp and hugs. (P.S. She wasn't pregnant after all.)

Swiss herbalist Rina Nissim says: "**Clay works wonders**, but may increase breast pain initially."

• Pure essential oil of **orange peel** (*Citrus reticulata*) or **lavender** (*Lavendula vera*) is said to dissolve breast lumps and stop the replication of abnormal cells. Some women dilute 20–50 drops of either one in an ounce/30 ml of olive oil, and apply it morning and night for several months. Essential oils of **rose geranium** (*Pelargonium* species) and **Roman chamomile** (*Anthemis nobilis*) can also be used: 5 drops of each, or 10 drops of either one–diluted in a large spoonful of olive oil–is applied daily to cysts in the breasts. (**Caution:** Essential oils can irritate the skin; *see* pages 63-64.)

• If your lump doesn't respond to simple remedies, you may want to try using **Powerful Poultice Powder** (recipe, page 304).

• Regular use of aluminum salts (as in commerical antiperspirants or those "natural" clear stones) can contribute to breast lumps, especially when applied to skin abraded by shaving. Think it's not enough to make a difference? Women are advised not to wear antiperspirant when going for a mammogram, as it interferes with breast imaging. Try herbal vinegar splashed in the armpits instead.

Step 4: *Internal Remedies to Stimulate/Sedate*

★ Isla Burgess, founder of the Waikato School of Herbal Studies in New Zealand, relies on internal use of lymphatic stimulating **poke root tincture** when seeking to resolve breast lumps. She says best results come when the dosage of poke tincture is increased daily by 1–2 drops until a response occurs (such as sensation of heat, soreness, tingling, or queasiness). She continues with that dosage for a week, supporting the internal remedy with ginger compresses or cabbage leaf poultices.

• Eliminating **methylxanthines**–found in coffee (even decaffeinated), regular and diet colas, chocolate, black tea, kukicha, green tea, and medications such as Midol, Anacin, Extra Strength

Excedrin, Sinarest, and Dexatrim—may eliminate benign lumps and slow the growth of abnormal cells.

Six weeks of abstinence is enough to bring about dramatic improvement if you're sensitive to methylxanthines. It's worth a try, though some women find it doesn't make a bit of difference. (To ease coffee withdrawal headaches, try 5–20 drops of skullcap tincture. For that "wake-up-and-get-the-bowels-moving" effect, try clover-mint infusion as your morning beverage.)

• There are excellent Chinese herbal formulas used to relieve breast lumps, some of which may be effective against very early cancers. Beware of packaged over-the-counter herbal remedies from China; they may contain drugs and heavy metals. Consult a practitioner skilled in Traditional Chinese Medicine for a formula of herbs you can brew at home if this seems right to you.

**Step 5a.** *Use Supplements*

★ Six weeks of daily use of 1–2 tablespoons/15–30 ml (4–8 capsules) of **flaxseed oil** (rich in omega-3 fatty acids) or **borage, black currant, hemp**, or **evening primrose seed oil** (rich in gamma linoleic acid) can diminish breast lumps, especially those initiated by hormonal imbalances. Clinical studies confirm this as an effective treatment for women at all stages of breast cancer.[13]

• Iodine, as **aqueous iodine or iodaminol**, taken daily for years, is exceptionally good at eliminating breast cysts, dissolving interior scar tissue in the breasts, relieving breast tenderness, and reducing cancer risk. Other forms, such as potassium iodate and kelp, are less effective. The daily dose is quite high, 5–20 mg (RDA is only .15 mg). Side effects may include a sore throat or sore neck glands. Iodine is as effective as Danazol (see Step 5b), far cheaper, and much safer.

• **Vitamin E** (**succinate** is especially favored) taken before bed (800 IU is the usual dose in this case) has helped some women resolve breast lumps. **Caution:** Women with diabetes, high blood pressure, rheumatic heart conditions, visual disturbances, or on digitalis or anticoagulants need to consult a trained healer before using vitamin E supplements. Vitamin E supplements may feed some cancers. To increase vitamin E without supplements, eat sunflower seeds, grind your own flours, and use cold-pressed oils.

• Women troubled with breast lumps also reported using supplements of calcium, selenium, vitamin A, vitamin C, and the B vitamin complex—especially $B_6$. (Food sources are listed on page 53.)

**Step 5b.** *Use Drugs*

• **Some drugs can cause breast lumps**: digitalis-derived drugs, Tagamet (cimetidine), Compazine (chlorpromazine), and high blood pressure medications, including beta-blockers.[14] Supplemental estrogen can cause tender, tense, painful, and nodular breasts.

• **Thyroid hormone supplements** are reported to shrink cysts and eliminate breast pain.

• Wild yam-based **progesterone creams** (e.g., Progest) may soften and dissolve breast lumps during the fertile years, but ought to be avoided by pre- and post-menopausal women, whose breast cancer risk increases with increasing exposure to progesterone.

• Diuretic drugs are prescribed for women with breast lumps, but their hormone-like effects can increase pain and lumpiness.

• Danazol (danocrin) is prescribed for women with multiple painful cysts in their breasts. But it costs $200 or more per month, loses effect as soon as you stop taking it, and can cause acne, weight gain, voice deepening, facial hair growth, and disruption of menses.

• Parlodel (bromocriptine) is occasionally prescribed for women with very lumpy breasts. Side effects include seizures, fatal strokes, heart attacks, and psychiatric illness.

• You have choices about the kinds and amounts (including none) of **sedatives** and **anesthesia** you receive if you choose a biopsy. (*See* Step 6.) Relaxation techniques, such as breathing or listening to trance-inducing music, can be used instead of immune-suppressing drugs for closed biopsies. Even open biopsies can be done with local anesthesia and deep relaxation. If you feel strongly about the risks of anesthesia, discuss this with your doctor. You may need to insist on what you want, or even get a different surgeon or anesthesiologist. *See* "Choosing Anesthesia," page 125.
     The Physicians Desk Reference (available at libraries) is the resource doctors use to check on the dangers and side effects of drugs, including anesthesias. Ask friends (or friends of friends)

who've had surgery what they liked and didn't like about their general anesthesia. Tell the anesthesiologist what you want, and don't want, before the procedure. Is it important to you that you're not in pain when you wake up? Not sick to your stomach? Able to remember what happens to you? Able to think clearly?

• You'll probably be given a **tranquilizer** before an open biopsy, which you can refuse (it does depress immune system functioning). If you drink a cup of **oatstraw** infusion every day for a week before the surgery, or take 10 drops of **motherwort** tincture daily for the same period—plus take 10–20 drops of **skullcap** tincture as near to the surgery as allowed—you'll not only be tranquil, your immune system will be strengthened and you'll be less stressed by post-surgical pain.

**Step 6.** *Break & Enter*

• A biopsy is the only scientifically accepted way to determine if a lump is cancerous. But a recent German study found that biopsies which cut into (or punctured) malignant masses shortened survival times.[15] Excisional biopsies do not cut into masses; needle biopsies (fine needle, Tru-cut, stereotactic) do. There are other problems associated with biopsies; research your options thoroughly before proceeding.[16-18] More about biopsies on pages 126–127.

• One million U.S. women had biopsies in 1994. Of those, 175,000 were found to have cancer. More biopsies are being performed as more women go for mammograms, for—unlike palpable lumps—mammographic shadows include a broad grey area between very suspicious findings (stellate calcifications correlate with cancer nearly half the time[19]) and clearly benign findings. This compels clinicians to perform biopsies both "for the safety of the patient and for the fear of litigation should a cancer be missed."[20]
  Learn as much as you can about your lump before having a biopsy. Take the time to get a second, or even a third opinion.[21] If you decide to wait on a biopsy, set a specific date in the future when you will reconsider having one. Meanwhile, read Chapters 7, 8, and 9 in this book. The choices you make now can have an immense impact on your future life and health.

• Women familiar with their own breasts can detect lumps and changes that are invisible to a mammogram. If you feel strongly that you want a biopsy, don't let anyone talk you out of it.

• For hundreds of years, topical remedies have been used to "burn" suspicious lumps out of the breasts. This procedure is as invasive as surgery, but does offer some advantages. *See* "Instead of Surgery," page 188.

• If you or your doctor feel a lump, diagnostic mammograms may be ordered. When the mammogram shows abnormal signs, one would expect to have a biopsy, and one is recommended. But there are so many false-negative mammographic reports (the mammogram is clear, but cancer is found if a biopsy is done) that you'll be urged to have a biopsy no matter what the mammogram shows. **If you know you want a biopsy, you can refuse the diagnostic mammogram.** (You may have to insist on your right.) You can also inquire if less invasive means of imaging your lump—such as sonography or thermography—are available. (Trans-illumination, C-T scans, and MRI have not been shown to have value in determining the nature of breast lumps.)

• Before having a lump biopsied you might consider a **high resolution digital ultrasound** scan of the suspicious area. With a 99 percent specificity rate (only 5 masses out of 400 deemed benign by ultrasound were cancer upon biopsy), a negative scan gives you six months (then it's time for a recheck) to work with the less invasive healing methods of Steps 0, 1, 2, 3, 4, and 5a.

• If you'd probably choose a lumpectomy rather than a mastectomy if your breast lump *were* cancerous, make that clear to your doctor and surgeon *before* you undergo an open biopsy. If the mass appears malignant, a wide margin of tissue around the lump can be removed, which may spare you further surgery.

• If you choose a biopsy, agree with your doctor beforehand on exactly what tests will be done with your breast tissue. *See* page 135.

• *See* page 180 for ways to prevent infection from an open biopsy.

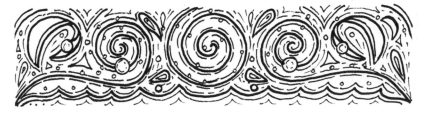

# Choosing Anesthesia

## Local Anesthesia

*Benefits*: Relatively safe.
  Less stressful to the immune system.
  Wears off quickly (usually in 1–2 hours).
  Less expensive.
 *Risks*: Surgeon must work quickly.
  Surgeon may feel uneasy with a conscious patient.
  Impractical for large areas needing careful suturing.
*Other Choices:* **Deep relaxation**, **controlled breathing**, and **self hypnosis** can separate you from sensations of pain as effectively as any local anesthesia—and improve the functioning of your immune system at the same time. I find these techniques so successful that I no longer use dental anesthesia. (It's tougher for the dentist than for me: He's been taught that only a shot can numb.) If you have these skills, talk it over with your surgeon. Is it acceptable to both of you for you to ask for a pain-killer at any time during the procedure if you do decide you need one?

## General Anesthesia

*Benefits*: Surgeon may be more comfortable.
  Wears off slowly; more pain-killing.
  You're less traumatized by conscious recollections.
  Allows for extensive surgery.
 *Risks*: One death per 5,000–10,000 uses.
  Depresses immune system.
  Aggravates asthma, lung and heart problems.
  Causes exhaustion for up to 5 days afterward.
  Can harm fetus if you're pregnant.
*Other Choices*: One of the classic uses of **acupuncture** is as anesthesia during surgery. If you want to have surgery, protect your immune system, and stay drug-free, find a surgeon willing to work with a skilled acupuncturist as well as an anesthesiologist.

# What is a Closed Biopsy?

In a closed biopsy (or aspiration) a hollow needle removes cells or tissue from a lump. Risk of infection is minor. A closed biopsy can be done in a doctor's office with or without local anesthesia. While less expensive and safer than an open biopsy, the results are not as reliable.

• **Fine needle** biopsies explore solid or fluid-filled lumps found by touch or mammogram. If the lump collapses during the biopsy, it is a cyst. If it survives, the sample is read.

Positive reports (cancer cells seen: 10 percent of samples) are usually correct, with only 0–1.5 percent false positives. Between one-sixth and one-third of all samples are non-diagnostic; they contain insufficient cells to determine whether cancer is present or not. But follow-up open biopsies on these find cancer only 2 percent of the time.

A fine needle biopsy takes such a small number of cells that there's always the chance of missing a small cancer. So negative reports (no cancer cells seen) are usually followed up by another biopsy. (These find cancer 3–16 percent of the time.) You can have a large needle biopsy to begin with, if that seems right to you; you can also choose to follow up on an inconclusive biopsy by using non-invasive treatments for several months before going for further tests.

• **Large needle** (Tru-cut or Trocar) biopsies remove a small piece of a lump, but one that is large enough to give a good reading. When read by someone with practice, there are no false positives. There is a high false negative rate (10 percent of follow-up biopsies find cancer), so, again, women with negative results are urged to have another biopsy. Compared to fine needle biopsies, Tru-cuts are more invasive, more painful, cause more infection, and may scar breast tissues, which makes subsequent lumps harder to detect.

• **Stereotactic large-core** biopsies use three-dimensional x-rays or sonograms to guide the insertion of the needle.

# What is an Open Biopsy?

An open biopsy is surgery, minor surgery, but surgery none-theless. An open biopsy is done in a hospital, under general or local anesthesia. The risk of infection from an open bi-opsy is 6–8 times greater than from a needle biopsy.

• Women with nonpalpable masses (such as calcifications on a mammogram) may have a **wire-localization biopsy**. High-dose x-rays monitor a hooked wire as it is inserted into the breast and positioned near the suspicious mass, which is then surgically removed. Internal scars are frequent; there is a high risk of infection. These open biopsies are being replaced with closed computer-guided stereotactic biopsies which reduce scarring, but still use high-level radiation. (Pro-tect yourself from radiation: Eat carrots, miso, and seaweed.)

As many as 90 percent of the biopsies done to follow up on suspicious calcification find no cancer. Yet, because the tissue sample is small, wire-localization and stereotactic bi-opsies can't totally rule it out, either. Non-invasive treatments are an alternative to repeated biopsies.

• Palpable masses (ones which can be felt) can be completely removed by **excisional biopsy**, or partially removed by **incisional biopsy**. If the mass is removed with a margin of normal tissue all around it (a **wide excisional biopsy**) fur-ther surgery may be avoided, even if the lump is malignant. Biopsied tissue is sliced and examined. Absolute diagnosis is not always possible–cells can be indeterminate–but open biopsies are considered reliable, so long as the sample is large enough, and fixed (not frozen).

Surgeons generally try to avoid incisional biopsies: Cut-ting open a tumor can spread cancer cells. If a tumor is large or awkwardly placed, chemotherapy, radiation, or alterna-tive treatments are used before surgery to try to shrink it.

• **Instead of surgery**, women have applied caustic herbs or minerals to burn out lumps; *see* page 188.

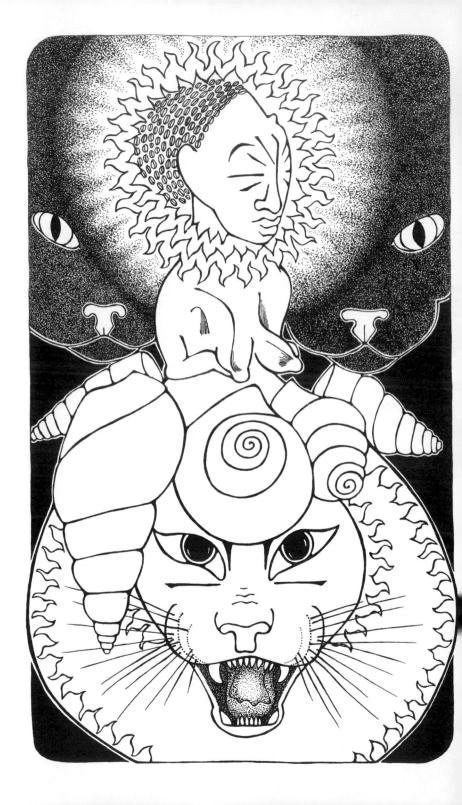

# section two
# For Women Dancing with Cancer

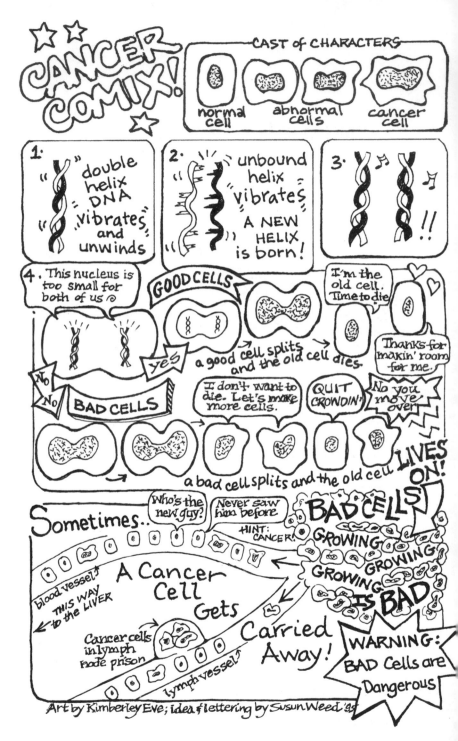

# 7.
# What is Breast Cancer?

**Breast cancer is unchecked growth of abnormal breast cells.**

• What causes cells to become abnormal and reproduce wildly? Damage to the DNA, the brain of the cell, which causes mutations and activation of oncogenes. Usually one mutation isn't enough; most cells must undergo several mutations before they become cancerous. (Sometimes the mutations must occur in sequence to create a cancer, sometimes random order will do it.) What causes DNA damage? Radiation, free radicals, genetic defects, electrical fields, chemicals, drugs, viruses, and metabolic stresses.

**Injury to the DNA initiates all cancer.**

• When mutations accumulate and oncogenes turn on, the cell is initiated. It is abnormal, but not cancerous. Initiated cells are diagnosed as atypia, dysplasia, or hyperplasia.

• Damaged cells alone offer no threat to long life. To become threatening, the abnormal cells must be promoted. Promoters bring the cells nutrients so they can reproduce. (One of the strongest promoters of breast cancer is estrogen.) Although promoted cells can disguise themselves so the immune sytem won't recognize them, most of them are seen and eaten, or encapsulated by the body so they do no harm. Promoted cells are called carcinoma *in situ.*

　　　According to Christiane Northrup, M.D., *in situ* cancer cells are frequently found in the breasts of women who die of causes other than cancer. And according to Susan Love, M.D., breast cancer specialist, *in situ* cells are reversible without invasive treatments and shouldn't be thought of as cancers.

**The cancer cascade: initiation, promotion, growth.**

• Promoted breast cells, no matter how many of them there are, are not classified as invasive unless they spread out of the tissues of origin and into the surrounding tissues. This is the growth phase. When promoted cells enter the growth phase, they begin to form a tumor and to recruit blood vessels to help supply their immense need for nutrients. (The tumor may grow so quickly that cells in its center die from lack of nourishment.) The diagnosis now becomes infiltrating or invasive carcinoma.

## The cancer cascade can be halted or reversed.

• Once a mass of abnormal, quickly replicating cells has created a network of blood vessels, individual cancer cells can separate from the tumor and travel to other parts of the body. Because the breast is not vital to life, a breast cancer that stays in the breast is not life-threatening. But if breast cancer cells get to the liver, lungs, bone marrow, or the brain and continue to grow, they can hinder the functioning of processes necessary for life. The body attempts to check this spread by locking breast cancer cells in lymph node prisons and by sending immune system cells out to eat traveling cancer cells. If cancer cells are found in the axillary lymph nodes, the diagnosis is aggressive or metastasized carcinoma.

## Ninety percent of cancer deaths are from metastases.

• Not everyone whose cellular DNA is damaged will get cancer. Why not? All cells have the capacity to repair themselves or to shut down if they are mutated or damaged. Good lifestyle habits and ordinary foods such as lentils also reverse DNA damage.

## Special immune cells eat potential cancers.

• The wear-and-tear of life gives rise to so many mutated, abnormal, initiated cells (even in a healthy person) that the immune system forms a constant stream of specialized cells to seek out and consume them. So long as the immune system is strong, and well supplied with nutrients, initiated and promoted cells can be harmlessly eliminated, checking the possibility of cancer.

## Cancer cells are immature yet reproduce without limits. Living long past their normal span, they appear immortal.

• Building powerful immunity isn't always enough, though. Cancer cells can trick the immune system into leaving them alone, and they can replicate so rapidly that they overwhelm the immune system with sheer force of numbers. One of the reasons breast cancer is so difficult to treat is that cancer cells are full of life. They no longer have the inner signal that tells them to die after reproducing. Like the sorcerer's apprentice, the woman with breast cancer finds herself with cancer cells that replicate unceasingly. Cancer cells never grow up and become productive members of their community. They simply take up space.

**Breast cancer is not one disease, but many.**

Because there are different types of cells in the breasts (e.g., ducts and lobes) and a variety of ways that a cell can be abnormal, there are many kinds of breast cancers and many possible treatments. Of the two dozen kinds of breast cancer known, the majority originate in the duct cells. (*See* illustration of duct cells, page 106.)

• Some breast cancers grow slowly, others quickly. Slow growing breast cancers double in size every 42–100 days or more. Quick growing breast cancers can double every 21 days. Pre- and perimenopausal women tend to have faster growing, more aggressive breast cancers (about 10–15 percent of all breast cancers).

• Post-menopausal women, who account for 60–80 percent of all breast cancer cases, usually have slow-growing cancers which rarely metastasize.

**Microscopic examination of cellular tissue is the only scientifically accepted way to diagnose cancer.**

• The first breast surgery most women will have is a biopsy. When there is a suspicious finding on a mammogram or a palpable lump, there is no way to rule out cancer unless a piece of breast tissue is removed and examined under a microscope by a pathologist. If there is a diagnosis of cancer and further surgery is done, the breast tissues removed then are also sent to the pathologist.

• The pathologist can see cancerous cells if they are present and can determine the type and state of the cancer by a variety of signs. These findings are collected into a pathology report which will, to a great degree, determine the treatment options that you will be offered. Pathology reports are based on opinion as well as fact, so many women have two, three, or even four different pathologists look at their tissue samples and give an opinion.

• To judge the "stage" of a cancer (*see* page 137), lymph glands are removed (excised) from the nearby armpit. Lymph gland excision always cuts some of the nerves to the arm. Removal of the lymph glands does nothing to treat or cure breast cancer, and may hinder the body's ability to deal with cancer. Lymph gland removal can cause numbness as well as pain, impaired circulation, swelling (sometimes severe and long-lasting), and a life-long risk of severe infection. The more lymph nodes removed, the more severe these side effects.

• Lack of cancer cells in the lymph nodes doesn't guarantee that the cancer hasn't metastasized (one-third of all women with negative nodes nonetheless have metastasizing cancer), but a positive finding does indicate that the cancer has metastasized and may be growing elsewhere in the body.

**It is difficult to determine if a cancer will metastasize.**

• Aggressive (metastatic) cancer requires more vigorous treatment than invasive (non-metastatic) cancer. And treatment is more effective if undertaken before the metastasized cells begin to form masses in critical organs. But micro-metastases and small clumps of cells are extremely dificult to find. What to do?

   Orthodox treatments include: Surgery to remove the primary tumor. Radiation to eliminate any other cancer cells in the breast tissues. Chemotherapy to kill any other cancer cells in the body. (But those that survive—and some always do—mutate and become invulnerable to further chemotherapy.) And hormones such as tamoxifen to check recurrence and metastatic growth.

   Alternative treatments include: Caustic herbs and pastes to burn away the primary cancer. Nourishing, tonifying, and stimulating treatments for building immune strength. And a variety of anti-cancer compounds used systemically to eliminate cancer cells in the breasts and elsewhere in the body. Exercise and a diet of healthy food, nourishing infusions, healing oils, and phytoestrogen-rich herbs to counter recurrence.

• Does survival after a diagnosis of breast cancer depend on orthodox medical treatments? Women who refuse such treatments do not die sooner than women who follow orthodoxy, according to an old (1977), but still valid, study by Hardin B. Jones, professor of medical physics. ("A Report on Cancer," is available at the library of the University of California at Berkeley.)

# Diagnostic Factors

*These factors indicate how aggressive the cancer is
and how likely it is to have metastasized.*

• **Microscopic Examination:** How do the cells look? Are their margins smooth (good) or jagged? Are the nuclei normal (good) or big? If there is a mass, are there dead cells present in the center?
• **ER/PR Assay:** Are there estrogen/progesterone receptors? (If so, the cancer may be easier to treat.)
• **DNA Index:** How much and what kind of DNA? (Diploid is normal; aneuploid/haploid are not.)
• **S-phase Fraction:** How many cells are replicating? (Fewer is better.)
• **Cycling Index:** How much proliferating cell nuclear antigen is present? (Less is better.)
• **Lymph Node Dissection:** Do the axillary nodes have cancer cells? How many? *Don't agree to have any nodes removed until you read pages 172–173.*
• **New Diagnostic Methods:**
   Very thin biopsy sections are examined for **angiogenesis**. In one study all women with 100 or more new blood vessels had recurrence in 3 years. In women with fewer than 33 vessels, only 5 percent experienced recurrence.
   Women with metastasized cancer have elevated urinary concentrations of **fibroblast growth factors** shortly after surgery; those with non-metastasized cancer do not.
   Women with negative nodes and aneuploid cancer cells who have a high level of **capthepsin D** are twice as likely to have recurrences as women who don't.
• **Grave signs of metastasizing cancer:**
   The cancer is more than 2 inches long.
   The skin near the cancer is swollen with fluids.
   The skin is red and hot near the cancer.
   The cancer has ulcerated through the skin.
   The cancer is attached to the chest wall and doesn't move.
   There are large swollen lymph nodes in the armpit and/or above the collarbone.

# Breast Cancer is Many Diseases

There are many kinds of breast cancers, and many stages that further distinguish each breast cancer. You can become the expert on your individual cancer, for–unlike healers and oncologists who must learn about all types–you can focus exclusively on your unique type of breast cancer.

• Breast cancers are divided generally into two types: lobular and ductal, but there are over 30 specific kinds known.
• More than three-quarters of all breast cancers are ductal. Most are found in an early stage. Included in this category are mucinous, papillary, and combination cancers.
• About 10 percent of all breast cancers are lobular. These are more difficult to treat.
• The remaining breast cancers are rare types such as Paget's disease and inflammatory carcinomas.
• Breast cancers that occur after menopause are generally less aggressive than ones that occur during the fertile years.
• Hormone-positive cancers are more responsive to orthodox treatment than horomone-negative cancers are. Most postmenopausal breast cancers are hormone-positive.
• The herbal and home remedies collected in this book have been used as primary as well as complementary medicines for a variety of types and stages of breast cancer.

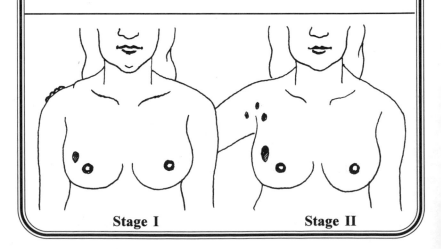

Stage I                              Stage II

**Breast cancer is staged,** in order of threat to life.

Early stages are 0 through II; late stages are III and IV.

Stage 0: *In situ.* Five-year survival with a ductal cancer is 95 percent; the majority never progress to invasive cancer. There is controversy about the best treatment at this stage.

Stage I: Tumor less than 2 cm (.8 inch) with negative lymph nodes. Five-year survival with a ductal cancer is 85 percent. Surgery is the usual treatment: mastectomy alone, or breast-sparing surgery with adjuvant radiation, tamoxifen, and/or chemotherapy.

Stage II: Tumor less than 2 cm but with positive nodes, or tumor 2–5 cm and nodes negative. Five-year survival with a ductal cancer is 65 percent. The usual treatment is surgery with chemotherapy, tamoxifen, and/or radiation.

Stage IIB: Tumor 2–5 cm with positive nodes, or tumor bigger than 5 cm. Five-year survival with a ductal cancer is 55 percent. The usual treatment is mastectomy plus adjuvant treatments.

Stage III: Tumor larger than 5 cm (2 inches) with lymph nodes positive. Five-year survival for those with ductal or lobular cancer is 40 percent. Aggressive surgical and adjuvant treatments are usual.

Stage IV: Cancer that has metastasized to a distant site (beyond the lymph nodes) or a primary occurrence of inflammatory carcinoma. Five-year survival is 10 percent. Extremely aggressive treatments are usual.

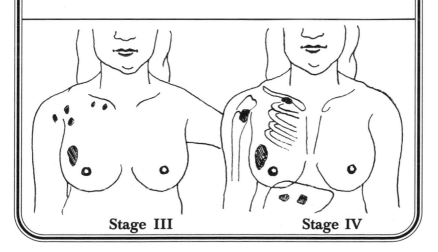

Stage III                      Stage IV

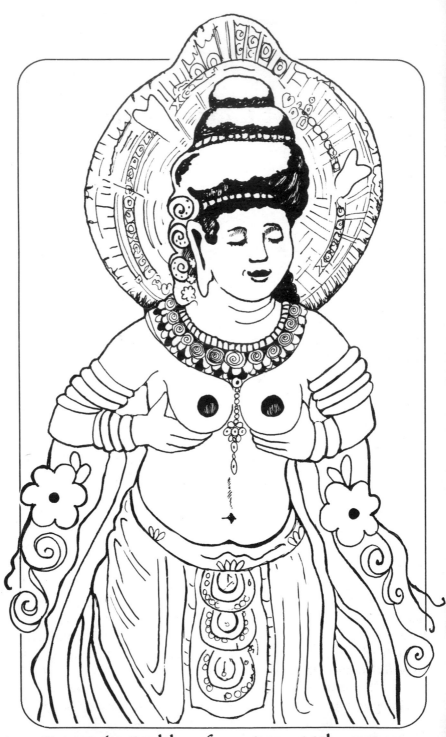

**138** *Fountain Goddess from Java, 11th century*

# Breast Cancer Stars

"We are the Ancient GrandMothers, ripe with wisdom and experience. We see the breasts as spinning energy, spiraling like galaxies. When the spiraling slows, the ether concentrates and curdles. A solid curd appears in the milky firmament of the breast. A light flares. A pulse of hot/cold vibrates. A star awakens.

"This curd of intense life is the star you call cancer. It is a star of light and life, like all other stars, but its radiance is trapped. It has lost the signal that tells it when and how to let go. So it grows and grows, becoming denser, brighter, hotter, colder as it gathers more and more into itself, believing itself alone, immortal, and perpetually young.

" This star of cancer draws into itself fine lines of energy and networks of blood vessels. Hormones and fats surround it, feeding it, making it richer and brighter, larger and tighter.

"When you focus exclusively on light, the star of cancer twinkles. When you neglect the quiet and refuse the nourishment of the dark, the star of cancer shines. When you fear multiplicity and begin to believe that there is only one right way, the star of cancer blazes.

"If you focus only on light – honoring it, seeing it as the ultimate goal, desiring it, consuming it, bathing in it, living with it always shining, using it to banish the dark and quell your fears – then ever-present light may call forth incessant action.

"If you focus on density – revering solidity, fixity, and permanence, fearing even the normal changes of age, trying to substitute correctness and concealment for honest confusion and personal truth – then density will lock up your energy, protecting you so well that even healing change can't touch you.

"If you avoid extremes, staying away from your edges, restraining your passion, always being polite and moderate, then your heated feelings will simmer below the surface, your deep frozen feelings will, glacier-like, push and strain. Balance becomes elusive.

"The energy speeds up, it is trapped, it overheats, it super-cools. A cancer star is formed. The heart of the star begins to pulse.

"Can you feel that very low frequency hum? It is the vibration the cancer star makes as it grows. It is the sound of light vibrating, a star song: a shivering hum of concentrated matter, the vibration of life, the rippling sound of a wave of hot/cold, the cease-less hum of cancer.

"Long ago, in the dark, in the quiet, there was little that hummed the songs of cancer. Long ago, when women walked wild gathering weeds and took nothing for granted, their humming and crooning was louder than the hum of cancer.

"But long ago has become today. A today of light-filled nights. A today lived by the clock. A today where fixity and repetition are the ideal, where health means sameness, and all is under control. A today that offers little support for those who would nourish their wildness, hone their edges, or live with passion. A today that vi-brates day and night with electrical wires that hum the cancer song.

"We are the Ancient GrandMothers. We speak for the dark. We speak for chaos. We speak for the far reaches, the edges. We are here to help you listen to your passionate, wild, eccentric nature. To help you nourish your darkness, your looseness, your timeless-ness, your unformed edges. We can teach you how to change the song your star of cancer sings. Teach you how to help it gently dis-appear, returning its energy to the vast spinning galaxy of your healthy/whole/holy breast."

# 8.
# The Diagnosis is Cancer

*"As soon as I heard it was cancer, I felt as if a time-bomb were ticking away inside my breast."*                              Sharon, age 49

When the diagnosis is cancer, there are voices from outside and voices from within telling you to make *immediate* decisions. Please don't. The advice of the women who shared their breast cancer stories with me, and the advice of many professionals as well, is: **You have time.** Treatment decisions need to be made, but not at once. You have time to collect information. The results of hasty actions are permanent. Regrets can last the rest of your life. You have time to devote to you, yourself, and only you. You have the time to let the path of your health/wholeness/holiness reveal itself to you.

Are you filled with the desire to tear off the offending part of yourself? Remember that breast cancer can recur even if you don't have a breast. Do you think it best if someone else (your doctor, for instance) makes the treatment decisions for you? This is a perfect opportunity for you to stop being the victim of life and begin writing your own story. Do you want to get the whole thing over with as fast as possible, with as little fuss as possible, with, hopefully, no one the wiser? One of cancer's gifts is that it forces us to ask for help, to bare our breasts.

**Give yourself the gift of time.** Set a date in the future when you will take action. (A month is reasonable unless you have a rare fast-growing breast cancer.) Don't consent to treatment from Steps 4, 5, or 6 until then. Use the time to pursue Steps 0, 1, 2, and 3. Do nothing. Collect information. Engage the energy. Nourish and tonify. Love yourself. You deserve it.

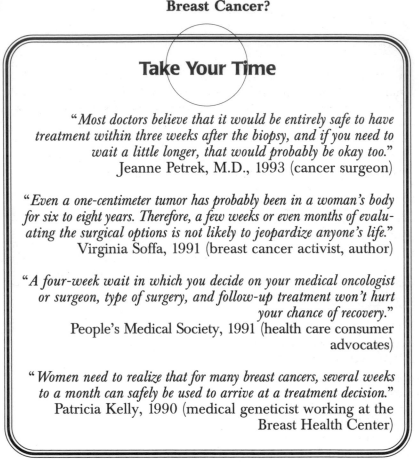

# Take Your Time

*"Most doctors believe that it would be entirely safe to have treatment within three weeks after the biopsy, and if you need to wait a little longer, that would probably be okay too."*
Jeanne Petrek, M.D., 1993 (cancer surgeon)

*"Even a one-centimeter tumor has probably been in a woman's body for six to eight years. Therefore, a few weeks or even months of evaluating the surgical options is not likely to jeopardize anyone's life."*
Virginia Soffa, 1991 (breast cancer activist, author)

*"A four-week wait in which you decide on your medical oncologist or surgeon, type of surgery, and follow-up treatment won't hurt your chance of recovery."*
People's Medical Society, 1991 (health care consumer advocates)

*"Women need to realize that for many breast cancers, several weeks to a month can safely be used to arrive at a treatment decision."*
Patricia Kelly, 1990 (medical geneticist working at the Breast Health Center)

**Step 0.** *Do Nothing*

• Relax with candlelight in warm, nicely scented water. Let yourself drift, let yourself float. If strong feeling or persistent thoughts come up, gently ask them to go.

• Hole up. **Turn off the lights**, unplug the phone, be swallowed by silence, **disconnect the clock**, live by your own cycles, retreat, withdraw, sink into **sleep**. Ask a friend to leave you food daily and help you out of your "holy cave" at a preset time.

• "Unexpected" survivors have this in common: a willingness to let go of the conscious, rational, controlling mind. They allow their inner wisdom to choose their treatment courses, and follow that, rather than anyone else's advice, no matter how informed or loving.

**Step 1.** *Collect Information*

★ What did the pathologist who read your biopsy see? With as many as 30 different kinds of breast cancer, diagnosis is complex. It is worth your time and effort to **get more than one opinion** on the tissue removed from your breast. And better if it is *not* someone your doctor recommends. Best if it's someone at a different hospital, perhaps even a different city. Some women recommend getting opinions from three or four specialists.

• **Reading** books—especially ones written by women who've been there—helps me gather all sorts of useful information and helps me understand my own healing journey with more clarity. My favorite books by breast cancer survivors (or their partners) are listed on page 168. I believe in the healing power of shared story so much that I asked my best friend, a cancer survivor of wit and wisdom, to share hers in this book; it begins on page 245.

• Descriptions of the **orthodox treatments** suggested for women with your diagnosis are available at no charge: Call 1-800-4-CANCER. Ask for the PDQ (Physician's Desk Query) State-of-the-Art Cancer Treatment Information fact sheets. Get the ones for physicians; they contain information not found in the patient set.

★ **Talking** with breast cancer survivors, healers, and doctors is an important way to collect information. *See* page 313 for organizations that offer information, networking, and help.

• Another way to collect information is to **pay attention to your intuition**. When the rational information you collect is enriched by your psyche, your personal path of healing emerges—not necessarily the "best" path, not necessarily the obvious path nor the one you "ought" to take, maybe not even the one you initially thought you wanted to take. It is, nonetheless, the path that leads to wholeness/holiness/health.

Use colors to make pictures of each of your treatment options. Write with your nondominant hand (left if you're right-handed), expressing your hopes and fears about each of your options. Visit your Wise Healer Within (*see* page 82). Ask an oracle. (My favorite: Pull two tarot cards for each of your options: One to represent your immediate response to each option and one to represent your life in five years if you opt for that treatment.) Ask for messages from your dreams. Consult a seer you trust.

# The Diagnosis Is *Carcinoma in Situ*

A diagnosis of ductal carcinoma *in situ* (**DCIS**) or lobular carcinoma *in situ* (**LCIS**) is frightening and confusing. There is no agreement in orthodoxy about the danger inherent in these conditions. Cancer specialist Susan Love, M.D., considers these not true cancers but *precancers*. Christiane Northrup, M.D., alerted me to the fact that over 40 percent of all normal breast tissues examined in autopsies have *in situ* cancer cells. With the widespread use of mammographic screening, more and more *in situ* carcinomas are found than ever before. A finding of *in situ* carcinoma increases the risk of later invasive breast cancer, but does not guarantee it. In fact, only a small percentage of *in situ* cancers progress to life-threatening cancer. Some remain stable for decades and some remiss without treatment.

Only 5 percent of all women diagnosed with LCIS will develop invasive breast cancer. Orthodox treatment is removal of *both* breasts (bilateral mastectomy) since invasive cancer–if it does occur–is just as likely to be in the breast without the LCIS as in the one with it. Women who choose this extreme treatment live no longer than women who elect frequent check-ups and care as called for.

Ductal carcinoma *in situ* is more likely to progress to invasive cancer. Modified mastectomy (removal of the breast and lymph nodes) is the "safe" treatment. However, women who choose this extensive surgery live no longer than women who choose lumpectomy (with or without adjuvant radiation) and frequent check-ups.[1, 2]

I have met and heard of many women diagnosed with DCIS or LCIS who treated themselves successfully using herbal remedies plus body work, energy work, and psyche work, as well as many who made use of minimal orthodox remedies in addition to Wise Woman ways.

• Go on a **vision quest**. Look for a vision of your health/wholeness/holiness. Traditionally this means spending three to five days alone in nature with minimal food and drink. But anything from a quiet walk at dusk to a ten-day wilderness adventure can serve to take you out of your daily routine and make room for your paradigm of healing to emerge.

★ **Define your paradigm of healing**. Caption your healing picture. When you define your own drama, it's easier to choose the best cast for your play. Are you a machine that needs to be fixed? Then hire the best mechanic. Is your cancer a deadly enemy? Engage a skillful general and fierce warriors. Do you have cancer because you did wrong, because you sinned? Confess, accept your punishment, and make amends. Are you the put-upon victim of a cruel world? Look for a savior or find a hero. Are you a soul eternally changing, aware that no answer is always right or always wrong? Seek the support of the wise women inside and outside of yourself. You can learn to fix your own machines, become your own general, accept your mistakes and forgive yourself, rewrite the script so you are the savior, accept your wildness, your chaos, and your darkness, and let cancer transform your life.

**Step 2.** *Engage the Energy*

★ When the diagnosis is cancer, you are offered an opportunity to **make yourself the priority**. Now. To make time for yourself, you need help: with meals, child care, elder care. Ask for it. Hire it. Take time off from work. The time you invest in yourself *this month* will make an enormous difference for the rest of your life.

• Cancer cells are immature. Cancer cells are greedy. Cancer cells aren't respectful. Cancer cells don't cooperate. Cancer cells are imperialists. Cancer cells are not neat and they aren't organized. What ways other than cancer do you have to express the immature, greedy, disrespectful, uncooperative, imperialistic, messy, disorganized parts of yourself?

• Focus on living. Be stubborn about it. Be "difficult."A 1985 article in *The Lancet* reported on a study of 57 women diagnosed with breast cancer in 1975. After ten years, recurrence-free survival was significantly higher among women who reacted with "fighting spirit" *or with denial,* than among those who reacted with acceptance, helplessness, or hopelessness.[3]

• The immune system is powerfully affected by emotions. Suppressed and unidentified emotions are known to depress immune system functioning, while strong feelings, even fear and anger, can strengthen the immune system if expressed with love and acceptance. (*See* "Dealing with Feeling" pages 163-165.)

★ One of the most powerful influences on how long a woman will live after her diagnosis of breast cancer is a high score for **joy** (on a standardized test). The correlation holds true even regarding women with metastasizing cancer: The greater the amount of joy, the longer the life. Indulge in pleasure. **Go for giggles!**

★ **Create a ceremony for yourself**. Call upon healing energies, forces, presences, the Great Mystery, God/dess. Act out your vision of healing. Do it alone, or—better yet—invite participants, witnesses, friends. Throw a healing party. Engage all your senses with color, smells, beautiful food, music, drumming, dancing, singing. Let yourself be the center of attention. Say out loud how you want to be helped in your dance with cancer. Open yourself to what others offer you. Allow yourself to deserve this help.

• **Keep a journal** of your feelings, dreams, experiences, observations, doodles. (In a real book with a pen, not on a computer.) Journaling helps us slow down . . . slow enough to write . . . slow enough to read our own writing . . . slow enough to catch the current of our own truth.

• Now's the time to make that **change**. Leave behind what you no longer need. Invite your inner child out to play. Set yourself on a new course. Go on a trip with only your toothbrush. Find a new style. Do what you really want to do with your life.

• Cancer can be the last straw for a love relationship: Almost half of the women who "lose" a breast, "lose" a mate, too. Cancer can also create intense **intimacy**, physically and spiritually, deepening a love relationship. Read *How Can I Help?* for help following the path of intimacy in the midst of a life-threatening problem.[4]

★ **Words are power.** "Don't call me a patient," she said; "I am a client." *Patient* is from *pathos*, to suffer, while *client* is from *cluens*, to hear. "I want to be heard. And I don't want treatment for my breast cancer, I want treatment for me. And I don't receive treatments, I choose them and I *take* them."

★ **Visualization** has a solid reputation for helping many women with cancer. One verified way to utilize healing imagery is the Simonton method, explained in *Getting Well Again*. *See* page 314 for a Simonton Center where you can learn the techniques.

• Nicki Scully, a woman dancing with breast cancer, wants to take you on a **guided healing journey**. Each of her two audio tapes–*Awakening the Cobra* and *The Cauldron Journey for Healing*–offers a healing visualization set to music on one side, and the same music without words on the other so you can create your own journey. Contact Nicki at PO Box 5025, Eugene, OR 97405.

• There are many **homeopathic remedies** used against cancer. Those that are specific for women with breast cancer include the potentially poisonous plants hemlock (*Conium*), poke (*Phytolacca*), and bloodroot (*Sanguinaria*), as well as harmless remedies such as red clover (*Trifolium*) and violet (*Viola*). Consult a homeopathic doctor for indications and dosage before using these remedies.
>    *Chimaphila umbellata*: mother tincture, fresh plant in flower
>    *Conium maculatum*: 6x to 30x
>    *Phytolacca americana*: 6x to 30x or mother tincture of root
>    *Sanguinaria canadensis*: fresh juice with alcohol
>    *Trifolium pratense*: mother tincture of fresh flowers
>    *Viola odorata*: mother tincture of fresh plant in flower

• Take off your bra. Stop shaving under your arms. Stop using aluminum-based antiperspirants. I'm not suggesting this will cure your cancer, but it can lessen the stress on your immune system.

**Step 3.** *Nourish and Tonify*

★ **Women with breast cancer who attend a support group live twice as long** as women with breast cancer who don't. Individual time with a therapist also improves longevity.

★ When dancing with breast cancer, wise women are particularly fond of **anti-cancer herbs** such as **astragalus, burdock, honeysuckle, nettle, red clover, Siberian ginseng,** and **violet**. These serious, effective, anti-cancer herbs are safe enough for the entire family to eat for dinner, yet powerful enough to counter *in situ* cancers. And they are important complementary medicines for women using Steps 5 and 6. *See* Materia Medica for more information, including dosages.

★ **Healing by nourishing** is hard to believe, so accustomed have we become to the idea that we have to poison the person to kill the cancer. But some foods have anti-cancer effects, some foods can mitigate the side effects of orthodox treatments, and other foods can help prevent recurrence and metastases. *See* Chapter 2.

I avoid alternative treatments that suggest that the answer to cancer is to cleanse. I believe that *fasting, colon cleansing, liver flushing, and similiar detoxifications are dangerous for women with breast cancer.* Most of the "bad press" attached to using non-orthodox treatments can be attributed to these treatments, which weaken vitality and may hasten death. *See* page 154.

• Rats fed diets rich in **calcium** show a significant reduction in primary and recurrent breast cancers. To get 2000 mg of calcium a day, I eat three things: one cup of organic yogurt (450 mg), two or more cups of nourishing herbal infusions such as nettle, comfrey leaf, oatstraw, violet, or red clover (300 mg per cup), and several big spoonfuls of mineral-rich medicinal herbal vinegars (300 mg per tablespoon).

• The *Essentials of Chinese Medicine* suggests pounding calcium-rich **dandelion** roots and leaves into a juice and drinking it diluted with wine to counter breast cancer. This is said to be especially effective against *in situ* cancers.

• Traditional Chinese Medicine has many formulas for helping women with breast cancer.[5] Ideally, a formula is created for you individually. Some of the many nourishing herbs that might be included are **astragalus**, **dandelion**, **ginseng**, **ginger**, **licorice**, **orange peel**, **self-heal**, **seaweed** (especially fucus), and **violet**.

• **Protein** intake has been shown in laboratory studies to have a direct effect on cancer. When calories from protein fall in the range of 20–25 percent of the diet (the average in Western industrialized countries is 25–30 percent), the initiation, promotion, and growth of cancer is enhanced. When protein is **under 20 percent** or **over 50 percent** of total calories, tumor growth is inhibited. Protein sources include beans, tofu, nuts, seeds, grains, and many greens, as well as meat, fish, eggs, cheese, yogurt, and milk. High sugar, low protein diets accelerate cancer growth, while low sugar, high protein diets slow it.[6] (Raw fruits and vegetables, especially when juiced, are high sugar, low protein.)

• Sunshine, moonshine, hugs, hope, a safe place to cry and rage–there are so many ways to be healed. Friendship, firelight, flowers, fantasies–there are so many ways to be loved. Clean water, organic food, massage, prayers, fresh air, satisfying work, and engaging recreation–there are so many ways to be nourished.

• Dr. Johanna Budwig, a German healer with extensive experience helping those with cancer, used **flax oil** and **fermented milk** protein as the basis of her approach to eliminating cancer. (*See* "Quark-Flax" recipe, page 311.) Dr. Budwig also recommended that those with cancer eat fresh rainbow trout as a source of EPA and DHA–fatty acids which potentize the treatment but are inadequately produced by those with cancer. (These fatty acids are also found in fresh, wild salmon, mackerel, sardines, tuna, and eel.) All other fats and oils were to be totally avoided until the tumor dissolved and health was reestablished. Dr. Budwig felt that vitamin and mineral supplements did more harm than good. She advocated a diet of at least 50 percent fresh raw vegetables, fruits, and nuts.

• It's vitally important to **nourish your immune system** when you have a diagnosis of cancer. A strong immune system is better able to stop recurrence and metastases, and help you heal from surgery and adjuvant treatments. *See* Chapter 4.

• **Immune strengthening therapies** measure their results differently than orthodox treatments. In successful immunotherapies the immune system may wall off the cancerous mass, preventing growth and metastasis, but leaving the size of the tumor undiminished. In contrast, orthodox medicine judges results strictly on the basis of tumor size and calls any shrinkage of the tumor a remission, even if the mass begins to grow again immediately following treatment.

• No matter how well you can take care of yourself, no matter how good you are at being fine-no-matter-what, you now need help and **support**. The more support, the better. Many women told me that they felt their support team had as large an impact on their healing as any treatment. Will someone go with you to meet with the doctors, oncologists, radiologists, surgeons, healers? Is someone willing to be a silent sounding board for you? You may want allies other than loved ones (who have their own needs and opinions).

# The Wise Woman Doesn't Ask Why

The Wise Woman asks "How?" She knows that "Why" leads to (and springs from) the erroneous belief that we can control our lives. "How" helps us remember that we can participate fully in our lives no matter how out of control they seem. "Why" points the finger of blame. "How" points to the places we need to nourish. The Wise Woman asks, **"How is this right?"** rather than, "Why is this happening to me?"

How can breast cancer possibly be right? How can breast cancer be an ally of health/wholeness/holiness? This is not an easy question to answer. And one can only answer it for oneself, never for another. Each of us has a different answer; each of us is unique perfection unfolding in her own way.

The part that is crying out for nourishment, the part that feels so unheard that it becomes a problem, is different in each woman. But it is always a part we deny. Perhaps the denial is total: We cannot see it, hear it, honor it, or nourish it, because to us *it does not exist.* Or perhaps the denial is partial: We see it and hear it, but don't think we have the time or the courage or the support to follow our dreams.

If I put my arm behind my back, eventually my shoulder will hurt. No remedy will ease my pain for more than a short while so long as I keep my arm behind me. It may seem obvious that if I release my arm, my shoulder won't hurt. But I can't see my arm back there, and I may not even be able to feel it. And I'll get angry if anyone suggests there is something behind my back. This is my denial.

Denial, by its nature, is difficult to see. Here's one Wise Woman way to find the arm behind your back.

First, ask: "What is the problem with my problem? What is the problem with having breast cancer?" Write down at least three answers. **Let these statements begin with "I."** Read them out loud.

Then, rewrite your answers, starting each statement with "I want to" or "I choose to." You will encounter resistance here: There will be statements that you don't want to write, that you don't believe you'd ever think. Good. That's the point: to get in touch with parts of yourself that you dislike, to hear from parts you've kept gagged, to liberate parts you've locked up. Be light with yourself; tell yourself: "I don't have to take this seriously."

Read each changed statement out loud five or more times. Listen to what you are saying. These statements give voice to the part of yourself for whom having breast cancer is perfect. It doesn't mean that you chose to have breast cancer, but that there is a part of you that has chosen to speak through breast cancer. Can you hear it? What else does it have to say to you? How would you describe it? How do you feel about it? How can you nourish it? How can you claim it as part of you?

Some hear cancer speaking with the voice of the inner child, the one who didn't get her needs met long ago. Is she wild, reckless, high-spirited, and passionate; or tender, damaged, and afraid? Run with her, give her wild places; hold her, love her, listen to her. Can you find a way to give her what she needs and wants? Even if it's something you think is bad?

Others hear cancer speaking with the voice of the shadow, the hidden side, the part that can control us without our knowledge.

No matter how untamed, how damaged, or how fearsome this denied part of ourselves is, the task of the Wise Woman is the same: Nourish it. But if we nourish our shadow, won't our demons destroy us? The Wise Woman way says: It is only starving demons that we need fear. Fat, happy demons don't cause problems! Nourish your demons symbolically—with attention, dialogue, visualization, art, and ceremony. You aren't becoming your demons, you're accepting them as part of your wholeness.

Our problems offer us grounded, unbounded wisdom. They are the unruly, chaotic, unpredictable parts of ourselves: the Mother of All, fearsome, but offering growth and wholeness.

Whatever the diagnosis, the Wise Woman nourishes the problem, the inner child, the shadow self, the wisdom within. I'm not saying it will cure your cancer. But I do guarantee that, if you nourish every part of yourself, when you do die—whether from breast cancer, a bolt of lightning, or fatigue at the age of 150—you won't feel like a victim. You'll meet death as the final stage of growth, not as a sign of failure.

**Step 4.** *Stimulate/Sedate*

★ **Poke** root is one of the strongest anti-cancer remedies available without orthodox supervision. Its reputation rests on extensive folklore, recent scientific studies, and clinical practice.

In *Back to Eden,* herbalist Jethro Kloss says women with breast cancer successfully resolved tumors with poultices of freshly grated poke. Dr. Christopher, one of this century's most respected herbalists, also writes in his book, *School of Natural Healing,* about using poultices of freshly grated poke root against breast cancer. (Poultices are left on for three days, then replaced, for 4–6 weeks.)

The tincture (taken orally) is also a renowned anti-cancer remedy. The *Journal of Economic Medical Plant Research* reports that pokeweed antiviral proteins nourish white blood cells, quickly increase lymphocyte replication, and inhibit a wide range of viruses (including polio, influenza, and herpes simplex).

A woman who treated her non-metastasizing breast cancer (quite a large mass, too) with alternating poultices of freshly grated poke root one day and freshly grated comfrey root the next, said that the poke ate away at her as though it were burning the cancer out. The comfrey was a soothing relief after the rigors of the poke. In the late fall she put several roots into tubs of damp sand and brought them indoors so she could continue her treatment throughout the winter. (Unfortunately, she didn't stay in touch and I don't know the outcome.) Poke root ointment is gentler.

*See* Materia Medica for dosage and **cautions**.

---

Arnie's diagnosis was metastasized cancer; his prognosis, only a few months of life. He said his wife died "not of cancer but of the treatments" and that he didn't mind dying, but "not like that, tortured to death." Arnie chose to take poke root tincture (gradually increasing his dose until he was taking 15 drops a day) and to follow a macrobiotic diet. The active macrobiotic community in his town gave him unwavering support for following his own path of healing and told him he could heal himself of cancer. A year later, orthodox doctors declared his cancer in total remission. (And he's still alive today, 16 years later.) Although the poke root and the dietary changes were, no doubt, important in his remission, I believe that the support Arnie searched out, asked for, and accepted was the critical element in his miraculous cure from terminal cancer.

• Some anti-cancer herbal formulas used with success for the last 50 years or longer include: **Essiac, Hoxsey Elixir, Juzentaihoto,** and **Jason Winter's Tea.** (Recipes begin on page 293.) These combinations are considered safe enough to use—with caution—with orthodox treatments.

★ I am particularly partial to the **Hoxsey** formula, which has been in veterinary use for over 150 years and has a strong track record with humans, as well. Harry Hoxsey (1901–1974) devoted his life to helping those dancing with cancer. Two federal courts and numerous medical investigators upheld the therapeutic benefits of his formulas. One medical panel even found his treatments clinically superior to surgery, radiation, and chemotherapy. Hoxsey claimed the formulas were family secrets, but the elixir is a variation on a classic Eclectic Tradition formula, and the salve has been used for several hundred years. For more on Hoxsey's anti-cancer program, read *You Don't Have to Die*, Milestone Books, 1956. Recipes for Hoxsey Elixir and for Hoxsey Salve, reported to be especially effective on breast tumors, are on page 303.

• Can hormone-rich herbs (e.g. licorice and ginseng) stimulate breast cancer growth like ovarian hormones do? My observation is—and other herbalists working with women with breast cancer agree—**hormones in plants have cancer-inhibiting effects**. Research showing soybean hormones to be cancer-reversing substantiates this.

• **Rosemary** (*Rosmarinus officinalis*) contains two phytochemicals—carnosol and ursolic acid—which can slow or stop tumor growth. In laboratory studies it inhibited mammary tumors in mice. The dose is 5–20 drops of the fresh plant tincture, 2–3 times daily.

• **Limonene**, found in **orange peels** and **lavender**, can reduce and prevent human breast cancer according to *Science News*, May, 1993. More than half the mammary tumors in laboratory mice disappeared when their diet contained 2 percent limonene (perillyl alcohol), and virtually none of them had recurrences. Traditional Chinese Medicine has utilized the anti-carcinogenic properties of bitter orange peel for hundreds of years. *See* Materia Medica.

★ Nutritional deficiencies occur quickly in a person with cancer if food is withheld (as in a fast), severely limited (as in an overly strict vegetarian diet), or not tolerated (as a side-effect of chemotherapy or radiation treatments). Even in a vigorous person, if no solid food is eaten for 24 hours, the heart muscle begins to break down and liver enzymes which protect against cancer, such as hepatic glutathione, are reduced by 50 percent.[7]

**Step 5a.**  *Use Supplements*

• Contrary to current practitice, **I avoid vitamin and mineral supplements** and probably wouldn't take them if I had cancer. If I did choose supplements, I would limit my use to a short duration. Many nutrients have been shown to interfere with the promotion and growth of cancer—e.g., carotenes, vitamins A, $B_{17}$ (laetrile), C, D, E, coenzyme $Q_{10}$, folic acid, the amino acid arginine, germanium, melatonin, and selenium—but supplemental forms of some can spur the growth of malignancies. Carotenes in food prevent cancer; supplements of beta carotene increased lung cancer in smokers. Foods rich in tocopherols (vitamin E) help prevent cancer; alpha-tocopherol pills magnify it. Iron-rich herbs are notable anti-cancer herbs (e.g., yellow dock , dandelion, plantain); supplements of iron can accelerate cancer growth.

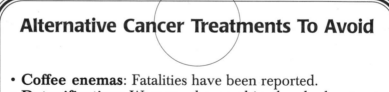

## Alternative Cancer Treatments To Avoid

• **Coffee enemas**: Fatalities have been reported.
• **Detoxification**: Women who combined orthodox treatments with a strict vegan diet augmented with carrot juice and vitamin tablets were twice as likely to die and three times as likely to have metastases as women who received the same treatments for breast cancer but no detoxification.[8] These results are similiar to those achieved with Gerson and other raw juice therapies.[9]
• **Fasting**: Can impair the functioning of the liver, immune system, nervous system, hormonal system, and the heart.
• **Injections of liver**: Fatalities have been reported.
• **Ingestion of goldenseal** (*Hydrastis canadensis*) **in large quantity**: Can damage the liver and the kidneys.
• **Long-term use of supplements**: Can promote cancer.

**Caution: Germanium** supplements have caused six deaths and many cases of kidney damage. Imports into the U.S. were banned in 1988 by the FDA. For safe sources, *see* page 49.

★ I get safe mega-doses of top-quality nutrients from herbal infusions, cooked greens, medicinal vinegars, mushrooms, seaweed, organic grains and oils, and yogurt.

★ Dr. Hans Nieper, a European herbalist who specialized in helping those with cancer, encouraged them to bring blood levels of **carotenes** to 6–8 mg per liter, or until their palms turned orange. Research points to several ways that carotenes counter cancer. Carotenes trigger genes that cause cells to mature and die: When cancer cells metabolize carotenes, they form retinoic acid as well as vitamin A; this acid is influential in promoting the production of proteins that initiate cell death. Plus, carotenes encourage macrophages and lymphocytes to secrete more of certain cytokines which are toxic to cancer cells. More on carotenes on page 47.

★ Clinical trials of **coenzyme $Q_{10}$** (390 mg daily) found it effective in shrinking primary tumors and capable of putting some women's breast cancers into complete remission. This naturally occurring substance also enhances immune response.[10]

• Very large doses of **vitamin C** (ascorbic acid) are frequently used by women dancing with cancer. But if taken with a mineral supplement high in iron, copper, and manganese, vitamin C supplements generate enormous amounts of cancer-initiating free radicals.[11] Vitamin C is optimally effective when ingested in fresh (not canned, bottled, frozen, or reconstituted) fruits and vegetables.

Linus Pauling, Nobel Prize winner and researcher into the effects of vitamin C, found that daily doses of 10 grams of ascorbic acid could increase the life span of those with terminal cancer. Further studies have failed to replicate his results, but there appear to be design flaws in those studies (such as limiting the length of time the vitamin was given, as opposed to Pauling's studies where the full dose was given until the person died). Pauling believed that taking large doses of ascorbic acid—and then stopping—might even hasten death in those with terminal cancer.

When women's daily intake of vitamin C was 2–3 grams, their T-lymphocyte activity increased and precancerous cervical cells (dysplasia) return to normal.[12] A diet exceptionally rich in antioxidants, including vitamin C, may help counter early-stage breast cancer.

• **Laetrile**, vitamin $B_{17}$ or amygdalin, is a simple compound that occurs in substantial amounts in the pits of apricots, peaches, cherries, berries, buckwheat, millet, and some peas and beans. When acted on (in the body or the laboratory) by beta-glucosidase–found in very high amounts in many cancer cells–laetrile becomes glucose, benzaldehyde, and hydrocyanic acid. Normal cells can safely metabolize a small amount of hydrocyanic acid, but cancer cells metabolize it into cyanide, which kills them. When fed laetrile, vitamin A, and pancreatic enzymes, 75 out of 84 mice with breast cancer had complete remission.[13, 14] (The others showed partial remission.)

For dosage, see page 29 or *The Physician's Handbook of Vitamin B-17 Therapy*, McNaughton, Science Press International, 1975. The Hospital Ernesto Contreras in San Ysidro, California claims to have treated more cancers with laetrile than any other facility in the world; you can contact them at 1-800-326-1850. **Caution:** Muscular weakness, dizziness, diarrhea, nausea, and respiratory difficulties can occur if excessive amounts of apricot pits are consumed. Young children who've eaten laetrile tablets have died.

• **Melatonin** (75 mg daily) is a powerful anti-cancer hormone found in all life forms from algae to primates. In humans, it is secreted by the pineal gland. In addition to its antioxidant abilities (which interfere with cancer initiation and slow free-radical damage), melatonin stops cancer promotion by altering the way other hormones are utilized. Melatonin may counter early stage breast cancer and is a complementary medicine. Taken before and after exposure to diagnostic x-rays, melatonin spared 70 percent of the cells that normally would have been damaged.[15]

Melatonin production can be increased by spending time in the dark, sleeping more, and perhaps by taking 125 drops/5 ml drops of the tincture of chaste tree (*Vitex*) daily. In clinical trials, pure melatonin in doses as high as 7500 mg a day caused no toxicity.

• **Selenium** is the anti-cancer mineral. Supplements of selenocysteine, selenomethionine selenium (1 mg daily), and sodium selenite (90 mcg) can slow or stop the growth stage of cancer and help prevent recurrence by suppressing cancer's ability to proliferate. Clinical and population studies have confirmed its ability to reduce cancer death rates, enhance immune system functioning, and prevent chromosome damage during radiation treatments. (More on selenium: pages 51–52.) **Caution:** Selenium may enhance cancer growth unless taken with vitamin E (at least 200 IU daily). Pure elemental selenium can be toxic. Sodium selenite, the most commonly available supplement, is potently anti-carcinogenic, but may be poisonous in doses over 100 mcg (.1 mg).[16]

• According to Nobel Prize winner, Otto Warburg, M.D., cancer cells use an anaerobic energy cycle which produces an enormous amount of lactic acid. Oral **hydrazine sulfate** blocks this process. So does **deep breathing**, such as loud, vigorous singing, done for 20 minutes, four times a day.

**Step 5b.**  *Use Drugs (or Drug-Like Herbal Preparations)*

★ The most frequently used—and seemingly most successful—alternative treatments available to the woman with invasive breast cancer are usually administered by injection: **714X, carnivora, sundew,** and **mistletoe.** *See also* **shiitake,** page 87.

• I'm impressed with the work of Gaston Naessens. His method of diagnosis—examination of living blood—is a radical departure from orthodoxy. His focus on nourishing the cancer, as well as the person, is clearly in the Wise Woman Tradition. **714X,** his treatment (which can be used at home) is injected into the lymph nodes near the cancer. It is designed to supply the cancer cells with nutrients (especially nitrogen), thus allowing the immune system to gain access to the nutrients it needs to make the specialized cells which can eliminate the cancer.[18] 714X is frequently (but not always) effective in slowing and reversing early stage breast cancers and has few side effects. For help acquiring 714X, *see* page 167.

• Carnivora, derived from **Venus's flytrap** (*Dionaea muscipula*) is highly effective against cancer. The preserved fresh juice of the plant reduces the growth rate of tumors, stimulates T-helper cells, increases macrophage activity, and alleviates pain, yet is completely nontoxic.[17] One woman credits carnivora for her total remission from inflammatory breast cancer, one of the most lethal type of cancers. Once treatment is begun, it is suggested that you remain on it for life. Both Yul Brynner and an ex-president are reported to have used carnivora. Some healers said they have occasionally seen remission from use of the tincture orally. Carnivora therapy is easily available in Germany. *See* page 167.

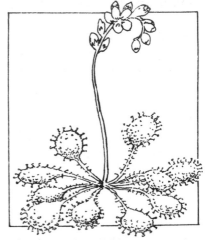

★ **Sundew** is highly recommended as a replacement for Carnivora, which is made from a plant that is not only rare in the wild, but difficult to grow. Sundew has the same anti-cancer properties, but is easily cultivated. ("Weed-like" says one source.) Better yet, it is as effective orally as carnivora is by injection. Dose is 30–90 drops a day. *See* Sources for Herbs, page 312, and Materia Medica.

• **Mistletoe** is a parasitic plant that looks and acts like metastatic cancer, spreading through its host tree and ultimately killing it. Rudolf Steiner, the creator of Anthroposophical medicine, processed mistletoe into Iscador. Iscador is meant, he said, to alarm the immune system and trigger it into dealing with the cancer.

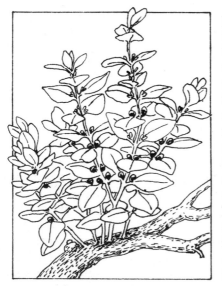

The more than 30,000 people who have used injections of Iscador or other mistletoe extracts (Helixor and Plenosol) consistently report that they are easy to tolerate, useful for inhibiting and shrinking tumors, and effective in preventing recurrence. (Injections can be done at home with an insulin needle.) Some healers report good results using tincture of mistletoe orally instead of injections. Those with late-stage cancers say mistletoe makes a dramatic improvement in general health. *See* Materia Medica for dose. (Mistletoe resources, page 167.)

• **Vaccine-like** preparations of killed bacteria stimulate dramatic activity in the immune system, including an increase in tumor necrosis factor which causes tumors to hemorrhage and liquefy. These preparations are currently being tested on women with breast (and ovarian) cancers.

• **Chemotherapy** is being urged on more and more women in earlier and earlier stages of breast cancer. (Like any treatment, it works best when the cancer is small and there are no metastases.) Read Chapter 13 before you choose chemotherapy.

> "*There is no logical reason to believe the people who recover after having major poisons assault their system, such as in chemotherapy, are not also instances of spontaneous remission; they too can be regarded as having gotten well because of their attitude and in spite of the treatment.*"
> Jeanne Achterberg, *Imagery in Healing*[19]

**Step 6.** *Break & Enter*

• **Removal of your breast does not guarantee a cure.** It is a common first reaction to the diagnosis of cancer to want the offending breast cut off. But cancer can recur even when both breasts are removed. The majority of women who make a hasty decision to amputate their breasts regret it. More and more women are choosing breast-sparing surgery (with and without radiation) and saving the mastectomy until later, if need be.

Some women find that removal of their primary cancer eases the stress on their immune system, giving them rapid improvement in health. Others find that surgery spreads their cancer or allows secondary tumors to grow. (Primary tumors can secrete substances which prevent the growth of other tumors.) For them, surgery is the beginning of endless rounds of trying to heal the damage caused by the previous cure. Read Chapter 9 before you choose breast surgery.

• **Laser surgery** uses a laser to vaporize or burn away cancer cells rather than physically cutting them out of the breast. This lessens the risk of cancer being "spread by the scalpel." Other advantages include less damage to normal tissue, less blood loss, less drainage after surgery, less pain medication needed, shortened hospital stays (1–2 days), less damage to lymphatic drainage, and fewer hematomas.[20, 21]

• **Lymph node surgery is more damaging than breast surgery**. The more nodes removed, the more severe the after effects. Removal of nodes slows normal lymphatic drainage from the arm, making it susceptible to swelling and infection. Consider keeping your lymph nodes, especially if your diagnosis is intraductal carcinoma (the most common type of breast cancer).[22]

• **Radiation therapy** can weaken the ribs, damage the lungs and heart, permanently change the color and texture of skin, and deaden sensation in your breast. Radiation therapy does little to increase longevity. Read Chapter 12 before choosing radiation therapy.

• **Electrochemical therapy**, as envisioned by Swedish professor Bjorn Nordenstrom, is currently used in Beijing hospitals to ionize and kill cancer tissues. Electrodes are placed through the skin into the tumor and current is introduced continuously for 3–4 hours. In addition to killing the primary tumor, this treatment sharply reduces rates of recurrence and metastases.

• In a similiar vein, electrodes implanted into a tumor are used to heat the cancer, destroying it. Another technique uses **microwaves** to increase the temperature of the cancer to a lethal 108° F. These techniques are said to be especially effective on breast cancers.

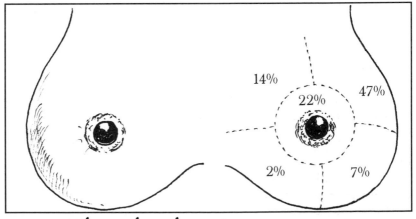

*Where does breast cancer occur?*

# Treatment or Overtreatment?

We are encouraged to think of breast cancer as one disease. Not so. Breast cancer is "a spectrum of diseases from *in situ* lesions with minimal malignant potential to extremely aggressive lesions, such as inflammatory carcinoma." How is a woman or her doctor to judge where on this spectrum her cancer lies and what treatment is needed? It isn't easy. And so the tendency is to overtreat.

Primary breast cancers, no matter how large, rarely cause death. Metastasized breast cancers, no matter how small, almost always do—though sometimes not for quite a long time. (It is rare, but possible, to die from breast cancer metastasis when no primary tumor can be found.)

As soon as a diagnosis of breast cancer is made, the riddle of "Has it metastasized?" begins. The answer seems to promise the difference between life and death, between moderate treatments and invasive ones.

Since it is the metastases, not the primary cancer, that can cause death, it is essential that we find out how likely it is that our cancer has metastasized. The more likely metastasis is, the more reasonable it becomes to use aggressive, even life-threatening treatments. The less likely metastasis is, the safer it is to use non-invasive natural treatments.

To help determine the likelihood of metastasis, you're likely to be "staged," a process that groups various signs of breast cancer by measures such as size of tumor and lymph node involvement. (Breast cancer cells have a special affinity for lymph nodes and will often be found there if they are metastasizing.)

Each stage implies a lesser or greater likelihood of metastasis. But staging is a good guess at best, and there is no way to say for certain that the primary tumor has *not* shed cells. Many premenopausal women whose lymph nodes show no signs of breast cancer cells nonetheless have metastasized breast cancer.

The riddle of metastasis is worthy of a fairy tale, for it has no solid answer. Without an accepted orthodox means to rule out the possibility of metastasis, we wind up with a system where most women are overtreated in an attempt to treat adequately the few women who need aggressive remedies.

Overtreatment of women with breast cancer is not a new problem. Many women diagnosed with breast cancer in the decades from 1930–1970 were told that their best choice for longevity was radical mastectomy: removal of the entire breast, all the lymph nodes near it, and the chest muscle underlying it. When put to the test, though, radical mastectomy gave no greater lifespan than mastectomy with radiation or simple mastectomy; all yielded the same mean survival time of 15 years.

Radical mastectomies are now used less and less as more women are given orthodox support to choose simple mastectomies and lumpectomies. (Women who choose breast-sparing surgery also have a mean survival of 15 years.)

But where we gain one place, we lose another. Women who choose breast-sparing surgery are told that they must also use radiation or chemotherapy. It is not unusual for a woman to be told that if she refuses these, her doctor will refuse to treat her. But these therapies are hazardous and overused. When longevity statistics are compared, it is clear that chemotherapy and radiation are not as much help to women with breast cancer as they are made out to be.

Looking back, we can see that radical mastectomies harmed women and were ineffective in preventing metastases and recurrences. Candace Pert, who's spent her life studying the immune system, prophesies that we will look back in horror at the use of chemotherapy and radiation to treat people with cancer. Twenty-first century treatments, she suggests, will counter cancer through manipulation of brain chemicals such as melatonin.

Some women deal with the riddle of metastasis by agreeing to whatever treatment the doctor urges (and this is true whether it's an alternative doctor or an orthodox doctor). Other women deal with it by seeking healers who will help them build health and wholeness, who will support them in using less-invasive treatments, and who are willing to deal with an empowered person who wants to decide on her own treatment.

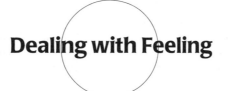

# Dealing with Feeling

Feelings arise at the mention of breast cancer, feelings we usually don't want to feel: fear, terror, shock, rage, grief, despair, depression, betrayal, humiliation, to name but a few. Like finding you're pregnant when you don't want to be, a diagnosis of cancer can infiltrate every thought and dream, echo behind every action, fill the mental screen at every break.

*I still feel a shock of pure terror every time my breast is touched, even if I touch it.*

Dealing with cancer is compounded by dealing with feelings—our own and the feelings of others. It is easy to feel out of control in the face of such seeming betrayal on the part of our bodies, such confusion among the experts over how best to treat the cancer, and the unpredictable upwellings of powerful emotions.

*I wanted to run away from my breast; I thought it was going to kill me.*

*I was more terrified of chemotherapy than cancer.*

*I was more embarrassed about being fat [from the chemotherapy] than I was about having one breast.*

Grief is a healthy part of healing. Avoid compulsion—which goes over and over the same thing endlessly with no resolution—but allow the chaos of grief, which runs its course and ends.

*A deep shattering in my personality had to be dealt with.*

*Facing reality instead of denying it gives me the courage to go on.*

When you find yourself obsessing about your breast cancer, think of a big orange pumpkin. Let that pumpkin fill your mind until everything is orange, orange, orange (the color of strong immunity). Feel your mind relax.

*Challenge the cancer, don't fight it. Dissolve it, banish it, replace it, but don't kill it or destroy it. Remember, it is part of you; it grew from your cells.*

This treatment will benefit any woman: Seek the support and encouragement you need to think independently, to self-actualize, to listen to your body, and to respond to its needs.

*When I walked out of there I was myself again, because I knew I had a choice.*

*A doctor who is there for you is a form of support and adds a dimension that's immeasurable.*

Depression is always lurking after a diagnosis of cancer. Depression (even with thoughts of suicide) is understood, in the Wise Woman Way, as a desire to transform—radically—ourselves and our lives.

*I was fine through the treatments, then I got very depressed; I really didn't want the treatments to end.*

*Mutilation produces anger. I learned to replace that anger with humor.*

**Bach flower essences** are special vibrational remedies for the emotions which help us be at ease with difficult feelings.
When you feel fear–*Aspen.*
When despair predominates–*Gorse.*
When you're filled with guilt and blame–*Pine.*
When there is persistent terror–*Rock Rose.*
When there's panic or mental shock–*Star of Bethlehem.*
When resentment and bitterness are heavy–*Willow.*
When you feel disgusted by your diagnosis, are filled with shame, and want to keep it a secret–*Crab apple.*

*Cry with a friend.*

*Learn to say to yourself "This is a bunch of b.s.," when they tell you you're going to die if you don't do it their way.*

*Keep a journal.*

*Join a support group.*

**Homeopathic remedies** can also help you cope with the overwhelming emotions that arise when the diagnosis is cancer:

When the fear is overwhelming and you can't cope–*Baryta carb.*

If you're anguished and turn totally inward–*Cannabis indica.*

When you feel you're as good as dead–*Hyoscyamus.*

When you feel hysterical but deeply depressed–*Ignatia.*

If you feel deeply wronged, abandoned, victimized–*Lyssin.*

When everything seems unreal; you're angry, overstimulated, restless, unable to stop, super-sensitive–*Medorrhinum.*

If you're plunged into despair and so intensely anxious that all familiar things seem strange–*Morphium.*

When you vacillate between terror and rage–*Stramonium.*

If you feel restless, agitated, and despairing–*Veratum album.*

My favorite herbs for easing the emotions:
- **motherwort** tincture (10–15 drops as needed)
- **oatstraw** (a cup of infusion or 25 drops of the tincture)
- **marijuana** (*see* page 233)

For more Wise Woman ways to deal with grief, depression, thoughts of suicide, rage, crying jags, oversensitivity, anxiety, fear, and other emotional uproars, see my book *Menopausal Years, The Wise Woman Way.*

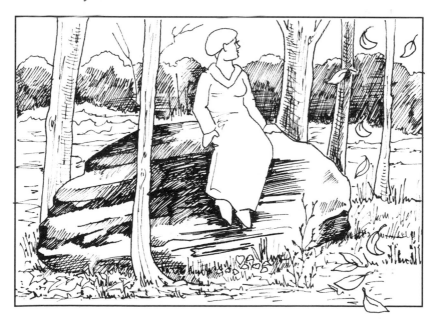

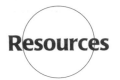

# Resources

## Non-Orthodox Options for Women with Breast Cancer

### Books & Newsletters
- *Alternatives in Cancer Therapy: The Complete Guide to Non-Traditional Treatments,* R. Pelton and L. Overholser, Fireside, 1994
- *Beating Cancer With Nutrition,* P. Quillin, NTP, 1994
- *Choices in Healing, Integrating the Best of Conventional and Complementary Approaches to Cancer,* Michael Lerner, MIT Press, 1994
- *Cancer Therapy: The Independent Consumer's Guide to Non-Toxic Treatment,* Ralph Moss, Equinox, 1993
- *Options: Alternative Cancer Therapies,* Richard Walters, Avery, 1993
- *BCA Newsletter* and books by mail—Breast Cancer Action, 1280 Columbus Ave, #204, San Francisco, CA 94133; 415-992-8279.
- *Options: Revolutionary Ideas in the War on Cancer* and books by mail—People Against Cancer, PO Box 10, Otho, Iowa 50569; 1-800-662-2623
- *Equinox Newsletter,* books by mail—Ralph Moss, 1-800-929-9355

### Help with Herbs
- Alternative Association of Naturopathic Physicians: 206-323-7610
- American Herb Association, PO Box 1673, Nevada City, CA 95959
- Bastyr Naturopathic College: 206-523-9585
- Herb Research Foundation: 1-800-748-2617
- Homeopathic Educational Services: 1-800-359-9051
- Southwest College of Naturopathic Medicine: 602-990-7424

### And
- Cancer Control Society, 2043 N. Berendo St, Los Angeles, CA 90027; (213) 663-7801: Can connect you with women who've treated their breast cancer alternatively; also, offers a directory of non-toxic therapies and by-mail diagnostic tests.
- **Bach Flower Remedies** distributed by Joel Packman, 111 W. Mt. Airy Ave., Philadelphia, PA 19119; 215-242-3706

## Carnivora
• Helmut Keller, The Chronic Disease Center, Am Reuthlein 2, D-8675, Bad Steben, Germany; 011-49-9288-5166; fax at 011-49-9288-7815

## Mistletoe
• Physicians Association for Anthroposophical Medicine, (P.A.A.M.) PO Box 66609, Portland, OR 97290
• Lukas Klinik, CH-4144 Arlesheim, Switzerland; 011-41-61-701- 3333
• *Clinical Studies on Mistletoe Therapy*, Helmut Kiene, available from 241 Hungry Hollow Rd., Spring Valley, NY 10097

## 714X
• C.O.S.E. Inc., 5270 Mills, Rock Forest, Quebec J1N 3B6, Canada; 819-564-7883; fax at 819-564-4668
• Genesis West-Provida, PO Box 3460, Chula Vista, CA 91902; 619-424-9552
• Dr. Dietmar Schildwaechter, PO Box 16602, Dulles International Airport, Washington, DC 20041; 703-430-7789

## Videos
• *Cancer Doesn't Scare Me Anymore!* Lorraine Day, M.D., 2 hours, $19.95 from Rockford Press, PO Box 852, Rancho Mirage, CA 92270; 1-800-574-2437
• *Hoxsey: When Healing Becomes a Crime*, $19.95 from People Against Cancer, PO Box 10, Otho, IA 50560; 515-972-4444
• *Self Healing*, Norman Cousins; *Vitamin C*, Linus Pauling; and *What Your Dr. Won't Tell You About Cancer* from Malibu Video, 6955 Fernhill Dr., Suite 14, Malibu, CA 90265; 310-457-0833

## Vision Quests
• Circles of Air, Circles of Stone, Sparroe Hart, PO Box 48, Putney, VT 05346
• Earthrites, Leav Bolender, 1550 S. Pearl St., Suite 203, Denver, CO 80210; 303-733-7465

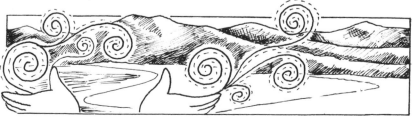

## Books to Read When the Diagnosis is Cancer

- *Breast Cancer: What You Should Know (But May Not Be Told) About Prevention, Diagnosis, and Treatment,* Steve Austin and Cathy Hitchcock, Prima, 1994
- *Dr. Susan Love's Breast Book,* S. Love, M.D., Addison-Wesley, 1990
- *Everyone's Guide to Cancer Therapy,* M. Dollinger, M.D., E. Rosenbaum, M.D., and G. Cable, Somerville House, 1991
- *The Journey Beyond Breast Cancer, Taking an Active Role in Your Own Healing,* Virginia Soffa, Healing Arts, 1994
- *Love, Medicine, & Miracles,* Bernie Siegel, M.D., Harper, 1986
- *Patient No More,* Sharon Batt, Gynergy, 1994
- *Spontaneous Healing,* Andrew Weil, M.D., Knopf, 1995
- *Women's Cancers, How to Beat Them,* Kerry McGinn, R.N., and Pamela Hay, R.N., Hunter House, 1993

## Women Share Their Stories of Breast Cancer

- *Breast Cancer Journal,* Juliet Whittman, Fulcrum, 1993
- *Breast Cancer in the Life Course: Women's Experiences,* Julianne Oktay and Carolyn Walter, Springer, 1991
- *Cancer as a Woman's Issue,* Midge Stocker, Third Side, 1991
- *Cancer Journals,* Audre Lorde, Aunt Lute Press, 1983
- *Examining Myself,* Musa Mayer, Faber & Faber, 1993
- *First You Cry,* Betty Rollin, New American Library, 1976
- *Grace and Grit,* Ken Wilber, Shambhala, 1991
- *Journey Through Illness,* Brenda Lukeman, Steppingstones, 1994
- *Love, Judy: Letters of Hope and Healing for Women with Breast Cancer,* Judy Hart, Conari, 1993
- *Minnie: Rest in Peace, Mom,* Nancy Ford-Kohne, Trimtab, 1986
- *My Breast,* Joyce Wadler, Addison Wesley, 1992
- *No Less A Woman: Ten Women Shatter the Myths About Breast Cancer,* Deborah Kahane, Prentice Hall, 1990
- *Refuge,* Terry Tempest Williams, Vintage, 1991
- *Stories of Hope and Healing,* Leslie Strong, M.D., Equinox, 1994
- "Surviving Breast Cancer, Seven Extraordinary Women Talk About Going On," *McCalls,* October 1993

# She Who Holds the Knife

"I have heard that a wild animal caught in a trap will chew off its leg to gain freedom. Is cancer a kind of a trap? Will you chew off your leg – no, your breast, to be free of this trap? Many women have, many still do, and many more will. There's something so definite, so final, so absolute about cutting off the part that has cancer and throwing it away. There's something so primitive and powerful about choosing the knife.

"Is it a sacrifice? A breast for a life? Are you caught in a steel-jawed trap? Will you free yourself of cancer by removing the offending breast(s)? It seems so simple, so obvious, so necessary.

"But you are not a wild animal, GrandDaughter. You have thumbs: You can release the trap. You have the ability to reason: You can open the trap. You can collect information from others who've lived through their ensnarement; you can learn ways to free yourself.

"Let me explain. Cancer is not the trap your stories make it out to be. Oh, no. There is a trap here, and you may be caught in it, but the trap is not cancer, precious GrandDaughter, the trap is your fear. Do you feel its teeth? The vise-like grip it has on you? The way your primal survival urge thrashes about, not caring what is hurt so long as you live on? This desperation, this frantic desire to survive, this adrenaline-driven panic, this is the trap.

"And though it may seem that this trap is of your own making, your own choosing, I tell you clearly, this is not true. Cancer exists; it has a life of its own. Fear exists; it, too, has a life of its own. They are unwanted house guests, family you can't say 'no' to, come to help you celebrate.

"You did not create the trap. You are not out to trap yourself. These things exist, and so do you, and now your paths have crossed.

"At the crossroads you meet. Will you let yourself be led by fear? Will you follow the path that seems to lead away from death only because it leads away, without ever looking where you are going? Some feelings are wise, GrandDaughter, but fear is not one of them. Fear is not careful; fear is not observant. Do you begin to understand how easy it is to blunder into the trap set by fear?

"Easy to fall into the trap. Easier still to be pushed into it. Not only will your own fear beckon to you, urging you away from your truth, but the fears of those around you will do so, too. And with very persuasive voices. Your family and friends don't want to lose you. They don't want you to die. They don't want you to change radically. They are afraid of cancer. They may insist you do things you'd rather not.

"And you may be pushed by the fear of your doctors, who fear the worst and have learned only one song: 'There is but one way and it is our way, and if you don't do it our way, you'll die.' But cancer urges you to choose life, your life, your way, not theirs, no matter how well-meaning their admonitions and their fears.

"There will be many times in your dance with cancer when you feel buffeted by the storms of emotion within and without you. We offer you a quiet space, a place where you can love even that which you choose to cut away. We love you, GrandDaughter. And we offer you this wisdom:

"It is not enough to cut off your breast; you must also nourish your wholeness. It is not enough to give up your breast; you must also give up the patterns that manifested as cancer. It is not enough to offer your breast as an appeasement to fear; you must also open yourself to realms greater than fear.

"The task we set before you is arduous and difficult. You must hone yourself. You must make of yourself the cutting edge, the sharp scissors, the steel razor. With your own hand you must grasp the knife and say, 'I cut this out.' You must honor your ability to give death, just as you honor your ability to give life. You must dare to cut cleanly and deep, to pare away all that is not you, not your truth, not your beauty, not your path."

# 9.
# Choosing Breast Surgery?

Will you choose breast surgery? How much breast tissue will you have removed? Who will do the surgery? The stitching? What kind of anesthesia will be used? Will you choose reconstruction? When—now or later? What are the after-effects of surgery? Can they be mitigated? How can you help yourself heal? Are there alternatives to surgery? Wise Woman ways can help no matter what choices you make.

### Is surgery the only way to remove breast cancer?

The earliest record of breast amputation dates to the first century (by the Greek physician, Leonides). But until the twentieth century, surgery as a cancer treatment was rare: Surgery was as life-threatening as the cancer.

What was used instead were a variety of caustic herbs and minerals. These treatments may still be safer than surgery. "Cutting into cancer spreads it and makes it grow," says Dr. George Crile, Jr., emeritus surgeon of the Cleveland Clinic. "Sometimes when you remove an original cancer, the secondary cancers grow faster," says Judah Dolkman, M.D., professor of surgery at Harvard Medical School. Overuse of surgery in the treatment of breast cancer has been a documented problem for over 60 years.[1] Although most orthodox doctors urge immediate surgery after a diagnosis of cancer (or if there are very suspicious mammographic findings), the majority of women can safely wait two weeks or more before scheduling their surgery.[2] (For more information on burning away cancer, *see* page 188.)

### How much breast tissue should I have removed?

Until the mid-'60s, all breast cancer surgery removed the entire breast—nipple and skin included. Since then, breast-sparing surgery has gained in respectability and popularity. This is why:

Mastectomy confers no advantage over wide excision lumpectomy and radiation in the treatment of women with early stage breast cancer, according to the National Breast Cancer Clinical Trial. The treatment option is "entirely up to the woman as the studies consistently show that each has exactly the same survival rate."[3] This holds true for tumors up to 4 cm.

Women who choose a mastectomy live no longer than women who choose wide excision lumpectomy, with or without radiation, according to the National Cancer Institute's National Surgical Adjuvant Breast Project. Ten-year survival rates were the same (70 percent) in all three groups. Recurrence in those who used radiation was 10 percent; in those who did not, 40 percent. Recurrences are generally treated with mastectomy (though some surgeons will do a second wide excision). Simple recurrence is not inherently life threatening.

Neither complete nor radical mastectomy conferred an advantage over partial mastectomy—with or without adjuvant radiation—in a group of 1,843 women with breast cancer. Longevity, freedom from recurrence, and freedom from metastases were equal in all groups.

Women who choose breast-sparing surgery are no more anxious about recurrences than women who choose mastectomy, according to a recent study. Some women choose a mastectomy because they are afraid of radiation treatments, but you can have breast-sparing surgery without choosing radiation, if you wish. You can choose the specific treatments you want, no matter what's recommended. (You may have to change doctors.)

*"Whether you irradiate or don't irradiate, whether you lumpectomize or take the breast off, there is no difference for survival."*
National Surgical Adjuvant Breast Project

### How many lymph nodes do I want removed?
Lymphedema affects nearly all women whose lymph nodes are removed—no matter how few are taken. The swelling may be mild (rings and sleeves feel tight) and self-limiting (resolving within six months), but about half of all women who choose mastectomy plus radiation—and a third of those who choose lumpectomy with deep excision of lymph glands plus radiation—have more severe problems: painful swelling of the arm, hardening and discoloration of the skin, and muscular weakness—for the rest of their lives.

One way to prevent lymphedema is to refuse adjuvant radiation. Another is to refuse to have your lymph nodes removed. Because breast cancer staging usually relies on microscopic examination of lymph tissue, you will have to fight to keep your lymph glands. But it is a fight you can win, easily, if you find a doctor or a hospital willing to pay heed to the recommendation that lymph nodes be left alone if the diagnosis is intraductal carcinoma (5 cm or less) or ductal carcinoma *in situ*.[4] Or to the fact that tumor size, grading, and overexpression of the c-erbB-2 oncogene and of lamine receptors is a more accurate way to stage breast cancer than examination of lymph nodes.[5] And it's worth the fight.

### Who will do the surgery?

You deserve the best. You deserve someone with whom you feel confident and comfortable. If the most highly recommended surgeon seems cold and uncaring to you, or if you leave the oncologist's office feeling upset, keep looking. Hospitals and helping agencies (*see* page 313) have lists of surgeons who are cancer specialists. Be sure the M.D.s you choose are board certified.

Once you find the right surgeon, you aren't done yet. Unless you specifically state, in writing, and have it signed, that all of your surgery will actually be done by him/her, you may be operated on by your surgeon's associates, assistants, or students.

And don't neglect the closure of your wound; sewing is a different skill than cutting. For a minimal scar, hire two surgeons: one to cut, and one (usually a plastic surgeon), to sew.

For a detailed, well-illustrated look at lumpectomy and radical mastectomy, consult *The Surgery Book*.[6]

### When should I have surgery?

Retrospective studies trying to gauge the impact of breast cancer surgery done at different times of the menstrual cycle give support to the idea that women should avoid surgery just before and during the week of their menses (bleeding). In one sample of 40 women, 71 percent of those who had surgery between the 7th and 20th days of their menstrual cycle were alive after ten years, compared to 27 percent of the women operated on at other times. In another, of 249 women, 84 percent of those on days 13–28 of their cycle were alive after ten years, compared to 54 percent of those whose surgery was on days 3–12 of their cycle.

### Do I really want reconstruction?

You may be pressured to make a decision about breast reconstruction at the same time as your initial surgery. In general, I found that women who resisted this were happier with their subsequent choices, whether they ultimately decided for reconstruction or not. Immediate reconstruction may have long-term health consequences and may prevent the grieving process needed when one loses (or gives away) a breast.

Reconstruction surgery is not safe. Some women survive cancer only to die from reconstruction. Reconstructive surgery often requires numerous surgeries, each one longer and more difficult (for you and the surgeon) than a complete mastectomy. For a matching reconstruction, your other breast must be cut and shaped as well. If you want nipples, that means more surgery. Healing from reconstructive surgery can be painful and lengthy. Unexpected follow-up surgery may be needed to deal with painful scars, to remove leaking saline bags, to loosen encapsulated silicone bags, or to make the breasts match better.

If you choose reconstruction, note that silicone implants (and saline implants in silicone bags) are implicated as a cause of immune system dysfunction, and, as such, may not be appropriate for women dancing with cancer.

You may be surprised to find you like yourself one-breasted or flat-chested, although, admittedly, it takes some getting used to, and you may have little or no support for your decision.[7, 8] But you aren't restricted to choosing between reconstruction and *au naturel*; there are breast forms. Not one woman that I've met wears her commercially made one more than a few times a year. Some felt they increased lymphedema, others found them cumbersome and uncomfortable. Audre Lorde recommended a puff of lamb's wool: soft, sexy, and natural. Some women swear by nylons stuffed in their bras. Most dress so no one can tell.

Women who lose a breast are Amazons. "A" means "without" while "mazon" refers to mammary, that is, breast, so Amazon means "without breast." Lore surrounding historical Amazons tells us they removed a breast to increase their archery skill. Can breast surgery give your life better aim?

### Should I have a prophylactic mastectomy?

Probably not. Removal of one or both breasts to prevent primary (or secondary) cancers has yet to prove itself superior to rigorous clinical surveillance with high-quality tests.[9, 10] Numerous studies show that this procedure is often recommended or chosen because of the woman's anxiety or the physician's fear of lawsuits, not because it is effective.[11]

# Breast Surgery Problems

Whether for a primary tumor, a recurrence, or a reconstruction, breast surgery can cause side effects ranging from the **after-effects of anesthesia** (nausea, sore throat, headache, impaired concentration, memory loss, and fatigue) to **scars, infection, pain, lymphedema,** and–for some women–**depression**. These Wise Woman ways can help you prevent and alleviate most of the problems associated with breast surgery.

## Before Surgery

★ With preparation, your entire hospital stay can aid your overall healing. What material support will you want before, during, and after surgery? Music and meditation tapes? Homeopathic *Arnica*? Nourishing food? Infused herbal oils? An herbal pain-killer and an herbal anti-infective? Zinc? **Gather your healing resources**.

• General anesthesia is easier to induce and maintain (and thus less dangerous) if you **stop smoking tobacco** for at least two weeks prior to surgery. (And you'll heal more quickly if you don't start smoking again after the surgery.)

★ **Choose your anesthesiologist** as carefully as you choose your surgeon. You life will literally be in their hands. (For more information on anesthesia, *see* page 125.)

• If you're having a mass removed, **decide beforehand which tests you want done on the tissues**. (*See* page 135.)

• **Donate your own blood** as far before surgery as you can. This ensures you of matching (and disease-free, in so far as you are) blood in the event you need a transfusion.

• **Increasing the iron level of your blood** prior to surgery slows blood loss during, and protects from fatigue and infection after, surgery. My favorite iron tonics: two or more cups of nettle infusion daily or 10–25 drops of yellow dock root tincture daily.

• Avoid supplements of vitamin E and C for several weeks before and after your operation; they increase your risk of blood loss during surgery. But **supplemental zinc**, taken with food for a few weeks after surgery, can help speed healing.

• **Essiac** (*see* pages 276 and 301) is said to check metastases. Nurse Caisse, creator of the formula, used 2 ounces/60 ml daily for a week before surgery and three months afterwards.

★ Create **an environment that nourishes you**–no matter where you are. Words of advice from women who've been there:

"*Being in the hospital is so dehumanizing. I refuse to wear their gowns and robes; I bring my own.*"

"*What I want when I'm in the hospital is for someone to bring me home-cooked food, real food, whole grains and greens, yogurt smoothies, food made with love, made with care for me.*"

"*I was eternally thankful that someone suggested that I take a small tape player and headphones and my favorite music to the hospital with me. The healing sounds I filled myself with made all the difference in my recovery, I'm sure.*"

"*I bring my own blankets and pillows.*"

"*I don't take anything with me, because I don't stay in the hospital. I have all my pre-op tests done on an outpatient basis the day before. I arrange for someone to drive me to the hospital and to come get me after the operation. Most hospitals will let you go (sometimes with grumbling) as soon as three hours after the operation, or as soon as you're ready to leave the recovery room.*"

"*I took photographs of all my friends and covered the hospital wall by my bed with them.*"

"*I listened to a chanting tape during my surgery. Afterwards I used meditation tapes to deal with the pain.*"

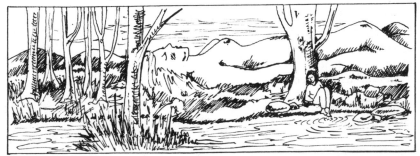

## After-Effects of Anesthesia

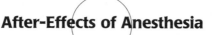

• Wise Woman ways can help prevent and relieve the common after effects of general anesthesia: sore throat, nausea, headache, constipation, memory loss, and impaired judgment. (For help with fatigue, another common side effect, *see* pages 218 and 239.)

• Until your intestines recover from the relaxing effects of anesthesia, you will be limited to a few ounces of water a day. Homeopathic remedies, which can be dissolved in the mouth without water, are especially useful says Carolyn Dean, M.D., author of *Complementary Natural Prescriptions for Common Ailments*.
 To help clear the effects of anesthesia–*Phosphorus* 6x
 To lessen pain, shock, and swelling–*Arnica* 30x
 To speed recovery from surgery–*Veratrum album* 6x

• A teaspoon of **olive oil** twice a day or several **slippery elm** tablets a day re-establishes bowel function smoothly and quickly.

★ **After-Surgery Lozenges** combine the healing powers of slippery elm with **ginger** for warmth after the chill of the operating room, a boost to intestinal movement, and quick relief from nausea (the most frequent side effect of general anesthesia) and sore throat (from intubation). Recommended by several doctors, these lozenges are easily made at home and may safely be dissolved in the mouth—even when the order is "nothing p.o." or "nothing by mouth." (The recipe is on page 301.)

• Another way to stop vomiting and nausea is to pinch (hard!) the **anti-nausea point** in the muscles between your thumb and first finger. Try several places until you find a tender spot: That's it.

• To relieve **headaches**, I usually use 5–15 drops of **skullcap** tincture. After surgery, however, the headache may be from an overburdened liver processing the various drugs you've been given. In that case, I'd use 10–20 drops of liver-supportive **dandelion** root or **milk thistle** seed tincture in a tiny spoon of water, repeated as needed.

• General anesthesia can fog your brain, leaving you with impaired judgment for 3–7 days afterwards and no memory of visitors, instructions, or anything else that happened. This can happen even if you feel fine. Take it easy. Avoid decisions, driving, and other demanding tasks for at least a week. And try memory-enhancing **ginkgo** tincture, 25 drops several times a day.

• **Local anesthesia** can collapse small blood vessels. As it wears off, they can hemorrhage, causing swelling and discoloration. To prevent or treat this problem, wet a washcloth with drugstore witch hazel and lay it on the incision. For a stronger effect, soak the cloth in an infusion of **witch hazel** (*Hamamelis virginiana*) or **oak** bark.

## Healing Wounds and Bruises Minimizing Scars

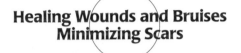

**Step 1.** *Collect Information*

★ The extent of your scar is determined largely by how the incision is closed. Staples make big scars. Little subcutaneous stitches make nearly invisible scars. **For minimal scars after breast surgery, hire a plastic surgeon to close the wound.**

• It generally takes 2–3 weeks for incisions to heal and bruising to dissipate, but 2–5 years for the scar to fully mature and fade. Regular use of **infused herbal oils** (e.g., calendula, comfrey, St. Joan's wort—*see* pages 61-67) can minimize scarring and discoloration.

**Step 2.** *Engage the Energy*

• **Ceremony** helps us mark important changes in our lives, such as breast surgery. It can be as simple as lighting a candle or as complex as a theater piece witnessed by many people. Let your imagination loose. Create a special time and space to honor your loss.

• **Homeopathic remedies** can help heal wounds and bruises.
      To prevent and heal bruises and speed healing—*Arnica.*
      For deep wounds to the muscles—*Bellis perennis.*
      The remedy of choice if the area around the incision is cold or numb—*Ledum.*

• Subtle physical manipulations (e.g., Alexander, Feldenkreis, and Rosen techniques) and energy work (e.g., Muriel or Reiki sessions) are important allies in reconnecting body-mind after the disruption of surgery.

**Step 3.** *Nourish and Tonify*

• Healthy skin scars less and heals more rapidly. Good nutrition, with special emphasis on **winter squash, sunflower seeds, seaweed, olive oil**, and **leafy greens**, creates healthy skin.

★ External applications of **calendula** blossoms, both as a tincture and as an oil or ointment, offer a superb wound dressing that is highly antiseptic and counters scar formation. I use the tincture frequently until the wound is sealed, then the oil once or twice a day for the next month. Women who tend toward **keloid scars** claim that calendula is especially effective for them, decreasing the size and hardness of the scar when healed.

★ **Comfrey leaf** is a superb ally for wound healing. Comfrey's reparative powers go deep into muscles, tendons, ligaments, and skin. It has an almost magical ability to speed healing, prevent and dissolve hematomas, and reduce scarring. Comfrey poultices produce the most dramatic healing, but ointment works well too.

• **Yoga** and **tai chi** are extremely beneficial after surgery. They restore tone to cut muscles, flexibility to stressed connective tissue, and a means of learning how to move in your altered body.

**Step 4.** *Stimulate/Sedate*

★ Some women have intense **itching** in the incision or where skin is stretched by reconstruction. **Plantain** ointment not only calms the itch, it also promotes rapid healing and reduces scarring.

• Those who smoke commercial tobacco heal more slowly and have more (and more severe) complications after breast surgery.

**Step 5a.** *Use Supplements*

★ **Zinc** is essential for wound repair, being a co-factor for more than 200 enzymes used in cell division, protein synthesis, and DNA replication. Major surgery decreases blood levels of zinc by up to 60 percent for eight days or more. A supplemental dose of 100 mg daily, with a meal, is considered safe, but high doses of zinc may suppress the immune system. Zinc-rich foods include pumpkin seeds, dulse, and nettle infusion.

★ **Carotenes** are critically important for wound healing. Food sources include carrots, kelp, dandelion greens, and violet or nettle leaf infusion. A supplemental dose is 10,000 to 100,000 IU daily for 3–4 weeks.

• **Avoid** supplements of vitamins E and C before surgery; they thin the blood and increase risk of hemorrhage and hematomas. But they can be taken beginning a week after the operation to help hasten healing. Usual daily dose is 1–6 grams ascorbic acid and 200–400 IU vitamin E, or six servings of fresh, raw fruit or vegetables and half a cup/125 ml of sunflower seeds.

• **Papaya enzymes** (5 tablets 3 times a day, or half a fruit daily) minimize scar tissue when taken for several weeks after surgery.

## Infections

• The risk of infection increases when the lymph nodes are removed or if  reconstruction is combined with mastectomy.

★ Hospital-bred infections are often antibiotic-resistant. I avoid them with the help of **echinacea, usnea,** or **St. Joan's wort** tinctures. For complication-free healing, I'd use a protective dose of 25–50 drops of any one daily for up to a month (or even a few days) before surgery. To keep immunity strong, I'd take the same dose, 2–3 times a day, while in the hospital. If there were active infection, I'd take more, plus 1–4 drops of poke tincture.

★ **Fever** is the body's normal mechanism for dealing with infective organisms. (Neither bacteria nor viruses can reproduce at temperatures over 100° F.) It is reasonable—and possibly even very healthy—to run a slight fever after surgery.

• The blood loss that inevitably occurs during surgery contributes to lack of resistance to infection. Transfusions add further stress to the immune system. **Nettle** infusion, several cups a day, or **yellow dock** tincture, 10–25 drops daily, builds blood quickly.

## Pain, Numbness, and Discomfort

### Step 0. *Do Nothing*

• Stop resisting the pain. Sink into it. Feel it. Accept it as part of you. It's amazing how well this soft approach diminishes pain.

### Step 1. *Collect Information*

• Breast surgery is not too painful, as surgeries go, though healing from a radical mastectomy can be. Whether you've chosen to have part or all of your breast removed, the tissues will be traumatized and your nerves will definitely tell you about it. For some women the pain is moderate and behind them in a matter of several weeks; other women feel pain for months; a few (mostly after mastectomy) are left with painful tightening across the chest which lasts for years.

• **Numbness** in the underarm tissue is a common side effect when deep layers of lymph glands are removed, since nerves must be cut to harvest the glands. (If done with care, removal of one layer of lymph nodes shouldn't result in numbness.)

### Step 2. *Engage the Energy*

★ Homeopathic *Arnica* is a powerful ally for preventing pain after surgery. Homeopathic *Hypericum* is specific for easing nerve pain. Use lavishly both before and after surgery.

### Step 3. *Nourish and Tonify*

• Nerve-nourishing **oatstraw** infusion is a wonderful addition to the daily routine of those dealing with chronic pain. Oats and oatstraw increase the insulating sheaths of the nerves, diminishing pain.

★ **St. Joan's wort tincture** is one of the best allies a women can have after breast surgery: It relieves pain, eases muscle cramps, counters depression, nourishes the immune system, shrinks enlarged lymph glands, and prevents viral and bacterial infections. (It may help prevent recurrences, too.) A dose of 25–50 drops taken up to 10 times a day is a specific remedy for injuries (including surgery) where the pain is throbbing, deep, aching or burning. It also heals and eases nerves that are severed or jangled.

★ After surgery you may be extremely sensitive to movement or touch. (Some women find anything tight around the chest unbearable.) What green ally can heal nerve endings, reduce hypersensitivity, bring ease to the armpit and upper chest, and help prevent lymphedema? St. Joan's wort again, but this time as **St. Joan's wort oil/ointment**. Frequent applications to the entire arm, shoulder, armpit, and chest area are especially useful for easing "pins and needles," phantom pain, and other darting, prickly sensations.

• Women who've had a breast removed often sit hunched over in a protective, shielded way so characteristic of this surgery that medical literature mentions it. Gentle **yoga** or **tai chi** stretches at least once a week help you remember to stand with your shoulders back. (And St. Joan's wort used internally will keep your muscles cramp-free so you can stand tall without pain.)

**Step 4.**   *Stimulate/Sedate*

• When I hurt, I reach for **skullcap** (*Scutellaria lateriflora*) tincture. For minor pain: 4–10 drops. For pain that keeps me from falling asleep: 10–25 drops. For severe pain: 25–50 drops. I repeat the dose, small or large, every 15 minutes until the pain lifts.

★ **Hops** (*Humulus lupulus*) and **valerian** (*Valeriana officinalis*) are favorite nutritive painkillers. Sleep-inducing hops tea mellows jangled nerves and relieves general angst from low-level persistent pain. Valerian tincture, 20 drops diluted in water, eases pain from intense muscle spasms, and overwhelming physical/emotional distress, as well.

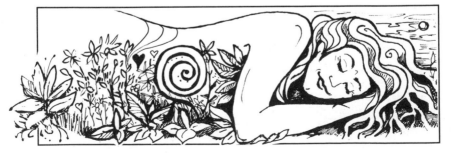

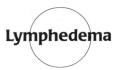

# Lymphedema

**Step 0.** *Do Nothing*

• Lymphedema is one problem that you need to **act swiftly** to counter. After lymph node surgery, the lymph drainage remains unstable, leaving you susceptible to lymphedema indefinitely. Preventive measures (see steps 2 and 3) need to be initiated immediately after surgery and continued for the rest of your life.

**Step 1.** *Collect Information*

• Mild, short-term lymphedema affects virtually every woman whose lymph nodes have been disturbed. Lymph node removal damages the lymphatic drainage, so body fluids flowing into the arm can become trapped, causing swelling so extreme that it can limit movement. In addition, the trapped fluids are loaded with proteins—nourishment for infection-causing bacteria—making severe infection an ever-present risk.

• Symptoms of lymphedema include swelling, heaviness, hypersensitivity of the skin, loss of feeling in the affected limb, redness, weeping rashes, itchiness, and pain, ranging from dull to throbbing.

★ **Don't ignore** the slightest suggestion of **swelling, redness, hardness,** or **warmth** in your arm. Tissues that become engorged with fluid become damaged, making it harder and harder to drain them and to relieve the pain. The sooner you act, the less your chances of severe complications: Only half of those who wait until their arms have swollen two inches improve significantly, while 85 percent of those who start before the arm has swollen one inch improve.[12]

• In the early stage of lymphedema, pressing on the swollen flesh leaves a pit. If lymphedema becomes chronic, the flesh can become more and more firm, and can, without constant tending, harden into lymphostatic elephantiasis. In extreme instances the affected arm becomes so swollen that standing is impossible, and sitting or lying down is quite awkward as well.

• Women with limited mobility, and those who are affected by diabetes, rheumatoid arthritis, chronic phlebitis or gout, are more vulnerable to severe lymphedema. These conditions are sufficient reason to keep your lymph nodes and perhaps to refuse adjuvant radiation as well.

• Lymphedema can be mildly annoying or a constant, lifelong difficulty. It can occur soon after surgery or many years later. It can serve as an awful reminder of what you've lost. Or it can be a warrior's mark that gives you pride in being alive. There is no known cure for lymphedema, but consistent home care can greatly reduce the severity.

• For more information: **National Lymphedema Network**, 2211 Post St., Suite 404, San Francisco, CA 94115; 1-800-541-3259.

**Step 2.** *Engage the Energy*

★ **Elevate**, elevate. Gravity pulls fluids down; use it to your advantage by raising your arm over your head. Set aside specific times every day to elevate your arm. The more you put your arm up, the more you reduce your chances of severe lymphedema. Elevating your arm as soon as you notice swelling does more to counter lymphedema than any remedy used later. When you aren't elevating, keep your arm moving, change your arm's position frequently, and don't let it dangle down or remain motionless in your lap, especially when traveling.

• **Envision** the fluid in your arm flowing while you're elevating it: moisture soaking into the earth which filters it down to deep underground rivers where it is carried away. Flowing, ever flowing.

• **Wear loose-fitting clothing**, and limit or eliminate constricting apparel such as tight rings, heavy bracelets, underwire bras, clothing with tight armholes, and heavy purses.

• **Homeopathic** *Silica* is the remedy used by those with swollen lymph nodes, skin infections, and cold extremities. The symptoms that *Silica* treats often develop slowly and leave one feeling confused, tired, and very vulnerable.

• **Manual Lymph Drainage**, a slow, spiraling, gentle massage that barely touches the skin, is very effective for treating mild lymphedema. Gentle, non-invasive energy work such as Reiki or polarity therapy is also useful in the early stages of lymphedema.

## Step 3. *Nourish and Tonify*

• **Exercises** to loosen your arm and help prevent lymphedema (such as creeping your fingers up the wall) will probably be taught to you in the hospital after your surgery. If not, ask for a Reach to Recovery volunteer to visit you, or take a beginners' **yoga** class within two weeks of surgery.

★ **Massage**, massage to prevent lymphedema. Regular massage encourages strong circulation, making swelling much less likely. Massage of the arm and back can begin a few days after surgery. Include the front of the chest as soon as the incisions seal. Massaging with infused herbal oils (such as calendula or dandelion flower) helps lessen the formation of scar tissue, keeps muscles and fascia unconstricted, and encourages good lymphatic flow.

• **Massage**, massage to deal with lymphedema. An electric, vibrating massager can be used on the affected arm twice a day or more. Or massage with pressure can be used cautiously. The preferred technique is a long slow stroke of the flat palm. The **pattern** to use is quite specific.[13] First massage the chest and front of the shoulder, working up. Then the back of the shoulder, working up. Still working up, massage the front and then the back of the upper arm. Massage the front of the lower arm with upward strokes, then massage the back of the forearm. Finally, massage the hand, from fingers to wrist, palm first, then the back of the hand. Use a gentle but firm pressure. Apply your compression sleeve, if you wear one, immediately after the massage. And elevate your arm for as long as you can afterward.

★ **Moisturize and examine** the skin of your arm daily; it will respond quickly to being lavishly anointed twice a day with healing herbal oils/ointments. **Poke oil** reduces swelling, **comfrey oil** strengthens skin, **St. Joan's wort oil** counters numbness as well as sensitivity, **calendula oil** helps keep infection in check. While anointing yourself, make a good visual check for skin integrity. Apply **plantain, yarrow, or comfrey** oil/ointment to any breaks, abrasions, red areas, weepiness, or rashes.

**Step 4.**  *Stimulate/Sedate*

• A **compression sleeve** is a tight tube of elastic worn on the arm to keep lymph fluids from pooling when the arm isn't elevated. Take time to get one that fits properly; too much pressure will backfire, leaving the fingers painfully swollen. If you anoint your arm with infused herbal oils before you go to sleep, wash it well before redonning your compression sleeve in the morning; residual oil can damage the sleeve.

• Eliminate or **cut back on smoking**, **alcohol**, **coffee**, and **salt** to decrease occurrence of lymphedema and reduce its severity.

• Recommendations for preventing lymphedema-associated infections: **take meticulous care of your arm and hand**, protect them from overuse, and protect the skin from injury, burns, insect bites, scratches, intense sun, and all household chemicals. The more at risk you are, the more important it becomes to: use gloves when gardening (or anytime you might injure your hands), use a thimble when sewing, use an electric razor if you must shave under your arms, avoid carrying heavy objects, avoid intense heat, wear rubber gloves when doing the dishes, and  remember not to receive injections or have blood pressure taken on that arm.[14]

★ Tincture of **cleavers** (5–100 drops a day) or **poke root** (1–8 drops a day) has been used with excellent success to treat and prevent lymphedema. *See* Materia Medica.

• One hundred years ago **Sichert's Lymphatic Ointment** was used to relieve lymphedema. The mixture, made from extracts of hemlock (*Conium maculatum*), foxglove (*Digitalis*), autumn crocus (*Colchicum autumnale*), henbane (*Hyoscyamus niger*), and May apple (*Podophyllum*), was applied morning and night to relieve pain and reduce swelling. (A purified extract of hemlock–coniine–is currently used as a drug to alleviate cancer pain.)

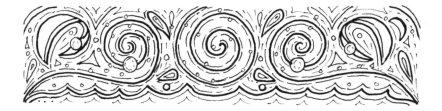

• **Compression pumps** (or sequential gradient pumps) are like having a tireless—but insensitive—massage therapist who can provide hours of rhythmic pressure to force lymph fluids back into circulation. (This can hurt.)

• **Caution: Hot water**, saunas, hot tubs, hot compresses, and sweat lodges can make lymphedema worse, or precipitate it if you are at risk. They are definitely contraindicated in chronic lymphedema where the skin is fragile and easily damaged by heat.

• **Caution: Air travel** seems to aggravate lymphedema.

**Step 5a.** *Use Supplements*

• The nutrients most critical to fluid flow in the lymphatics are **vitamin C, vitamin A**, and **folic acid**.

**Step 5b.** *Use Drugs*

• **Infections** in the arm affected by lymphedema can be sudden and severe. Women at risk often keep antibiotics handy for immediate treatment of any infection. See page 180 for information on anti-infective herbal allies.

• **Steroids** such as cortisone may be suggested if the lymphedema seems to be caused by obstruction to rather than removal of the lymphatics. Long-term use of steroids increases risk of severe osteoporosis and may encourage or promote cancer.

• **Diuretic drugs** may cause complications by mobilizing fluid everywhere but in the affected arm, resulting in dangerous electrolyte disturbances, dehydration, and low blood pressure. Herbal diuretics, like nettle infusion or dandelion root tincture, do not leach minerals from the body. They nourish and help maintain electrolyte balance while encouraging fluid flow.

**Step 6.** *Break & Enter*

• An operation to ease the pressure of lymphedema is risky. The affected arm heals slowly, and the result may be worsening of the lymphedema.

# Instead of Surgery?

Very few women with breast cancer refuse surgery. There are, however, options for those who want to remove a lump without surgery and anesthesia. Carefully prepared salves containing herbs and alkaline minerals—as well as some individual plants such as celandine (*Cheladonium majus*) and stinkhorn mushroom (*Phallus impudicus*)[15]—can selectively destroy malignant cells while hardly affecting normal tissues. These treatments can, however, cause severe pain and leave scars, so proceed with caution. Take the time to read *Cancer Salves and Suppositories* by Dr. Ingrid Naiman, available from the author at 29 Brisa Circle, Sante Fe, NM 87501.

• **Poke root poultices** are the most frequently used herbal application for "burning away" cancer. Literature and folklore confirm many successes. Freshly grated root is applied every 2–3 days, and a poultice is worn continuously throughout the course of treatment, 4–6 weeks. *See* page 299.

• **Tea tree oil,** full strength, topically, is said to be especially effective at eliminating ulcerated cancers.

• **Escharotic Salves** usually combine one or more caustic herbs and a mineral, e.g., zinc chloride, in a fatty base. The salve is applied thickly to a bandage which is then taped over the site of the cancer and left for 24 hours, even if the area becomes hot and painful. These salves are said to dissolve or pull out cancerous masses. They may blister and discolor the skin over the cancer, which, as it dies, will form a series of scabs. These scabs must be kept moist with salve, but allowed to come off naturally. Treatment is complete and salves are discontinued when no more scabs form. A feeling of heaviness at the site of the tumor and a foul odor may accompany the treatment. **Black Ointment**, page 304, is a classic example of an escharotic salve. **Caution:** The area of application must be kept tightly taped.

• Sometimes a soothing second salve, such as **Yellow Salve**, page 302, is alternated with the escharotic salve.

• Some breast cancers are successfully resolved with therapeutic radiation plus very high doses of beta-carotene.

• **It is important to use internal remedies too.**

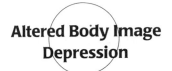

## Altered Body Image
## Depression

One of the after effects of surgery that no words can really prepare you for is the first sight of your altered body. For some women the alteration is so traumatic that they put off looking at themselves for weeks, months, years. For others the urge is to look and keep looking until the reality sinks in. For some women the loss of a breast may bring up feelings of worthlessness and sexual neutering.[15] Whether a part of your breast, a breast, or both breasts are gone, there is loss; there is grief. Even a woman who feels great relief that her cancerous breast is gone will still grieve her loss.

Grief is a difficult emotion. After breast cancer surgery it may be mixed with rage, fear, and relief. It's normal to be angry that you've had to undergo surgery, perhaps had to sacrifice a breast. And, paradoxically, fear of cancer may surge up when the operation is safely over. When our grief lacks expression in color, form, sound, movement, or words, it seethes within us, weighing us down, making life meaningless, making us depressed.

"Curse!" she said, when I asked about her favorite cancer therapy. "Angry women don't get depressed." Depressed women who find a safe space for their anger get better faster. You don't have to scream; talking about your anger helps too.

"Make art!" Let your feelings manifest as drawings, songs, poems, quilts, stories, dances, drumming.

"Make love!" to the chaos of life. Surrender to the charming (and alarming) unpredictability of life's current. Touch life. Touch your feelings. Touch your scar. Allow the emptiness. Welcome the new flesh. Touch the altered you. Be touched. Know that you are, and always were, whole.

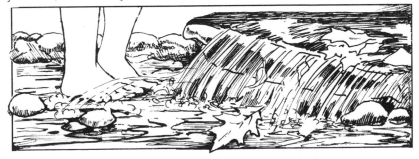

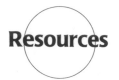

# Resources

• *Recovery in Motion: An Illustrated Guide to Lymphedema for the Breast Cancer Patient,* available from Breast Cancer Physical Therapy Center, 1905 Spruce St., Philadelphia, PA 19103

★ *Women Talk About Breast Surgery,* Amy Gross & Dee Ito, Harper Collins, 1991

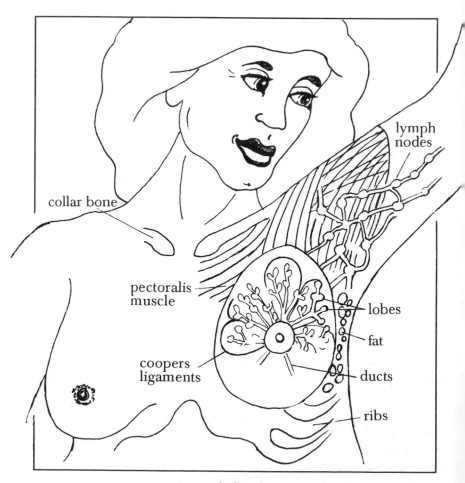

## Anatomy of the breast area

# The Call of the Dance

"The events of the cancer cascade – the initiation in your DNA, the promotion of the wild cells, and your immune system's inability to check their growth – these events may have manifested as a mass in your breast, GrandDaughter, but they have affected the other cells in your breasts as well. That fierce intensity, that hot/cold light, that wildness called cancer has become visible in one place, but may be invisibly present in other sites as well.

"Your attention is focused on your lump, but what if there are cancer cells elsewhere in your breasts? What will you do about them? How do you feel about them?

"Let yourself imagine these cells. Come with us to visit them. Sink with us into your breast, softly, like the faint hum you hear. See the cells that could become local recurrences. They have been initiated and promoted, but they aren't yet growing. They still acknowledge the larger life that contains and sustains them; they still sing in harmony with the whole.

"What happens to these cells when you feed them fear? Experience it now. See how their vibration intensifies. And when you feed them fear of death, see how they hope to please you by trying to fend off death with the unbounded life-force of cancer – killing you in the process. What else can you feed them? What if you feed them love? What if you offer them acceptance? What if you take them to heart? Experience that now.

"Come with us deeper, into the hidden places, to touch any cells that could grow into recurrent cancer. Offer your ears. Offer your compassion. Sit and listen for a while.

"Do not be afraid, GrandDaughter, to discover how very different you have become now that you are dancing with cancer. Hasn't your dance swept you into new steps? Into trying ancient ways of healing: herbs, energy, prayer, massage? Haven't you reached deep inside yourself to call forth healing? Haven't you allowed others to reach into you as well? With a tender touch and a comforting word? With sharp knives? With radioactive rays? With chemicals and drugs? With pointed questions?

"Do you long for your life to return to normal? To heal over without a scar, without a trace of all that has happened? This will not be. Your life must never return to what it was, precious GrandDaughter. For when you long for return, you call out to recurrence. Having survived cancer, you dare not return. If you return yourself to the state you inhabited before your diagnosis of cancer, you may return yourself to a state which calls forth cancer. To return is to deny your changes, and that is the road to recurrence.

"There is no return for a woman who has passed through the initiation of breast cancer. Like menarche, like childbirth, like menopause, once a woman is initiated by breast cancer, she is forever changed, forever set apart, forever different from the way she was before. Just as you are changed beyond return by your first blood, marked permanently by pregnancy, and transformed by the hot flashes of menopause, cancer changes you, marks you, transforms you.

"Cancer brings fear, grief, and anger – and the inner stillness that comes when one accepts these difficult feelings. Cancer demands that you give away parts of yourself, even essential parts – and offers you the opportunity to give up that which constricts you, to cut out that which makes you small, and to abolish all that narrows your view of yourself. Cancer asks you to love yourself, even the ugly parts, even the out-of-control parts.

"There is no return, GrandDaughter, for you are now much, much more than you were before. Though you may have lost a breast, you have gained much. Your vision of yourself is larger; you no longer fit in your old view. No way to go back? Let us go on; let us continue. There are futures to plan."

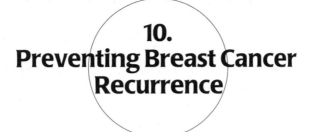

# 10.
# Preventing Breast Cancer Recurrence

Recurrence technically includes both simple local recurrence and metastasized recurrence. But this obscures a critical difference: Simple recurrence of breast cancer is not linked to shorter life span. Metastasized recurrence is.

Since recurrence can occur anytime after treatment, women are urged to use orthodox adjuvant therapies to prevent recurrence, and to have check-ups with invasive, expensive, and time-consuming tests for years afterward. But invasive tests and adjuvant therapies such as hormones (tamoxifen), radiation, and chemotherapy are themselves detrimental to health. And orthodox tests for recurrence are not reliable, nor do they improve longevity.[1, 2]

Preventing recurrence is much like preventing cancer, but with more emphasis on stopping the promotion and growth of cancer cells. A monthly visit with your Wise Healer Within and regular visits with a health care professional of your choice can spot recurrence if it occurs. And these Wise Woman ways can help prevent it.

**Step 0.** *Do Nothing*

• When you feel that your breast cancer treatment is complete, get away for a while. Get away from home; get away from your routine; get away from your responsibilities; get away from all the people who want you to return to "normal."

**Step 1.** *Collect Information*

• What causes local recurrence? There is no consensus. Surgery can spread cancer cells. Surgery may miss some cancer cells. And it is always possible that whatever initiated and promoted the primary cancer also initiated and promoted other cancers (of the

193

same or different type) which didn't grow until the primary mass was removed. (Primary breast cancers can secrete a substance which blocks the promotion and growth of other cancer cells.)

• Age appears to be a better marker for likelihood of recurrence than node status. **The older you are when diagnosed with breast cancer, the less likely you are to have a recurrence**.

• Post-menopausal women who choose wide excision lumpectomy rarely have a recurrence, whether or not they choose radiation.[3]

• Long-term studies of women who survive breast cancer show that adjuvant radiation *increased* their risk of recurrence about 1 percent a year after an initial short-term reduction of recurrence.[3]

• According to award-winning cancer investigator Ralph Moss, nine out of ten women with early stage breast cancer who limit their treatment to surgery will not have a recurrence.[4]

• Recurrence of breast cancer is of three types:
      **Simple recurrence** is a new mass, in the breast tissues or nearby muscle, of the same kind of cells as the original cancer.
      **Secondary recurrence** is a new mass, in any type of body tissue, of a different type of cells than the original cancer. Secondary recurrences can be caused by hormone therapy (liver cancer), radiation therapy (new breast cancers, blood cancers, lung cancers), chemotherapy (blood cancers, bone cancers), or the same processes that caused the original cancer.
      **Metastasized recurrence** is a new mass, anywhere but in breast tissues, of the same kind of cells as the original cancer. Breast cancer metastases occur in the lungs, liver, bones, and occasionally the brain. (Breast cancer cells that lodge in the lymph nodes are not inherently dangerous and are not considered recurrences.) Malignant breast cells spread to other organs and attempt to turn them into breasts! This interferes with vital life processes and can lead to death.

• Women with simple recurrence have excellent statistical life expectancies; their new lumps can be removed, just as their primary tumors were. For those with secondary recurrence, the prognosis and treatment depends on the type of cancer. But women with metastasized recurrence face a situation where no known treatments of any kind are reliable. They now begin a different kind of dance. Is it a dance into miraculous life or a dance into miraculous death? No one can say for sure, just as no one knows how long that dance will be. (*See* Chapter 15.)

• Simple recurrence is most likely to be seen within three years after the primary breast cancer is diagnosed and treated. Metastases can take as long as 8 years to become visible, but may occur at any time. Secondary cancers (including those caused by radiation and chemotherapy) take 10–40 years before they grow to a noticeable size.

• As with primary tumors, most recurrences are found by the woman herself, not by tests. Having an experienced healer check for recurrence on a regular basis is important, but you won't endanger your life if you refuse tests other than mammograms.[4a]

**Step 2.** *Engage the Energy*

• Recurrence is up to four times more likely if surgery is done during or around the time of the woman's menstrual period. Recurrence is twice as likely if the surgery is done during the first half of a woman's cycle rather than the latter half.[5] **Reduce risk of recurrence by having breast surgery done between ovulation and menstruation**. (*See also* page 173.)

• Regular breast massage with infused herbal oils is an excellent way to focus your loving energy on your breasts and avert, as well as be alert to, local recurrence. **Visualization, prayer, affirmation**, and **meditation** are used by M.D.s such as Larry Dossey, Deepak Chopra, Bernie Siegel,[6] and the Simontons to prevent recurrence. Breast cancer survivors Angela Trafford[7] and Linda Dackmen[8] share their stories, and their affirmations in their books.

• Read *Pathwork of Self Transformation*[9] or *Meeting the Shadow*[10] to help yourself explore and **reclaim your shadow**—the wild, lost, ignored, denied, feared, and loathed aspects of yourself. Many healers (and the Ancient GrandMothers) believe that cancer is a desperate attempt on the part of that inner wild child to get your attention and love. The Pathwork is profound psychological soul work, but any process that takes you deep within yourself will do.

*"If you barely recognize yourself after a year or two, the work you're doing is deep enough."*          Clove, tumor survivor, age 35

**Step 3.** *Nourish and Tonify*

★ Foods that help prevent cancer help prevent recurrence too. Some of the best are **apples**, **burdock**, **carrots**, **dark leafy greens**, **dried beans**, **garlic**, **kelp**, **soy products**, **sweet potatoes**, and **wild mushrooms**. When eaten regularly, these foods have been shown to check the growth of microscopic cancers in the breasts, repair damaged DNA, and return cancerous cells to normal.

• Sticky substances in apples (pectin), burdock (mucilage), and kelp (algin) trap chemicals, radioactivity, and other cancer-promoting substances, and remove them from the body. Eat one or more daily.

★ The legume family offers powerful allies for women who want to prevent recurrence: **Dried beans**, **lentils**, **tofu**, and the notable anticancer herbs: **red clover**, **astragalus**, and **alfalfa.** (In China, astragalus is the herb used most often to prevent recurrence.) In one study, eating beans five or more times a week was found to be as effective as chemotherapy in preventing recurrences.

★ Orange and green pigments in food are **carotenes**, anti-recurrence champs. Per 100 grams (3.5 ounces): **dandelion greens** supply 60,000 IU; **stinging nettles,** 15,000 IU; cooked **carrots,** 8,000 IU; raw carrots, 5,000 IU; and **sweet potatoes,** 6,000 IU.

• **Echinacea** root tincture is said to have an inhibiting effect on recurrence if taken in small doses (3–5 drops daily) for long periods of time (3–6 months).

• Eliminating saturated and polyunsaturated fat from the diet, and reducing total fat intake sharply reduces risk of recurrence. For every 1 percent increase in fat consumed above daily needs, the risk of recurrence rises 10 percent, say researchers at the National Cancer Institute.

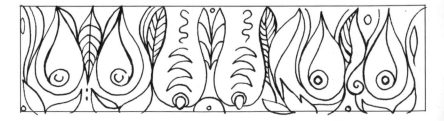

**Step 4.** *Stimulate/Sedate*

★ **Turmeric** (*Curcumae longa*), the root that gives curry its yellow color, is extremely effective at inhibiting recurrence in laboratory animals. Turmeric shows greater antioxidant abilities than vitamin C, vitamin E, or beta carotene. It is also strongly liver-protective and antimutagenic, making it a wonderful ally for women who choose chemotherapy or tamoxifen. Best way to use it? As a seasoning in food. Make your own anti-recurrence curry powder: Mix together freshly ground dried tumeric, cardamom, cloves, cumin, coriander, celery seed, and cinnamon. Use liberally to season rice, vegetables, and soups.

★ **Prevent weight gain** to prevent recurrence. Women more than 25 percent over their ideal weight have a 30 percent higher risk of recurrence according to the *Medical Tribune*, October, 1992. Copious amounts of fresh **chickweed** (or 75–100 drops of the tincture daily) can stimulate metabolism and lower weight.

• Essential oil of **lavender** contains several components that prevent the formation of tumors and may help prevent recurrences. Essential oils are concentrated and may cause side effects, so I use them externally only and go slowly, gradually adding larger amounts (starting with 4–5 drops) to an ounce of infused herbal oil and anointing the breasts at least once a day.

**Step 5a.** *Use Supplements*

• Supplemental antioxidants in large, and potentially harmful, daily doses—such as 100,000 units **beta-carotene**, 350 mg **coenzyme Q₁₀**, 100 mcg **selenium** (sodium selenite), 200 mg **germanium**, 100,000 units **vitamin A**, 1,000 units **vitamin E** (increased slowly from 400 units a day), and 10,000 mg **vitamin C** (in several doses)—are used by some women to prevent recurrence of breast cancer.[11] **At these dosages, supplements can impair health**. (See especially germanium caution, page 155.) Before deciding you need supplements, be sure you are eating a healthy diet of whole grains, beans, vegetables, fruits, and only organic oils and animal products. Supplements can prevent deficiency diseases, but they don't make up for a poor diet, and may stress those dancing with cancer more than they help. Whole foods nourish the complexity and wildness of your entire being, supplements don't.

**Step 5b.** *Use Drugs*

• **Tamoxifen** is the adjuvant hormone most widely prescribed for preventing breast cancer recurrence. *See* Chapter 11.

• **Chemotherapy** immediately after surgery is an aggressive way to try to prevent recurrences. *See* Chapter 13.

• According to the February1982 *New England Journal of Medicine,* women taking a full dose of **digitalis** for heart conditions are unlikely to have recurrence of breast cancer.

• Chemotherapy may be used less if there is success with the clinical trial (begun in 1994) of a **vaccine** made from breast cancer tumor antigens (covering 40–60 percent of breast cancers). It is hoped that the vaccine will provide a great degree of protection from recurrence with little side effect.

**Step 6.** *Break & Enter*

• **Say "no" to bone scans.** C-T scans (used to monitor possible metastatic recurrence to the bones) have a false positive rate of 90 percent, making them more likely to harm you (with high doses of radiation and by ringing false alarms) than help you.

• **Say "no" to surgical removal of noncancerous breast tissue.** Removing your breasts may seems like a logical way to prevent recurrence, but experience shows logic the liar. One-fifth of the women who choose complete removal of both breasts still have a recurrence. A woman who chooses to have all her breast tissue cut off offers only hard-to-remove tissues (such as the chest muscle or skin) as sites for recurrences, while a lumpectomy leaves easy-to-remove breast tissues as sites for recurrence.[12] Furthermore, local recurrence within the breast is more responsive to treatment than recurrence in the skin after mastectomy.[13]

• **Say "no" to adjuvant radiation.** The March 1992 issue of *The New England Journal of Medicine* reported that the risk of recurrence significantly increased among women under 45 who chose adjuvant radiation.

# Hormonal Harmonics

"Dear GrandDaughter, come with us into the dark, into the deep. Come with us into the pulsing, spiraling flow of your blood. Close your eyes and listen to the sounds. Like the oceans, these waters are filled with singing, sounding life – beautiful life, ephemeral life, changing life.

"That sound . . . do you hear it? So fierce, so energetic, so filled with vitality. Come closer. Listen. That is the symphony of the hormones. Listen to the unique hum of each hormone. And the way they all play together to make one swelling, ebbing, ever-changing flow of sound. So lovely. So filled with emotion. So rich and colorful. No wonder that many cancers love them and thrive in their company.

"Cells change when touched by these vibrations. The hormonal orchestra awakens, quickens, and invigorates each cell with its rhythms and melodies. And every cell responds with its own vibration, subtly altering the whole. Each hormonal sound not only delivers special frequencies, but also collects the unique vibrations from each cell and takes them to the pituitary. There, deep in the brain, the hormonal conductor listens, engages different instruments, modulates the rise and fall of the different hormones, and tunes your body to your own song, as well as to the mysterious movement of life's great symphony.

"Can you hear the sounds of individual hormones? Each one, like an oboe, a flute, or a violin, has a signature sound. Those slow, sonorous ones are testosterone. The sweet, lulling ones, progesterone. And those swelling, evocative tones are the estrogen chorus.

"But those, those high-pitched whistles – they are the calls of the hormone-mimics: You call them pesticides, bleach, pollution. Their vibrations are exotic and beautiful, but, like plants brought to an environment where they have no predators, they have over-run your inner ecosystem and deafened your inner conductor to the hums of your own hormones.

"How can you create change here? Can you prevent cancer cells from using hormones to grow? Will you purge the 'bad' vibrations? Retrain the conductor? Replace the musicians or the instruments? Yes, but you must proceed with great care. Changing the hormonal harmonics not only affects cancer, but many other aspects of your health. Purge that which is 'bad' and you inevitably weaken yourself and make yourself less whole. But nourish the best, and the least falls away. Focus on what is optimally functional and what is not working will change.

"If you remove your ovaries (or mute their vibrations with radiation or chemicals) their vital notes in your orchestral composition will become silences. If you take hormones to prevent recurrence, you may find you have avoided one kind of cancer, only to fall into another. There are unknowns along with the best scientific certainties. Risk accompanies benefit. Abrupt change can bring discord and arrhythmias.

"If you choose hormonal therapies, let us help you tune their harmonies so they resonate with your most perfect wholeness. Let us hum the melodies of healing for you. Let us sing your perfect pitch. Accept these plant hormones, and let them hum in your blood, too. Open your heart to the universal vibration and embrace your treatment in all its holy/healing complexity. We can guide you. We want to help you. You are precious GrandDaughter, and your life is of immense value."

200

# 11.
# Choosing Tamoxifen?
## or Other Hormonal Therapy

Exposure to estrogen has long been recognized as an important factor in the promotion of breast cancer, so orthodox medicine has focused a great deal of attention on preventing recurrence by reducing ovarian production of estradiol. Rendering the ovaries nonfunctional with high doses of radiation or chemotherapies, or surgically removing them, accomplishes this. Until the mid-'70s, oophorectomy was a common orthodox adjuvant treatment for premenopausal women with estrogen-sensitive breast cancers. Then hormonal drugs such as DES and tamoxifen were found to provide the same benefits with fewer side effects. Their use in preventing recurrence has increased every year since.

Tamoxifen is now recommended for all premenopausal women with hormone-positive cancers, as well as for most postmenopausal women with breast cancer, and for a growing number of premenopausal women with hormone-negative cancers. Tamoxifen is currently used by more women with breast cancer than any other drug. And a large-scale study is under way (despite protest) to determine if tamoxifen can prevent breast cancer as well as recurrence. Despite such widespread use, there are many unresolved questions about tamoxifen and its benefit-to-risk ratio.[1, 2]

*". . . the value of many drug therapies in breast cancer is ambiguous. The use of tamoxifen and other hormonal agents is even more debatable."*
M. DeGregorio, professor of medicine, and V. Wiebe, assistant professor of medicine and pharmacy, University of Texas[3]

Tamoxifen is a synthetic nonsteroidal compound with hormone-like effects, many of which are poorly understood. Although it does counter breast cancer recurrence, it promotes particularly aggressive uterine and liver cancer, and can cause fatal blood clots. Tamoxifen causes the same abnormal changes seen in the cells of women taking estradiol or DES.[4]

# Relief from
## Side Effects of Hormone Therapy

*For specifics on preparation and dosages of each of these plant allies, see Materia Medica. In general, I use 1–4 cups of infusion, 1–3 large spoonfuls of vinegar, or 10–30 drops of tincture daily. Any one ally will work alone, but they can be used together.*

*(Percentages refer to number of women taking tamoxifen who experience this side effect.)*

- **Blood clots**: *See* thrombophlebitis, page 203.
- **Bone marrow suppression**–decreased platelets, red blood cells, white blood cells (2%): *See* pages 229-230.
- **Cancer** (Some studies show a 50% increase in new cancers among women treated with tamoxifen.[16]): Preventing liver cancer, page 205; preventing uterine cancer, page 206.
- **Depression**: St. Joan's wort tincture, 25–30 drops, 1–4 times a day.
- **Endometrial polyps**: *See* uterine problems, page 206.
- **Eye problems** (6%): *See* page 205.
- **Fatigue**, lethargy: *See* pages 218-219.
- **Fluid retention**, edema (16%): Nettle infusion, burdock root vinegar/tincture, dandelion in any form.
- **Headaches** (5%): 10–20 drops skullcap tincture plus 25 drops St. Joan's wort tincture every 15 minutes for up to three hours; 25–30 drops dandelion tincture; sleep.
- **Hot flashes** (20%): 25 drops milk thistle seed tincture, dandelion root tincture, or motherwort tincture.
- **Irritability**: Motherwort tincture; oatstraw infusion.
- **Liver damage, liver cancer** (1+%): *See* page 205.
- **Menstrual irregularities, menopause** (90%): 30 drops motherwort, ginseng, or chaste tree tincture, 3 times a day.
- **Nausea/vomiting** (10%): After-surgery lozenges, page 301. More remedies are on pages 231-234.
- **Thrombophlebitis** (15%): *See* pages 203-204.
- **Uterine problems, polyps, cancer** (2-10%): *See* page 206.
- **Vaginal dryness**, bleeding, itching (20%): *See* page 241.
- **Vocal cord damage**: *See* page 206.
- **Weight gain**: *See* pages 240-241.

Despite tamoxifen's proven ability to reduce recurrence in postmenopausal women, major studies have shown that tamoxifen reduces death from breast cancer only marginally.[5] The majority of women who take tamoxifen live no longer than women who refuse it.[6] Furthermore, some breast cancers learn how to use tamoxifen to stimulate their growth.

The National Institutes of Health Consensus Statement on Early Stage Breast Cancer states that the overall benefits from tamoxifen outweigh its problems—for postmenopausal women—but, especially for premenopausal women, the long-term consequences are uncertain. And, while tamoxifen causes less acute toxicity than chemotherapy, "no statement is possible regarding chronic toxicity or comparative efficacy."[7]

The benefits of tamoxifen are limited. Virtually all women who take it become resistant within five years.[8,9] (Once resistance occurs, a different hormonal agent—such as aminoglutethimide, halotestin, megestrol, or leuprolide—can be used, but the cancer cells soon become resistant to them.) In fact, cancer cells become resistant to every chemotherapeutic and hormonal drug used in the treatment of breast cancer, requiring ever-changing strategies to try to keep ahead of them.

Tamoxifen resistance was once attributed to a diet high in phytosterols, but this view has been discredited. I strongly suspect that women with a phytosterol-rich diet resist recurrence as well as women taking tamoxifen. Daily use of beans, lentils, soy products, astragalus, and red clover keep phytosterol levels high.

Tamoxifen and other hormonal therapies—whether used alone, in combination with, or immediately after chemotherapy—cause a variety of side effects. The list on the previous page gives some remedies, but serious side effects are easier to prevent than treat, so don't put off reading what follows.

## Thrombophlebitis

Tamoxifen irritates the walls of the veins. Inflammation (a natural healing response to irritation) follows. This constant irritation and inflammation weakens the veins causing bleeding, clotting, thrombophlebitis, and—in the worst cases—obstruction of the blood vessels serving the lungs, which can be deadly, and can occur with little warning. The incidence of thrombophlebitis in women using oral contraceptives is generally regarded as significant (1 in 2,000). With tamoxifen, it's 30 times greater.

★ These herbal allies nourish and tonify the veins, reduce irritation and inflammation, and help prevent blood clots:

**Garlic** is renowned as a protector of the blood vessels.

**Red clover** and **nettle** (equal parts) infused with a pinch of **horsetail** gently thins the blood, strongly counters inflammation, and is said to restore the veins to youthful vigor.

**Hawthorn** (*Cratageus* species) berries, leaves, and flowers have long been used as tincture (75–100 drops a day) or infusion (1–2 cups/250–500 ml ) to relieve inflammation of the blood vessels.

**Willow** (*Salix* species) and **wintergreen** (*Gaultheria procumbens*) contain the same active ingredient as aspirin, and are excellent anti-inflammatory blood-thinners. I steep fresh willow bark or wintergreen leaves in apple cider vinegar for six weeks and use a teaspoonful/5ml of the resulting brew instead of two aspirin tablets.

★ Any **exercise** which improves circulation helps prevent thrombophlebitis. The value of walking a mile a day cannot be overstated, not just to prevent the side effects of hormone therapies, but to invigorate the immune system as well. Inverted postures, such as **yoga** shoulder stands or head stands, strengthen the veins and help prevent irritation.

★ I get rapid, reliable results using very small doses (1–8 drops a day) of **poke** root tincture to counter a variety of inflammations. Since it is highly anti-cancer as well, it is an excellent choice.

• **Symptoms of thrombophlebitis** that may indicate an immediately life-threatening situation include generalized swelling of a leg or arm, localized warmth, sudden pain (especially in the chest), abrupt but persistent shortness of breath, or a bloody cough. Seek help without delay.

• Orthodox treatment for thrombophlebitis depends on chemical blood thinners (e.g., heparin or warfarin). **Herbal blood thinners** include cleavers, sweet woodruff (*Asperula odorata*), alfalfa, willow, and wintergreen. Dose is 10–25 drops of one tincture or 1–2 cups/ 250–500 ml of infusion of one herb. Vitamin E and ascorbic acid (vitamin C) also have blood-thinning effects. **Caution**: Do not use these herbs or vitamins while taking blood-thinning drugs.

## Liver Problems

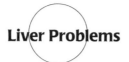

Liver damage has occurred in every animal given tamoxifen. The latest human studies show a six-fold increase in liver cancer among women taking tamoxifen for more than two years. Liver failure and tamoxifen-induced hepatitis, although rare, have been reported.

•Vinegars or tinctures of **dandelion**, **burdock**, or **yellow dock** roots, or **milk thistle** seeds nourish and strengthen the liver, as well as protect it from damage. (*See* Materia Medica for doses.)

## Eye Problems

Irreversible corneal and retinal changes can occur in those taking 20 mg of tamoxifen twice a day (twice the usual dose). These changes may have no immediate effect on visual acuity, but they may predispose the eyes to later problems including cataracts, according to the *Physician's Desk Reference* entry on Nolvadex (tamoxifen). Blindness has been reported as a side effect of very high doses (240 mg daily).

★ Traditional Chinese Medicine connects the eyes with the liver. Since tamoxifen damages the liver, it's no surprise that it causes eye problems, too. Protect your eyes with liver-loving herbs (see above) and **carotene-rich foods** (see page 47).

• **Fennel seed tea** is reputed to strengthen and nourish the eyes.

★ **Palming**, an exercise taught as part of the Bates Method of vision improvement, keeps energy and blood circulating through the eyes, protecting them from damage. Here's how to do it: Sit comfortably outside. Close your eyes and let the sun shine on your lids. Rub your palms together briskly until they feel warm. Placing your elbows on your thighs, let your head fall into your hands, eyes coming to rest on the palms, fingers on forehead. Rest like this with your eyes closed for a minute or two. Release the palms softly, noting how relaxed your eyes feel.

## Abnormal Uterine Changes

Uterine growths such as polyps, tumors, endometrial thickenings, and cancers occur in a significant number of women taking tamoxifen. One study detected abnormal endometrial cells in subjects the day after the first tablet was taken.[10] Precancerous uterine and endometrial changes were seen in 10 percent of the women taking tamoxifen in a recent study.[11]

      The higher the dose of tamoxifen, and the longer it is taken, the greater the risk of these changes. Women taking the standard dose of 20 mg daily for two years run a risk of uterine cancer that is 2–3 times greater than normal. After five years, the risk is 6–8 times greater than normal.[12, 13]

• If you are taking tamoxifen and have any **signs of uterine cancer** seek help promptly: abnormal menstrual bleeding, abnormal vaginal bleeding, change in vaginal discharge, pelvic pain, ache or pressure in the abdomen. Tumors and cancers that develop during tamoxifen therapy can be extremely aggressive and, even if caught early, are more likely than usual to be fatal.[14, 15]

• These daily allies help prevent tamoxifen-induced uterine changes: pelvic-strengthening **yoga** postures, **soy products**, **lentil** soup, **red clover** infusion, and **burdock** tincture.

## Vocal Cord Damage

Changes to the vocal cords resulting in impairment of singing and speaking abilities are occasionally caused by tamoxifen.

• **Slippery elm** lozenges (page 301) or several cups of warm **comfrey** leaf infusion are two of my favorite allies for soothing and strengthening the vocal cords.

• **Osha** root (*Ligusticum porterii*) is chewed or taken as tincture (a dose is 3–5 drops) for fast, dependable relief of inflamed throat tissues. That's why some people call it "singer's root."

# Fighting Fire With Fire

"I sense that you are attracted to the high energy of radiation, GrandDaughter. I hear the words they offer to reassure you that it is safe. Will you trust the shattering frequencies of x-rays? Will you thread your breast with pearls of radioactive light? Let us talk.

"When high energy x-rays shake the very nuclei of your cells, you are alone in the room. When radioactive pellets nestle in your breast, you are alone in the room for days. Your healers will hide behind lead shields, slide your food in through a slot in the door, and tell you this is safe.

"You know that cancer cells are moving rapidly, replicating and growing at a fevered pitch. A pitch which is closely matched - in both intensity and nature – by the energy emitted by radioactive materials. Fighting cancer with radioactivity seems absurd at first, knowing, as we do, that radiation causes healthy cells to die, to mutate, and to become cancerous. It's fighting fire with fire: battling cancer with that which causes cancer, like blowing up a burning oil well to put out the fire. Radiation therapies increase the vibration of that which is already too fast and add more to that which is already overloaded. If the fire can be made big enough, fast enough, it will consume itself and die.

"When the energy of radiation joins the energy of cancer, the cancer cells can blow apart like supernovas. Tremendous energy is released in your body from the dying cancer cells and the high-frequency vibrations of the x-rays. This energy can disturb and distort the frequencies of all your cells, especially those that are reproducing, for that is when cells are most vulnerable to changes in the energy matrix.

"Remember the teachings of energy, my dear: Energy must move. Let it flow and all are nourished. Try to hold it and you'll be pushed, maybe damaged. Keep the energy of radiation moving

207

through your being; do not let it linger.

"Come with us now to the center of your being, the center of the universe, where opposites unite and the Moebius loop turns, where all is all, and yin-yang becomes yang-yin. Come with us to the place which holds the wisdom that will allow you to choose this raging radiating fire, to embrace it as part of your health/wholeness/holiness, and move it through your being.

"Here in the center we can help you stoke your inner fire, GrandDaughter. We can help you fan your commitment to healing. We affirm your right to be alive. We bring nourishment for your heated nature. We urge you to let your passionate self emerge. Allow yourself to radiate the brilliance of your unique beingness and meet the radiation from these machines as an equal. When the center point is touched, the harmonic waves slide into synchrony and radiation cancels cancer, leaving you untouched.

"Claim your own radiance, GrandDaughter. Find your own source of x-rays. Passive reception of radiation opens your energy field to permanent damage. Participate actively. To use radiation well and wisely requires an enormous output of energy from you. But it can be done, and we are with you, no matter what you choose."

*"I received my 'radiation therapy' from my friends. Every day for six weeks they all sent ten minutes of radiant energy to my breast. And my own radiant energy went out to meet theirs! The only side effects were feelings of love and peace and a* knowing *that the cancer cells were maturing and moving into a normal cycle of life and death."*
Joy Craddick, M.D., breast cancer survivor

208

# 12.
# Choosing Radiation Therapy?

To prevent local recurrence, women who choose breast-conserving surgery, and women with diagnoses that warrant it, are urged to choose adjuvant radiation. Radiation following lumpectomy does seem to reduce the rate of recurrence, especially during the first few years following surgery. But adjuvant radiation does not increase longevity and it carries considerable risks. Acute and chronic side effects from radiation include severe lymphedema, heart damage, and initiation of secondary cancers.

*During an average 43 month follow-up, 91 percent of the women treated for breast cancer without adjuvant radiation were alive, as were 92 percent of those treated with adjuvant radiation.*
Journal of National Cancer Institute, May 1992

Different types of breast cancer respond to radiation differently. The most strongly affected are invasive intraductal cancers (*not* ductal carcinoma *in situ*). But a meticulous wide excision with clean edges generally prevents recurrence to the same extent that radiation does. And a Wise Woman anti-cancer lifestyle offers many ways to stay cancer-free and prevent recurrence should you decide against adjuvant radiation.

If you do choose radiation, it will most likely be a six-week course of therapy, and it can only be done once. (It is considered unsafe to use radiation therapy on the same breast twice). Radiation therapy can cause DNA damage, skin injuries (burns, discoloration, and permanent texture changes), nausea, appetite loss, hair loss, exhaustion, chest pain, pneumonia, and permanent damage to the lungs, heart, and ribs (known as late-stage injuries). These Wise Woman remedies offer safe and effective ways to prevent as well as deal these problems, so don't wait: Read this now, before you begin treatments.

# Relief from
## Side Effects of Radiation Therapy

*For specifics on preparation and dosages, see Materia Medica.*

• **Appetite problems**: Sip nourishing herbal infusions, eat with friends, eat often. *See also* pages 215-216.
• **Chest pain**: Violet leaf infusion. *See* pages 219-221
• **DNA damage** (cancer initiation): Drink black tea; eat foods rich in carotenes before each treatment, drink miso seaweed soup afterward. *See also* pages 211-212.
• **Exhaustion**: Sleep, exercise, laugh; ginseng. *See* page 218.
• **Hair loss**: Nettles, seaweed, exercise. *See* pages 216-217.
• **Heart protection**: Garlic; tincture of hawthorn or motherwort, 30 drops 3 times a day.
• **Late-stage injuries**: Life-threatening damage to chest tissues can build up over the course of the radiation treatments. Tissues damaged by radiation (evidence of this is visible within 15 minutes of a treatment) become irritated and inflamed, and gradually thicken and build up scar tissue, causing severe late-stage problems if blood vessel, lung, and heart tissues are affected. Inhibiting inflammation for several hours immediately following treatment can forestall late-stage radiation injuries. Anti-inflammatory drugs are used in orthodox medicine; herbalists use willow or wintergreen. Osha and poke roots are my favorite anti-inflammatories; they're both anti-cancer and they don't inhibit healing, as do many anti-inflammatories. I use 3 doses of 5 drops of osha tincture or 3 doses of 1 drop of poke tincture, hourly, for one hour before and two hours after each treatment.
• **Lung protection**: Comfrey leaf infusion. *See* page 221.
• **Nausea, vomiting**: Tiny spoonfuls of plain yogurt, slippery elm lozenges (page 301), smoke of dried cannabis flowers. *See also* pages 231-234.
• **Skin damage**: Aloe vera gel, comfrey leaf poultice, St. Joan's wort oil (really, even if you aren't supposed to use oil); all externally. *See also* pages 212-215.

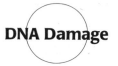

# DNA Damage

**Step 1.** *Collect Information*

• DNA damage from radiation therapy can initiate cancers that won't manifest until 15–20 years after the treatments.

**Step 2.** *Engage the Energy*

• Journey with your Wise Healer Within (page 82) to let your cells know what's happening. Ask them if there is a way you can protect them from damage. (One woman wrapped herself in psychic lead, allowing only the cancer to be touched by the x-rays.)

• Listen to Stephen Levine's tape, *In the Heart Lies the Deathless,* available from Warm Rock, PO Box 108, Chamisal, NM, 87521.

**Step 3.** *Nourish and Tonify*

★ Japanese researchers found that diets high in **carotenes** significantly reduced DNA damage in humans exposed to radiation. Supplements of beta-carotene (or of vitamins C or E) did not show this effect. Some oncologists recommend that women stop taking antioxidant supplements prior to radiation therapy. But you can still eat lots of orange and dark green foods to protect yourself from radiation-induced cancers. *See* carotenes, page 47.

• Guinea pigs bombarded with radiation lived a lot longer if they were also fed **broccoli** or **cabbage**. You aren't a guinea pig, but those cabbage family plants don't mind; they'll be glad to protect your cells from the damaging effects of radiation, too.

★ **Miso** broth is the classic food for prevention of radiation damage. There's twice the protection if a quarter-ounce/5 grams of dried **seaweed** is added to the soup. In scientific studies, seaweed was able to neutralize radioactive isotopes in the human body. Researchers at McGill University say radioactive strontium binds to the algin in brown seaweeds to create sodium alginate, a compound easily and harmlessly excreted. Common **black tea** exhibited the same anti-radiation effects in several Japanese studies.

★ **Burdock** root removes radioactive isotopes from the body. Dose is 4 ounces/120 grams of cooked fresh root, or up to a pint of dried or fresh root infusion daily for the duration of the treatment.

• Eating any amount of **reishii** reduces damage from radiation. *See* page 86.

• **Dried beans**, especially lentils, eaten throughout the treatments, can reverse DNA damage done by radiation.

• Anti-Radiation Easy Meal (page 308) is a tasty way to get all seven of these protective foods (carrots, cabbage, seaweed, miso, burdock, reishii, and beans) in one bowl.

• **Selenium** protects DNA from radiation damage. The best sources are nettles (2200 mcg per 100 grams), kelp (1700 mcg/100 g), burdock (1400 mcg/100 g), catnip (*Nepeta cataria*), ginseng, Siberian ginseng, milk thistle seeds, garlic, astragalus, green or black tea, and shellfish. Minerals are not extracted into tinctures; prepare herbs as vinegars or brew into infusions. (See pages 294, 296.)

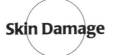

## Skin Damage

**Step 1.** *Collect Information*

• Radiation can be extremely damaging to the skin; that's why people wear sun-block. Radiation treatments are far more powerful than the radiation from the sun and can cause your skin to: display sunburn-like heat and redness; age prematurely; become permanently discolored in minor and severe ways with red, purple, and brown splotches; be prone to recurrent bouts of shingles; lose elasticity, smooth texture, and flexibility; and be impaired in its ability to heal from wounds, including subsequent breast surgery. Discoloration of the skin may not become obvious until up to two years after radiation treatments are over.

**Step 2.** *Engage the Energy*

• Choose an image, an icon, a plant, anything meaningful to you, as a focusing agent for those who want to help. Ask them to put their affirmations, blessings, **prayers**, visualizations, and healing love into the plant or image, which you can access whenever you need their help.

• **Homeopathic remedies** are taken before and after each treatment.

When you want to prevent and relieve hardness, tenderness, extreme sensitivity, darting or tearing pains, burning sensations, and redness in the breasts–*Belladonna*.

When you feel overwhelmed by the radiation and need protection–*Plumbum* (lead).

**Step 3.** *Nourish and Tonify*
Use external and internal remedies together.

Step 3: *External Remedies to Nourish and Tonify*

• Most doctors recommend that only **water-based** preparations be used on the irradiated area. The ultimate water-based skin care ally is also a superb healer of burns: **aloe vera**. And there's no better way to use it than fresh. I cut off a piece of the fleshy, slightly barbed leaf, slit the skin open and scrape out the clear gel, which slowly dissolves when spread gently on the skin. Aloe also relieves and repairs irritated, seeping, and discolored skin.

★ Water-based recommendations aside, women who used a light application of **St. Joan's wort oil** on the entire chest, before and after every radiation treatment, were uniformly thrilled with the results: supple, normal-colored, new-looking skin. I use this oil as my only sunscreen, and find it not only immediately effective, but even more protective with continuing use over years. I suspect it also helps prevent late-stage radiation injuries by preventing inflammation of the irradiated blood vessels.

• **Infused oils** of **comfrey, calendula, St. Joan's wort**, or **yarrow**, used in the days or weeks before radiation treatments begin, will strengthen the skin and help it resist injury.

★ After the course of treatments is completed, infused herbal oils/ointments made from the flowers of **St. Joan's wort, calendula**, or **dandelion** can be used several times a day on the irradiated area to promote skin flexibility and suppleness, and to lessen darkening and scarring. Many women said regular use of these oils prevented their irradiated skin from becoming dry, brittle, and hard, and that made it much easier to go through subsequent breast surgery (therapeutic or cosmetic).

★ **St. Joan's wort oil** is an extraordinary ally for women with **shingles**. They use the oil externally—as many times a day as possible—and take 25–40 drops of tincture in some water every couple of hours until the pain is gone. Most continue for at least a week more, some for several more weeks, but using only 3 doses a day.

• "Bend over in the shower and flap 'em," is the advice given by one radiation veteran. "It keeps your breast skin resilient and more capable of taking the radiation without damage."

Step 3: *Internal Remedies to Nourish and Tonify*

★ **Comfrey** leaf helps heal the skin from the inside out, protects the lungs, and has a reputation for preventing cancer recurrences. A cup or two of infusion daily for 6 weeks is a marvelous green ally for the woman choosing radiation therapy.

★ **Burdock** seed infusion (a small spoonful of seeds steeped in a cup of boiling water for 30 minutes), sipped frequently throughout the day, is noted for helping to prevent skin damage from severe burns. Added benefits include protection for the lungs and DNA from radiation damage, and burdock's scientifically established "tumor-growth-inhibiting factor."

• **Selenium** promotes tissue elasticity, helps prevent damage to the skin surface, and discourages recurrences. Keep the selenium level of your diet high: Eat one-half ounce/15 g **kelp**, or 2 ounces/ 60 g fresh **burdock** root, or 1 cup **yogurt** made from organic, hormone-free milk daily. (For more food sources, *see* page 53.)

**Step 4.** *Stimulate/Sedate*

• Keeping underarms fresh-smelling can be difficult during radiation therapy, and afterwards, too, since the skin is likely to react to deodorants and perfumed soaps. What to use instead? Add 5 drops of essential oil of **lavender** and/or **roman chamomile** to one cup of water. Put it in a sprayer, spritz, and wipe. Or put a spot of drugstore **witch hazel** on a wash cloth and wipe your underarms with that. It feels great, lessens perspiration, and kills bacteria that make you smell.

• Choose your clothing carefully during the time of your treatments. You will probably be most comfortable if you forgo bras altogether. Loose-fitting, natural fiber shirts are ideal. Treat yourself to a shirt of butter-smooth **silk** or **pima cotton,** or a soft-as-sin **cashmere** sweater; let it glide across your skin and help you glow with health/wholeness/holiness.

• For healthiest skin, **avoid** these things during and for six months after radiation therapy: direct sun on your affected skin, immersion in chlorinated water such as in a swimming pool (use a filter for your shower if your water is chlorinated), tight or chafing clothing, harsh cleansers, cover-up creams, cosmetics, rough or heavy necklaces. Massage is fine but must not abrade the skin in any way.

## Appetite Problems

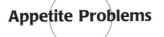

**Step 3.** *Nourish and Tonify*

★ It's important to keep yourself well nourished while undergoing radiation therapy. Your need for **protein** and **minerals**, especially **potassium** and **zinc**, is heightened. Make a really big pot of **Immune a Go Go Soup** (recipe, page 309) and freeze it in small containers so you'll have easy, nourishing, healing meals at hand.

★ High-protein, mineral-rich **nourishing herbal infusions** made from comfrey leaf, nettle, violet, or red clover can be frozen, cracked into chips, and slowly sucked to relieve nausea. Or warmed and taken with honey. Some say a pinch of mint in the brew settles your stomach even more; some say it is upsetting.

★ I rely on **yogurt** (organic, please) to keep me nourished when my appetite is asleep. You can have it plain, or fancy like this: **Yogurt Fruit Freeze**—Whir together in a blender one cup of yogurt, one cup of frozen fruit (peaches, apricots, strawberries, raspberries or pitted cherries), plus maple syrup (or sweetener of your choice) to taste.

★ For nourishment without eating, I dissolve sweet, soothing **After-Surgery Lozenges**—made with or without ginger but definitely with the strongest, darkest honey I can buy—slowly in my mouth, one after another. There's no overdose. Recipe, page 301.

• **Baby yourself** with applesauce, porridge, mashed banana, mashed potatoes, almond butter, and graham crackers to allay nausea and add nutrients. If very nauseated, give up on meals. Instead, take little bites and sips of foods several times an hour.

• Yes! Eat **chocolate**, in moderation, and of the highest quality you can afford. Chocolate is one of my favorite sources of iron. And specific fats in chocolate protect against breast cancer. The sugar isn't any more of a problem than the sugar in fruit. (All sugars, no matter where from, slightly depress the immune system for several hours after ingestion.) For organic chocolate, *see* page 222.

★ **Hops** (*Humulus lupulus*), as a tea, an infusion, or in all-natural, alcohol-free beer, is a classic remedy for those with little appetite. It is also a noted sleep-inducing herb, so don't drink it for breakfast. Her relative, marijuana, is an infamous appetite improver.

## Hair and Scalp

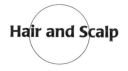

**Step 1.** *Collect Information*

★ The **crown chakra** (the energy center at the very top of the head) is connected to the hair and scalp and is affected by radiation and chemotherapy. Opening it as wide as possible allows the intense energy of radiation to flow through, preventing damage to the scalp. (To protect your hair, scalp, and life force during *chemotherapy*, close the crown chakra tightly.)

**Step 2.** *Engage the Energy*

• During, before, or after a radiation treatment, go inward and begin to breathe evenly, bringing your attention to your crown chakra. Imagine a **lotus** flower with a thousand petals opening on top of your head. As you breathe in, let the radiant energy of your treatment flow in. As you breathe out, let the fire flow out of your head and toward the sun.

• **Reiki** energy focused on the scalp can prevent or slow hair loss from radiation or chemotherapy without helping the cancer cells.

**Step 3.** *Nourish and Tonify*

• Drinking **nettle** infusion (up to a quart a day) can work wonders for hair and scalp. I like mine over ice. It's also nice hot with tamari or miso. It also works externally: Pour leftovers right on your head and let it soak in.

• **Burdock seed oil** is a Russian favorite for nourishing the scalp, helping prevent hair loss, and nourishing regrowth of healthy hair. Here's how to do it: Rub the oil in generously, cover your hair and head closely with a towel, shampoo an hour or so later.

• All **seaweeds** are noted for nourishing the hair follicles. People often remark at the glossy hair my animals (and I) have. "Seaweed," say I. And what a happy coincidence–seaweed removes radioactive isotopes from the body. I'm not talking about an occasional sprinkle of powdered kelp, I mean a half-cup serving of seaweed as a vegetable, or cooked into rice or beans or soups, at least every other day while receiving radiation. (Recipe books, page 237.)

**Step 4.** *Stimulate/Sedate*

• An ice pack "hat" that slows blood flow to the scalp can protect hair follicles from damage (especially from chemotherapy). It's offered in some hospitals–or you could bring your own. (Some oncologists maintain that this could allow metastasized cancer cells to live in the scalp.)

• A brisk massage with an infused herbal oil like burdock seed or dandelion flower feels great on the scalp and increases circulation, hastening the day you'll have hair again.

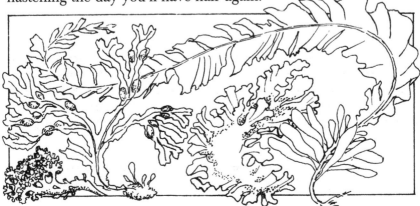

**Step 0.** *Do Nothing*

• Sleep.

• Be irresponsible.

• Be. In nature, if possible.

• Allow more time for everything.

**Step 1.** *Collect Information*

• Radiation, anesthesia, chemotherapy, and vomiting—together or individually—cause fatigue. If you're very tired, that's normal.

• When I don't have as much energy as I'm used to, or as much as I want, or as much as I think I ought to have, I stop . . . and pay attention to myself. I stop . . . and ask myself what's using that energy. The GrandMothers are quite clear that radiation (and chemotherapy) treatments require our active participation and an extensive expenditure of energy—reason enough to feel exhausted.

**Step 2.** *Engage the Energy*

★ Keep your body **moving** even when you feel tired. Light exercise (swaying to music, strolling a few blocks, gently stretching, or doing tai chi) gets your blood flowing and gives you energy.

• If you feel too tired to do anything: **Laugh!** Read funny comics. Look at humorous videos. Do something silly. Laughing is good exercise, and you'll be following in the famous footsteps of Norman Cousins, who laughed himself out of two incurable diseases.

**Step 3.** *Nourish and Tonify*

★ **Astragalus** improves energy, protects the adrenals, improves bone marrow activity, and augments interferon. See Materia Medica.

★ **Siberian ginseng** increases energy, builds stamina, protects against stress, strengthens the immune system, and improves one's sense of well being. *See* Materia Medica.

★ **Ginseng** is another energy-promoting herb; it helps protect you from the side effects of radiation, too. (*See* page 85.)

• To build stable, reliable energy, I use **nettle** infusion, **dandelion** root vinegar, or **yellow dock** root tincture daily.

**Step 4.** *Stimulate/Sedate*

• **Wheat grass, barley greens, mint infusion,** and **fresh carrot juice** are stimulating, short-term allies for increasing energy; they help prevent recurrence, too.

## Chest Pains

**Step 1.** *Collect Information*

• Radiation therapy can weaken the ribs, causing them to ache, feel sore to the touch, or throb. Radiologists told me that chest pain after radiation treatments is inevitable, and that it is likely to persist for years, sometimes forever. Many women mentioned how unexpectedly painful the treatment itself was. Some had sensations of nearly intolerable heat, others of being shattered or exploded.

• Chest pain from radiation therapy appears to be more pronounced in those who already have chest problems, such as heart disease, asthma, or allergies which affect breathing.

**Step 2.** *Engage the Energy*

★ **Homeopathic** *Hypericum* is a specific for pain caused by burns which disrupt the nerve endings, e.g., radiation burns.

★ If you can **transmit the energy** of the radiation out into the world, you can help stop it from giving you a pain in the chest. Imagine it as a hose spraying diamond bright healing out of your shoulders. Feel it as a wind of peace blowing through your breast. Experience it as loving flares from the ends of your fingers. Feel its passionate intensity and let it go. Let it bring brightness and warmth to all those in need. Use your own images. Keep the energy moving. Breathe it out.

• Bernie Siegel, renowned and beloved cancer surgeon, suggests that we harm ourselves when we choose therapies that we consciously or unconsciously believe are deadly. He relates two stories: one of a woman who saw her adjuvant radiation as a death ray and who got very ill from her treatments, the other of a woman who saw the **radiation as a healing ray** and had virtually no ill-effects from her treatments.

**Step 3.** *Nourish and Tonify*

• Radiation therapy has been described as "soulless." It is certainly done in cold, sterile, heartless, often isolated and isolating circumstances. It's enough to make anyone's chest ache. How can you nourish your heart during this therapy? How can you **touch the soul** of this energy? Is there a special nurse or technician or doctor who's compassionate and there for you?

★ Soothing, nourishing infusions of **oatstraw** or **comfrey** leaf (up to a quart/liter of either per day) help calm pain from damaged, overheated nerves while nourishing regeneration of damaged bones, lungs, and muscles.

★ **Violet** leaf infusion (the liquid in your stomach, the leaves on your chest) is the ally that gives fast relief from throbbing pain after radiation treatments.

• Encourage new bone growth in the ribs during and after radiation therapy by exercising, eating mineral-rich foods (add horsetail herb to your infusions), and doing yoga, Qi gong, or tai chi.

★ I rely on **St. Joan's wort** tincture, 25 drops repeated as often as needed, to relieve pain from burns (as well as headache pain and muscle pain). And I delight in the fact that it helps keep my immune system strong, unlike immune-depressing pharmaceutical pain-killers.

★ **Hugs** were a highly recommended remedy for women with chest pain; gently, please.

**Step 4.** *Stimulate/Sedate*

• **Juzentaihoto**, a traditional herbal formula from Japan, accelerates recovery from radiation-induced injuries, eases pain, improves immune response, and stimulates spleen colony-forming units.[6] Recipe, page 300.

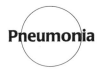

# Pneumonia

**Step 2.** *Engage the Energy*

★ Pneumonia is connected with **grief**. Has it all happened so fast that you haven't had enough time and space to grieve? When you express the sounds of your sadness, make the motions of your loss, find the symbols of your grief, and create images of your struggle you energize your lungs and your immune system.

**Step 3.** *Nourish and Tonify*

★ **Mullein** (*Verbascum thapsus*) or **comfrey** leaf infusions are favorite green allies for protecting and strengthening the lungs. Up to a quart/liter a day of either, sweetened with honey and mellowed with milk, if you like, is the usual dose.

★ **Carotenes** found in orange and dark green foods protect lung tissue from infection, heal lung damage, and prevent the formation of radiation-induced tumors.

**Step 4.** *Stimulate/Sedate*

★ **Elecampane** root tincture is a steadfast ally for resolving lung infections, including viral and bacterial pneumonias. A dose of 15–30 drops is used up to eight times a day, alone or with 75–150 drops **echinacea** or **usnea**. If you're vulnerable to lung infections, 25–50 drops of echinacea or usnea tincture, plus one drop of poke tincture, daily during treatments can improve your resistance.

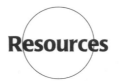

# Resources

• Rapunzel chocolate bars, made with organic chocolate and organic unrefined sugar cane juice, are distributed by Mercantile Food Company, PO Box SS, Philmont, NY 12565.

• Seaweed recipes in:
  *Healing Wise*, Susun Weed, Ash Tree, 1989
  *Macrobiotic Cooking for Everyone*, W. Esko, Japan Pub., 1980
  *Macrobiotic Cookbook*, Lima Ohsawa, Autumn Press, 1974
  *Sea Vegetable Gourmet Cookbook*, Lewallen, 1995 (to order by mail, see page 54)

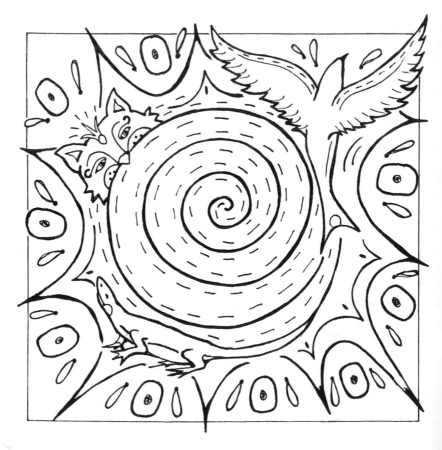

# The Poisoned Apple

"Who offers you poison as the cure for your disease? Do they tell you to take poisons to preserve your life, GrandDaughter? Do you trust them? Do you trust their poisons?

"These poisons are designed to seek out and kill all your fast-growing cells. Will they kill your quickness? Will they disrupt your rhythm? Will they attack your uniqueness and your wildness? Yes, GrandDaughter, these poisons will – unless you guide their actions with certainty and power.

"In this game of poisoning to create health, there is a little skill and a lot of luck. How much will you bet that your body can repair the damage done to it by these poisons? That your immune system can handle the cells mutated by the poisons? How much will you bet that the new poison, the new strength, the new combination will work better than the old one did?

"You've heard that there are those who can eat poison and be unscathed by it. It is true. And you can do it, too, if you choose. How? Nourish your deepness with sweet roots, with bitter roots. Invite your power; grasp the nettle. Gather your resources; take charge; command the forces of death that you invite into your bloodstream. Do not passively await their introduction.

"And let us help. We will sing for you the ancient songs. Songs of living, songs of liver, the spinning, spiraling songs of life. Some are sweet as candy, some bitter as these poisons you ponder. GrandDaughter, if you choose them, it is up to you to affirm your life, to sing a song of life. Your song will help you as you walk this path. Your song will help you stand in the spirit core of your being as you bite the poisoned apple. Through the storm that will rage within you if you do this thing, we will sing with you, GrandDaughter and, together, we will do what must be done."

# Relief from
# Side Effects of Chemotherapy

*Side effects are frequently seen with—but not limited to—the drugs in parentheses. Check Materia Medica before using an herb. See chart, page 243, for relief from side effects not included here.*

Note: 5-Flu = 5-FU; Adria = Adriamycin = doxorubicin; Cytoxan = cyclophosphamide; Methtrx = Methotrexate

• **Aching joints**, polyarthralgia: St. Joan's wort tincture; poke root tincture; or one dried poke berry, swallowed whole.
• **Bladder,** kidney stress (Adria, cisplatin, Cytoxan, Methtrx, mitomycin): Slippery elm; nettle infusion; 2 cups/500 ml infusion or 30–90 drops tincture of uva ursi (*Arctostaphylos uva ursi*) for 10 days will counter most bladder infections.
• **Reduced blood clotting time**: Nettle infusion.
• **Depression** (vincristine, vinblastine): St. Joan's wort tincture.
• **Fever** (Adria, Methtrx, mitomycin, Thiotepa): Yarrow or elder (*Sambucus*) tincture, 25 drops. Fever promotes remission.
• **Headache** (Methtrx,vinblastine): 5 drops skullcap plus 25 drops St. Joan's wort tinctures, every 15 minutes, as needed.
• **Heart damage** (Adria): Prevent with seaweed, garlic, oatstraw, vitamin E-rich oils, and tincture of motherwort or hawthorn, 3 doses of 30 drops daily.
• **Immune system damage**: Prevent with astragalus.
• **Nausea**, appetite loss, digestive woes: *See* page 246.
• **Liver distress** (Adria, Methtrx): Milk thistle seed tincture.
• **Lung problems, pneumonia** (Cytoxan, melphalan): Mullein, comfrey, elecampane. *See* page 221.
• **Memory loss**: Ginkgo leaf tincture, 25 drops 3 times daily.
• **Menstrual flooding**: 15-25 drops, as needed, even hourly, of witch hazel, lady's mantle, or shepherd's purse tincture.
• **Induced tumors** (Cytoxan, melphalan): Selenium prevents.
• **Nerve damage,** nerve pain, loss of reflexes, **hearing loss** (cisplatin, vincristine, vinblastine): Oatstraw infusion.
• **Skin discoloration** (Adria, Cytoxan, and 5-Flu): Infused herbal oils, e.g., comfrey, plantain; *see* page 61.
• **Sun sensitivity** (Methtrx): Infused oil of chaparral or St. Joan's wort. Chemotherapy can reactivate radiation burns.
• **Water retention**: Burdock, dandelion, or nettle.

# 13.
# Choosing Chemotherapy?

Adjuvant chemotherapy is used to kill cancer cells that have left the primary tumor (metastasized). But chemotherapy is designed to destroy *all* rapidly replicating cells, not just cancer cells. Thus, cells in the intestines, mouth, bone marrow, reproductive system, immune system, and scalp (and sometimes cells in the heart and the liver) are killed by chemotherapy, causing both acute and long-term problems. If your cancer hasn't metastasized, chemotherapy is more likely to harm you than to help you.

The benefits of chemotherapy are questionable.[1] Before choosing this therapy, become more informed: Do a Medline search (call 1-800-4-CANCER) or take a foray into the library of a medical school or large hospital. To make a truly informed decision, also read the books of Ralph Moss, M.D. and Steve Austin, N.D. (*See* Resources, page 244.)

The chemotherapy option circuit on the next page is inspired by the work of Austin and Cathy Hitchcock. Austin notes that most women with breast cancer won't die if they refuse adjuvant chemotherapy (but they will avoid its life-threatening side effects), while 75 percent of the women who, statistically, would die *without* chemotherapy, will die "on schedule" no matter what therapies they choose. His research shows that, for all stages and types of breast cancer, the only women who will benefit from chemotherapy are 25 percent of the ones who would have died (not 25 percent of the total). All others will receive no benefit at all.

Currently, lymph node involvement is the most commonly used diagnostic measure for deciding which premenopausal women ought to choose chemotherapy. (Chemotherapy has very little effect on the longevity of postmenopausal women and is rarely suggested for them.) If any cancer cells are found in any of the axillary lymph nodes, chemotherapy will be recommended. But this misses the many (over 30 percent) premenopausal women with clear nodes who are later found to have metastases. The orthodox solution is to urge all premenopausal women to choose

# Chemotherapy Option Circuit

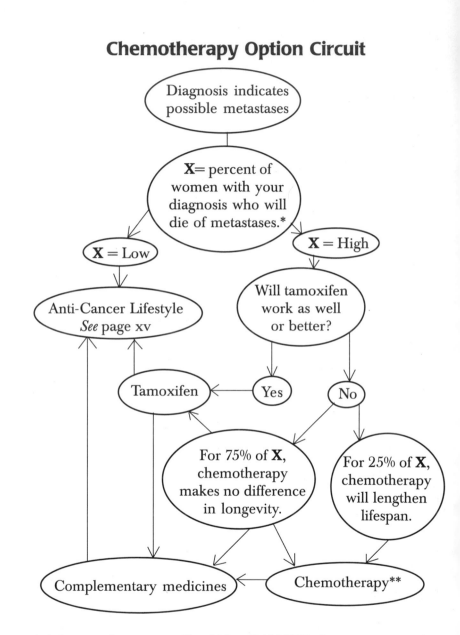

* Ask your doctor or call 1-800-4-CANCER (have your specific diagnosis at hand) for the answer to **X** for you.
** Aggressive alternative therapies can also be considered.

chemotherapy no matter what their nodal status. (Very important: If you are certain before your surgery that you do—or do not—want adjuvant chemotherapy, keep your lymph nodes.[2] )

A 1989 report from the U.S. General Accounting Office found no increase in longevity for premenopausal women who chose chemotherapy—as opposed to those who did not—as a treatment for stage II (or earlier) breast cancers.[3] Nor did chemotherapy improve survival for node-positive postmenopausal women.[4]

Most chemo horror stories are descriptions of last ditch attempts to slow the growth of multiple metastases. Your initial experience with chemotherapy may be much milder. And then again, it may not. "The whole lining of her gut, from one end to the other, was shedding. She was vomiting sheets of tissue. The doctors said this was the worst they'd ever seen, but still normal," reports Robert Distal of the Dana-Farber Cancer Institute, husband of Betsy Lehman, who died in 1995 from her early-stage breast cancer chemotherapy.

*"Most cancer patients in this country die of chemotherapy. Chemotherapy does not eliminate breast, colon, or lung cancers. The fact has been documented for over a decade [that] women with breast cancer are likely to die faster with chemotherapy than without it."*
Alan Levin, M.D., San Francisco Medical School (U.of California)

Although there are many Wise Woman ways to help prevent and heal the side effects of chemotherapy, it is still a therapy that carries enormous risks to future well-being. For instance, in a trial using prednimustine, Methotrexate, 5-Flu, mitoxantrone, and tamoxifen to treat advanced breast cancer, 13 percent of the women developed leukemic complications.[5] And, according to John Laszlo, the American Cancer Society's senior vice-president for research, recurrence rates are 25 times higher in women treated with both radiation and chemotherapy. For a list of the possible side effects of a particular chemotherapy, consult *The Breast Cancer Handbook*.[6]

Is chemotherapy worth the risks? Only you can decide. Let statistics inform you, but since so few women will be helped by chemotherapy, let your values and your intuition have the final say in your decision. If you do choose chemotherapy, study the rest of this chapter before beginning your treatments.

# For Women Choosing Chemotherapy

• Use the time—sometimes a month—between surgery and the commencement of chemotherapy to **strengthen your liver** (*see* below) and **build powerful immunity** (*see* Chapter 4).

• Adding **nettles** to your daily diet before and during your treatments will help prevent many common and dangerous side effects of chemotherapy: liver damage, breakdown of blood and veins, anemia, induced menopausal hemorrhage, fatigue, hair loss, depressed libido, water retention, and kidney damage.

★ The antioxidants selenium, vitamins E and C, carotenes, and glutathione not only help inhibit chemically induced tumors, but also protect the heart, liver, and blood, keep the veins strong, and increase the effectiveness of many orthodox cancer drugs. Carotenes and vitamin E encourage macrophages and lymphocytes to secrete more cancer-killing cytokines, and actually get the cancer cell to program its own death.[7] Food sources of these nutrients are discussed in Chapter 2.

## Protecting Your Liver

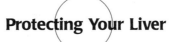

• Perhaps the single most important contribution herbal medicine can make to women choosing chemotherapy is to offer them ways to maintain strong liver function. **Dandelion**, **yellow dock**, or **burdock** root tincture, 20 drops, 2–3 times a day, will do, but my favorite liver ally is milk thistle.

★ **Milk thistle** is legendary for protecting the liver from damage. It is highly regenerative to liver tissue as well. In Europe it is used to treat liver degeneration (e.g., from cirrhosis, hepatitis, and chemical poisoning). Bloodwork and liver charts on women who take milk thistle seed tincture throughout their chemotherapy show strong liver function and good white blood cell count, unlike typical liver charts where the lines dip and dive.

For best results, 30 drops of milk thistle tincture (or **Silymarin** extract) is taken right before the dose of chemotherapy, or no later than 15 minutes afterwards. Milk thistle protects the liver, in part, by occupying receptor sites so hepatotoxins (liver damaging substances) don't have anywhere to grab hold.

Milk thistle also improves appetite, eases indigestion, and soothes mouth and tongue tissues without side effects. It can be used regularly for years if desired.

• **Ginkgo** (*Ginkgo biloba*) tincture—up to 100 drops daily—has been clinically shown to be extremely protective of liver function, non-interfering with chemotherapy, and an excellent antioxidant, adding further protection from chemotherapeutic damage.

• **Schisandra** (*Schisandra chinensis*), 90–100 drops tincture or up to a half ounce/15 grams of freshly powdered berries daily, has been clinically shown to prevent liver damage and liver necrosis from a wide range of hepatotoxins, restore the integrity of damaged digestive tissues, promote bile secretion, prevent ulcers, encourage sound sleep, and increase overall energy remarkably.

## Bone Marrow, Immune System, and White Blood Cells

One of the most problematic side effects of many chemotherapeutic drugs (e.g., Adriamycin, Cisplatin, 5-Flu, melphalan, mitomycin, Methotrexate, Taxol, Thiotepa, vinblastine, and vincristine) is depression of the immune system and the bone marrow, causing production of white blood cells to falter and lowering resistance to infections of all kinds. (Minor infections can get serious quickly.)

**Step 2.** *Engage the Energy*

• After receiving one dose of saccharine-laced Cytoxan, laboratory animals showed depressed immune systems whenever they tasted saccharine. Studies with humans show the same conditioned response (depression of the immune system) can be triggered by **smells** as well as **tastes** associated with chemotherapy. (Or, unfortunately, food you ate just before the chemo made you throw up.)

To counter this: Make a list of ten tastes and smells that give you a lot of pleasure. (Pleasure is immune-enhancing.) Experience as many of these as you can before beginning chemotherapy to build a library of immune-strengthening stimuli. Experiment with using your immune-enhancing stimuli (in reality or in your imagination) before, during, and after chemotherapy until you find the pattern that helps you build immune strength and overcome the automatic tendency of chemotherapy to depress immune functioning. One woman brought a bottle of vanilla extract to her sessions because she said the smell calmed her and her stomach.

★ When chemotherapies that depress the immune system are given in the **morning**, women recover faster from the side effects and are four times as likely to survive for five years as women whose doses are not timed.[8]

**Step 3.** *Nourish and Tonify*

• **Echinacea** and **usnea** tinctures are wonderful allies for women choosing chemotherapy. Both herbs promote the production of white blood cells and are proven anti-tumor agents. A protective dose during chemotherapy would be 25–50 drops of either herb (not both) 2–3 times daily. Do tell your doctor you're using these herbs as they can cause an abrupt upswing in your white blood cell count, which could be interpreted as a sudden infection or an indication that the chemotherapy dose isn't strong enough. (A lowered white blood cell count is considered an indication that an effective dose of chemotherapeutic agents is being given.) Or use other infection-preventing herbs, such as **poke** root, **St. Joan's wort**, or **Siberian ginseng**. *See* Materia Medica.

★ **Astragalus** root protects the immune system, restores bone marrow activity, improves interferon response, and protects the adrenal cortex during chemotherapy treatments. *See* Materia Medica.

• **Reishii** (exotic mushrooms) are used in Beijing hospitals to help those with cancer strengthen their immune systems, resist infections, and feel better while undergoing chemotherapy. *See* page 86.

★ **Honeysuckle** is another immune-protective herb frequently used in China by women choosing chemotherapy against breast cancer. *See* Materia Medica for specifics.

★ **Burdock** root, eaten as a cooked vegetable or taken as an infusion in any quantity, binds with cytotoxic agents after they have killed cancer cells and escorts them out of the body before they damage bone marrow. And it builds immunity by increasing the production of interferon. *See* Materia Medica.

## Step 4. *Stimulate/Sedate*

• To protect yourself while your immune system is depressed: Don't spend time with recently vaccinated children or adults returning from exotic ports of call; wear gloves when doing rough work; don't pick your nose or cut your cuticles; act promptly if you have any sign of infection such as a fever, a rash, or a tingling in your lips or vulva (an early sign of herpes infection).

## Step 6. *Break & Enter*

• One orthodox remedy used to try to stimulate bone marrow function is injection of human stem cell factor (produced by genetically engineered bacteria). When given to women using chemotherapy against breast cancer, it led to modest increases in white blood cell numbers, but stimulated allergic reactions and did not improve overall survival.

## Nausea, Vomiting, and Appetite Loss

## Step 1. *Collect Information*

• All chemotherapeutic drugs cause digestive disturbances.

## Step 2. *Engage the Energy*

★ The best **time** to take chemotherapy to protect the digestive tract differs from the best time for protecting the immune system. Heavy doses of Adriamycin, cisplatin, Cytoxan, 5-Flu (fluorouracil), melphalan, Methotrexate, mitomycin, and Thiotepa are better tolerated at night when the digestive tract cells are not replicating.[8] Programmable pumps can allow you to sleep through your session and awaken, if not refreshed, at least not nauseated.

★ Traditional Chinese Medicine uses **pressure on the P6 point—** about two inches above the crease of the wrist, in the center of the

inner arm–to quell nausea and vomiting. This works so well that
stretchy wrist bands with a bead affixed in the right place are now
sold in drug stores to stop seasickness and motion sickness. They
also prevent and relieve nausea if worn during or after chemotherapy sessions (surgery, too).[9]

★ **Homeopathic** remedies can ease nausea and digestive distress:
     When vomiting is sudden, severe, or repeated, especially
when accompanied by exhaustion–*Antimonium tartrate*.
     For those who also feel debilitated, restless, fearful, and
chilled–*Arsenicum*.
     When digestive distress is accompanied by fever, a flushed
face, and pain, especially on movement–*Belladonna*.
     When the vomiting is persistent, painful, or extreme and
brings no relief; the mood is irritable–*Ipecacuanha*.
     When the bowels are upset, the stomach feels filled with
lead, and there's no appetite; worse in the morning–*Nux vomica*.
     When the vomiting is violent and accompanied by pro-
fuse diarrhea–*Veratrum album*.

• The smell of **peppermint** tea or a whiff of essential oil of peppermint is a quick fix for an unsettled stomach.

• Write things you want to get rid of on small slips of paper. Put
them in a lovely container in the bathroom. Flush one down the
toilet instead of throwing up. **Study the art of giving away.**

**Step 3.** *Nourish and Tonify*

★ My favorite remedy for rapid relief of nausea and vomiting is
plain yogurt by the spoonful, slowly. Read more about it, page 234.

★ **Slippery elm** bark eases and heals all digestive disturbances,
from heartburn to colitis. After-Surgery Lozenges (*see* page 301)
are great after chemotherapy (and after radiation, too).

• **Liver-protective herbs** help reduce or eliminate nausea associated with chemotherapy (and radiation). *See* pages 228-229.

• **Seaweed** quickly restores a disturbed electrolyte balance and
heals digestive surfaces injured by repeated vomiting. If you're
too nauseated to eat seaweed by itself, boil some in a cup of water
for ten minutes and sip the liquid, or cook it with oatmeal.

**Step 4.** *Stimulate/Sedate*

★ **Marijuana** (*Cannabis sativa*) absolutely stops nausea and vomiting. One author claims that over 40 percent of practicing oncologists recommend marijuana to their patients.[10] Marinol–the prescription form of marijuana–is not as effective as inhalation of the smoke of the dried leaves and female flowers. Tincture of marijuana is not used: The active anti-nausea constituents are poorly extracted into alcohol, the effects of even good quality tincture are erratic, and it occasionally increases nausea. For similiar reasons, eating marijuana is likely to be counterproductive.

"Side effects" of the medical use of marijuana are generally helpful rather than problematic. They include increased appetite, more libido, heightened body awareness, enhanced creativity, and an enlargement of the mental perspective coupled with a feeling of peace which makes it easier to acknowledge and work with the difficult emotions that arise when the diagnosis is cancer.

Isn't smoking bad for the lungs? No. Smoking herbs from a pipe is a traditional medicinal treatment to open the bronchi and warm and tone lung tissues. Unless you're allergic to all smoke, your respiratory system will appreciate an occasional gentle "smoking."

Scientific studies of marijuana are scarce, making it difficult to know how it affects immune system activity. If the experiences of people with AIDS are any indication, however, immune function does not suffer when marijuana is smoked in moderation. Studies done in the early 1970s at the Medical College of Virginia showed that purified THC (tetrahydrocannabinol, the active ingredient in marijuana), when given to mice with breast cancer, extended their lives significantly.[11]

Marijuana is not addictive. Marijuana is not a drug. Marijuana is, at worst, benignly ineffective; at best, it is a powerful ally.[12]

**Caution**: This herb is illegal in the United States. You could be arrested and imprisoned (and have your car and house legally taken from you) if you grow or possess marijuana.

*"I never smoked until chemo. I was horribly affected by the drugs. I finally agreed to try some marijuana after a friend insisted it would help. It did! It put me in a euphoric state that held everything at bay, even the nausea, and let me relax for the first time since my ordeal began."*

• Many women felt that it was very important to drink a lot of **water**–as much as a gallon a day–while using chemotherapy, to dilute the drugs and wash them out of the body. This is recommended for those taking Cytoxan; for others it may stress the kidneys. As always, let your body guide you.

**Step 5a.** *Use Supplements*

• Be aware that taking multi-gram doses of ascorbic acid (vitamin C) during chemotherapy can cause diarrhea and weakening of your red blood cell walls. A mineral form (e.g., calcium ascorbate) is a better choice if you're resorting to supplements.

★ **Minerals** (including those needed to maintain powerful immunity) are leached from the body by repeated vomiting. A mineral supplement helps replace them, as do nourishing herbal infusions.

**Step 5b.** *Use Drugs*

• Orthodox medicine gives drugs such as Zofran (most expensive), Dexamethasone (a steroid), and Compazine (suppositories which are very strong but may suddenly become ineffective) before the chemotherapy dose to prevent and moderate nausea.

★ Stomach distress is the usual reason **cimetidine** is prescribed. One of its "side effects" is reduction in the production of C8 cells, which increase after surgery and suppress helpful T-cells. Another: It occasionally prompts remission of cancer.

## Diarrhea and Constipation

• Methotrexate, mitomycin, vincristine, vinblastine, and 5-Flu are especially likely to cause diarrhea and constipation.

★ Superb quality **yogurt**—even a single teaspoonful, but better to take more—not only checks diarrhea *and* relieves constipation, but settles queasiness, allays vomiting, and soothes stomach and intestinal pain . . . fast! Eating yogurt repopulates the gut flora (increasing the amount of nutrients you absorb) and strengthens the immune system (reducing your risk of infection).

★ **Slippery elm**, as tea or lozenges, stops diarrhea, relieves constipation, soothes abraded intestines, and eases sore throats.

• Home remedies for checking diarrhea include: strong **cinnamon** tea (a spoonful of the powder–the kind sold in the grocery store–in a cup of boiling water), a cup of **applesauce**, a **green banana**, or a cup of **oak bark** infusion.

## Mucous Surface Sores

*Nose, Mouth, Tongue, Gums, Anus*

The cells lining the mucous surfaces of the nose, mouth, and anus replicate on a daily basis, and are killed by chemotherapy (especially Adriamycin, 5-Flu, mitomycin, Methotrexate, melphalan, and vinblastine), leaving painful, raw sores. In most cases, this peaks about a week after a treatment.

★ **Comfrey ointment** is my choice for healing stubborn sores, anywhere. (Yes, it's fine to smear ointment inside your mouth, nose, and anus.) Comfrey root in a lanolin base is the form I prefer, but it's difficult to find for sale. The usual offerings, made from comfrey leaves, have excellent healing qualities but don't work nearly as well as ointments made from the fresh roots of comfrey.

If you have access to fresh comfrey, slit the stalk or the midribs of the leaves. The clear slime inside is an excellent soothing application, much like **aloe vera** gel when placed carefully and frequently on mucous surface sores.

A woman told me she suggested to her husband, who had stomach cancer, that he drink comfrey leaf infusion, an idea he didn't care for. But he was willing to put comfrey ointment on the sores that erupted in his mouth from his chemotherapy. And when he saw how quickly they healed, he began to drink the infusion by the jarful!

★ **Slippery elm** eases mouth sores, relieves sore tongues, keeps the mucous surfaces of the mouth, nose, and intestines moist, calms upset stomachs, and heals distressed intestines. Sucking on a slippery elm lozenge can counter strange (metallic, garlicky) tastes from chemo or bone marrow transplants.

"*The steroid spray that I had to use to stop the chemo-induced nose bleed made my shits so hard they tore up the lining of my rectum. That was a real low for me: ouch at both ends.*"

Sharon, age 39

• The **homeopathic remedy** *Ipecac* is said to relieve mouth sores.

• **Horsetail** tea (not infusion) strengthens gums if a cup a day is taken throughout the course of treatments.

• Infusion of green or red **garden sage** (*Salvia officinalis*), with or without honey, can be held in the mouth for a minute or so to help dry and heal mouth sores. It's okay if you swallow it. Infection in your mouth? Counter it with 5–10 drops of **myrrh** tincture in each mouthful of sage infusion.

• Avoid brushing or flossing your teeth and gums during chemo- therapy; this can cause mouth sores. Rinse well with myrrh tinc- ture in sage tea instead.

• If you have access to fresh **burdock root** (it's a common weed, and it's sold in some markets as gobo), see if holding the grated root in your mouth relieves mouth sores as fast as claimed.

• Help prevent and heal herpes outbreaks on your lips by using **St. Joan's wort** ointment as your lip balm.

• Here's a technique from kriya yoga to ease the pain of nose sores: Sniff **salt water** up your nose. Mix half a teaspoon/3 ml of sea salt and a cup/250 ml of warm water in a shallow bowl; put your nose into it, and *gently* draw the water in until you taste salt in your mouth; then let it drain out and down the sink.

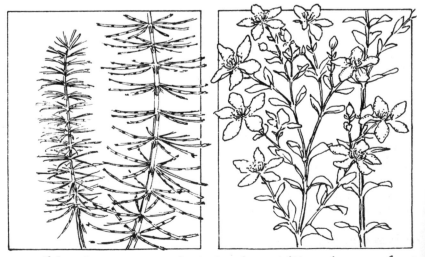

Horsetail (Equisetum arvense) · St. Joan's wort (Hypericum perforatum)

## Thrush and Anal Yeast

When the normal population of intestinal microorganisms becomes disrupted (by chemotherapy, antibiotics, preservatives in processed foods, or extended ingestion of chlorinated water), then one of those microorganisms, a yeast called *Monilia* or *Candida albicans,* sometimes reproduces rapidly in a desperate attempt to keep digestion going. It gets quite out of hand, however, and winds up proliferating so fast and so well that it spreads to the mouth and tongue (where it's called thrush), and down to the anus and vagina. Like most yeast infections, it is white, smells yeasty, and causes mild to severe irritation and itching.

Wise Women don't try to kill it; they know that *Candida* is needed for good health. Instead, they restore it to its (small) place in the dance by restoring healthy populations of all the other intestinal microorganisms. How? By eating small quantities of "food-quality" mold. From? Wild mushrooms; unwashed, unpeeled organic fruits (the skins harbor a variety of healthful yeasts and molds); naturally fermented and unpasteurized foods such as miso, sauerkraut, apple cider vinegar, chemical-free beer and wine, sourdough bread, and kombucha (actually, the vinegary brew the kombucha mother makes); and organic "moldy" cheeses, like blue or Camembert. Let your body be your guide; if one or more of these foods aggravates you, try something else.

★ **Yogurt** inhibits replication of *Candida,* provides soothing relief of symptoms, and improves the functioning of the immune system. A big spoonful of plain organic yogurt every hour while awake stops *Candida* overgrowth so quickly it's miraculous. To prevent thrush, eat a cup/250 ml a day throughout chemotherapy.

★ The dry ripe seeds and seed husks of the herb **plantain** (*Plantago*), soaked overnight in cold water (for use on the tongue) or cooked with oats (for intestinal healing) yield a mucilage that soothes oral and anal tissues, and eliminates yeast infections. I soak a big spoonful of seeds in a cup of water, or replace up to a third of the oats I'm cooking with plantain seeds and cook as usual. Metamucil contains the seed husks of a South American *Plantago.*

• **Pau d'arco** tea is regarded as a specific remedy against thrush.

## Maintaining Strong Veins

When cytotoxic drugs such as Adriamycin, mitomycin, vinblastine and vincristine are administered by IV or injection, they can burn the veins and leave them visibly dark. Repeated blood tests can leave veins with so many wounds that they collapse. The orthodox solution is to install a mediport, a surgically implanted access to a vein. This eliminates repeated needle sticks but increases the risk of infection—which can quickly become life-threatening, given that chemotherapy depresses the production of white blood cells.

★ **Nettle infusion** has a reputation for giving you veins as strong and resilient as a teenager's. **Burdock** root, **horsetail** herb, **hawthorn** berries, **oatstraw**, or **shepherd's purse** herb (*Bursa capsella-pastoris*) also help maintain the integrity of the veins, strengthening their connective tissues, and increasing their flexibility. I use them as infusions (a cup or more a day) or tinctures (10–25 drops up to three times a day).

## Anemia and Platelet Damage

Chemotherapeutic agents can kill platelets and red blood cells, opening the way to iron-deficiency anemia and hemorrhage.

★ **Yellow dock** builds strong blood. Daily doses of 5–20 drops of the root tincture will increase iron levels in the blood twice as fast as supplements. Yellow dock is tumor-suppressive and liver-strengthening. If you're experiencing diarrhea, use yellow dock with caution, as it may loosen the bowels. If you wish to avoid alcohol, soak chopped fresh yellow dock roots in vinegar to cover for 6 weeks and use 1 tablespoon/15 ml a day of the resulting medicinal vinegar instead.

• Other green allies that build blood health and keep iron levels high include dried **apricots, pau d'arco** herb, the roots and leaves of **dandelion,** and the leaves of **amaranth, collards, comfrey, kale, lamb's quarters, nettle, plantain,** and **seaweed**.

## Exhaustion

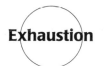

Exhaustion, normal during chemotherapy, is worse with mito-mycin. More remedies for fatigue are on page 218.

• Fatigue can be a symptom of anemia. (*See* page 238.)

• Remember Step 0. Give yourself permission to **do nothing**. Rest. Sleep. Take care of you.

★ Instead of herbal stimulants (e.g., coffee, chocolate, guarana, ephedra), I increase my energy by nourishing myself with green allies like **wheat grass** juice (an ounce a day), **nettle** infusion (up to a quart a day), **Siberian ginseng** (up to 100 drops a day), and **schisandra** berry tincture (up to 150 drops a day).

• **Dexamethasone** (Decadron) is a corticosteroid drug offered as an aid to dealing with the side effects of chemotherapy. It can make you feel too hyped up to sleep for days—and then so exhausted you can barely move. Let **oatstraw** infusion make the landing softer.

*"It took me a full year after the treatments were done to return to my usual self and my usual energy level. "*        Sherryl, age 34

## Hair Loss, Sore Scalp

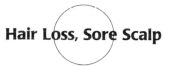

Hair loss isn't a side effect of every chemotherapy, but it's likely with Adriamycin, Cytoxan, 5-Flu, melphalan, Methotrexate, mitomycin, vincristine, or vinblastine. Hair usually starts to re-grow about six weeks after chemotherapy treatments end.

★ **Stinging nettle** infusion hastens regrowth of hair and dimin-ishes hair loss during chemo. There's a recipe for nettle hair tonic in my book *Healing Wise*. And more remedies on pages 216-217.

★ Even if you keep your hair, your scalp may become tender and sore. Soothe it with **burdock seed oil** or **St. Joan's wort oil**.

• Every book offering advice for women dealing with chemotherapy recommends a wig. But every woman I've met who's dealt with short-term hair loss said she preferred a scarf, a hat, being bald, **anything but a wig**. Wigs are easily available, if not in a nearby store, then by mail order overnight, so why not wait until the last minute to buy one? You might discover you don't want it after all.

## Induced Menopause

Induced menopause, whether from chemotherapy, surgery, or radiation, is harsher than natural menopause, but taking hormones is not the only way to ease symptoms and preserve your health. I know several women who refused them, ate well and exercised regularly, and are healthy and strong decades later.

★ **Chaste tree** berries help re-establish menses that have stopped prematurely as a result of chemotherapy. They also shrink cystic lumps in the breasts, restore hormonal sanity, and protect you against recurrence of breast cancer. The usual dose is 30 drops of tincture 3–4 times daily.

• Tincture of **motherwort** or **oats** (25 drops of either, once or twice a day) are favorite ways to help ease hot flashes, upset nerves, and a variety of other menopausal symptoms.

• Another ally for women with menopausal distress is **milk thistle** seed tincture, 25 drops on awaking and as desired throughout the day. See my book *Menopausal Years, The Wise Woman Way* for more ways to ease the myriad miseries of induced menopause.[13]

## Unwanted Weight Gain

The most common reasons for weight gain (typically 10–20 pounds, but sometimes much more) during and after chemotherapy include: use of tamoxifen, use of prednisone, sudden onset of menopause, and energy changes in the body.

★ **Superb nourishment** is critical during chemotherapy. This is not the time for a weight-loss diet. But **chickweed salad, fennel**

**seed tea**, and **bladderwrack soup** offer nourishing choices for women wanting to speed up their metabolisms, improve thyroid function, and lose some weight.

I have yet to find a limit to the amount of fresh chickweed (*Stellaria media*) that can be eaten when it's in season (spring and fall in most places). I cut it into inch-long pieces and eat it in my salads. Fennel (*Foeniculum vulgare*) tea–a spoonful of seeds steeped for 15 minutes in a cup of water just off the boil–is delicious hot or cold, sweetened or not. To make bladderwrack (*Fucus*) soup, I cover a handful of the dried bladderwrack seaweed with cold water and simmer it for 15 minutes, then drink a cup of the resulting liquid. (Put the leftover seaweed on your houseplants or compost it.) Best results accrue from daily use for 3 months.

★ The body can become dense when, to protect against harm from chemotherapy, the liver and the aura hold in energy. This density manifests as heaviness, that is, weight gain. **Meditations** or **shamanic journeys** can shift this heavy energy out of your physical body, helping you prevent unwanted weight gain, and offering you other ways to protect yourself.

## Vaginal Dryness

Sudden vaginal dryness and sexual dysfunction are especially distressing side effects of chemotherapy. They can strike another blow to a self-image already hit hard by cancer, magnifying fears of sexual undesirability, unlovability, even death.

• Many women report success increasing vaginal moisture with daily doses of 10–25 drops of **motherwort** tincture. For lots more remedies, see *Menopausal Years, The Wise Woman Way.*[13]

★ Here's the advice of one of the most extraordinary crones I've ever climbed a 14,000 foot peak with, Dolores LaChapelle, age 76. (Her book–*Sacred Land, Sacred Sex*–is a classic of woman-centered ecological awareness.[14])

"I insert **acidophilus capsules for vaginal dryness**. I have found over a period of years that I have to do this to sleep well, so once a week I do it. This is especially important for menopausal women. And it always works. There is a place to order them specifically for that. Along with your order comes a great plastic gadget to insert the capsules that makes it easier. They are expensive ($13.10 for ten Vagilac capsules plus the applicator), but you only need to order them once and then you'll have the inserter to use with any acidophilus capsules. I haven't found a U.S. distributor. Address: Rosell Institute, 8480 Boul. St. Laurent, Montreal, Quebec, Canada, H2P 2M6. Phone: 514-381-5631. I always send a Canadian money order."

## Your Sex Drive

Being scared to death is sexy for a few people, but for the rest it's a turnoff. Furthermore, stress, surgery, anesthesia, chemotherapy, and radiation directly interfere with libido by reducing minerals needed for hormone production, and by depressing the functioning of hormone-control glands.

★ These sexy herbs nourish libido and may help you find the mood again, even if you think you're beyond help: infusion of **oatstraw**, **burdock**, or **nettle** (up to a quart a day); or tinctures of **motherwort**, **chaste tree**, **ginseng**, **oats** or **Siberian ginseng** (25–75 drops a day); or–highly recommended–**marijuana**.

• Increase your libido by increasing the amount of **iodine** in your diet. Foods from the ocean–seaweed, fish, shellfish–are aphrodisiacs, say many writers (and lovers).

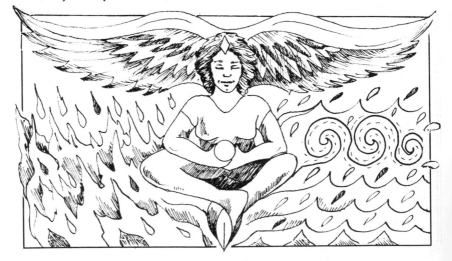

# Herbal Allies for Women Choosing Chemotherapy

| | astragalus | burdock | marijuana | comfrey leaf | dandelion | echinacea | kelp | milk thistle | motherwort | mushrooms | nettles | plantain | red clover | Sib'n ginseng | slippery elm | valerian | yellow dock | yogurt |
|---|---|---|---|---|---|---|---|---|---|---|---|---|---|---|---|---|---|---|
| adrenal help | ☆ | | | | | | ☆ | | | ★ | ★ | | | ☆ | | | | |
| anemia | ☆ | ☆ | | ☆ | ★ | | ☆ | | | | ★ | ★ | ☆ | | | | ★ | |
| anti-cancer | ☆ | ★ | ☆ | ★ | ★ | ★ | ☆ | ☆ | | ★ | ★ | ☆ | ★ | ☆ | | ☆ | ★ | ☆ |
| anti-drug* | | ★ | | | | ☆ | ★ | ★ | | ☆ | | | ☆ | ★ | | | | ★ |
| anti-infection | ☆ | | | | | ★ | | | | | ☆ | | | | | | | ☆ |
| anti-stress | ☆ | ☆ | ★ | | ☆ | | ★ | ☆ | ☆ | ☆ | ★ | | ☆ | ★ | | ☆ | | |
| appetite | ☆ | ☆ | ★ | ☆ | ★ | | ★ | | | ☆ | ☆ | | ☆ | | ★ | | ☆ | ★ |
| bone marrow | ★ | | | | | | | | | ☆ | | ☆ | | | | | | |
| constipation | | ☆ | ★ | ☆ | ☆ | | ☆ | ☆ | | | ☆ | ★[1] | ☆ | | | ★ | ★ | ★ |
| diarrhea | | | | ★ | | | | | | | | | | | | ★ | | ★ |
| energy | ☆ | ☆ | | ☆ | ☆ | | ★ | | | ☆ | ★ | ☆ | | ★ | ☆ | | ★ | ☆ |
| hair | | ★[1] | | ☆ | | | ★ | | | | ★ | | | | | | | |
| heart | | | | | | | ★ | | ★ | | | | | | | | | |
| heavy menses | | | | ★ | ☆ | | ☆ | | | | ★ | ★ | | | | | ★ | |
| hot flashes | | | | | ☆ | | | ★ | ★ | ★ | | | ☆ | ☆ | | | | |
| immunity | ★ | ☆ | | | ☆ | ★ | ☆ | | | ★ | ★ | | ☆ | | | | | ★ |
| libido | ☆ | ☆ | ★ | | | | ★ | | ★ | ★ | | | ☆ | ☆ | | | | |
| liver | | ☆ | | ★ | | | ★ | ☆ | | | ☆ | ☆ | ☆ | ☆ | | | ★ | |
| mouth sores | | ☆ | | ★ | | | ☆ | | | | | ★[1] | | | ★ | | ☆ | ★ |
| nausea | | ★ | ☆ | ☆ | | | ☆ | | | | | | | | ★ | | ☆ | ★ |
| pain | | | ☆ | ☆ | | | | | ★ | | | ☆ | ★ | | ☆ | | | ☆ |
| phytosterols | ★ | ☆ | ★ | ☆ | ★ | | | ☆ | | | | | ★ | ☆ | ☆ | ☆ | ☆ | |
| thrush | | | | | | | ☆ | | | | | ★[1] | ☆ | | ☆ | | | ★ |
| vagina, dry | | | | | | | ★ | | ★ | | | | | | ★ | | | ★ |
| veins | | ☆ | | ★ | | | ★ | | | | | ★ | | | | | | |
| vomiting | | | ★ | ☆ | ☆ | | ☆ | ☆ | | | | | | | | ★ | | ★ |

\* *stops poisoning without hindering cancer-killing effects*   [1]Seeds

☆ = **effective**     ★ = **very effective**

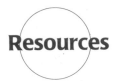

# Resources

• Chemocare, 231 North Ave.W., Westfield, NJ 07090; 908-233-1103 or 1-800-55-CHEMO; will connect you, at no charge, with a trained support person who has successfully completed the same chemotherapy (or radiation) treatment you have chosen.

• "Medical Use of Whole Cannabis: Statement of the Federation of the American Scientists," from F.A.S., 307 Massachusetts Ave. N.E., Washington, DC, 20002; 202-546-3300

• Suggested reading:
*Breast Cancer, What You Should Know (But May Not Be Told)*, Steve
    Austin and Cathy Hitchcock, Prima, 1994
*Chemotherapy Survival Guide*, Judith McKay, R.N., and Nancy
    Hirano, R.N., New Harbinger, 1993
*Coping with Chemotherapy*, Nancy Bruning, Ballantine, 1989
*Questioning Chemotherapy*, Ralph Moss, Equinox, 1994

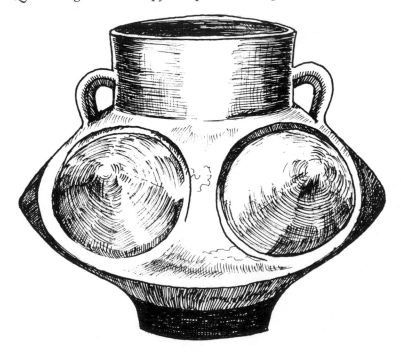

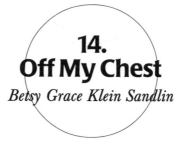

# 14.
# Off My Chest

*Betsy Grace Klein Sandlin*

I first found the lump 16 years ago. I was living in New York; I had a mammogram, and was told: Nothing to worry about, probably cystic.

Six years later, after the deaths of my closest college friend, my mother, my favorite uncle, and my husband of 11 years, and after moving to the desert with my seven-year-old son, the presence in my left breast began to grow perceptibly. For three months I drank violet infusion and used violet leaf poultices externally on the lump. And, when the lentil-sized lump in the inner right quadrant of my left breast did not stabilize or get smaller, echinacea tincture internally.

Knowing very little about breast cancer (although I remembered that my father's mother, Bessie, after whom I am named, died of it), I had the lump biopsied, and did some preliminary research in local libraries and bookstores. By then I knew that it was cancer, it was growing, and I needed to do something more aggressive than violet, and soon. I do believe that violet, my slimy friend, helped to keep my cancer in check, giving me time I very much needed. Time to do research, time to deal with the tricky elements of single-parenting my son, and time to prepare for the removal of my front porch.

In August of 1989 I gave both breasts to the first surgeon I encountered. Both, because statistically, the type of cancer I had, infiltrating lobular, had a 74 percent chance of appearing in my other breast within 14 months. Releasing my consciousness to anesthesia was the most stressful part of the surgery. I recovered quickly and went home as soon as allowed, to begin processing what it was to be a woman in her forties with no breasts. I learned much about being merciful to myself during this time; Stephen and Ondrea Levine's meditation tapes were helpful and reassuring. Family and friends gave me a center, a cup of tea, a tender hug, laughs, feedback, tears, comfort.

The pathology report after the bilateral mastectomy indicated that the lymph nodes were clear—no sign of metastasis—and that my cancer was estrogen-positive. Tamoxifen, among the most benign of the hormone therapies, was prescribed, 10 mg twice a day. It blocks estrogen by mimicking it at the receptor sites. I read about the drug, prayed at the pharmaceutical altar that I would survive its (for me, minimal) side effects, and took it. And still do, after a hiatus described later.

Breastless and well healed, I sought comfort in the bosom of cleavage. The first reconstructive surgeon I visited sat back in an elegant office, gracefully gesticulating with his hand about the perfection of "his" nipples. My heart started beating wildly, my mouth went dry. I left abruptly and never returned. This had occurred with the first oncologist I saw, too: I wouldn't let him examine me after we'd talked for about 15 minutes, and I left shaking and perspiring profusely. I thought I was playing some kind of wretched game with myself about not wanting to resolve this medical crisis I was facing, but I know now that it was gut-level politics, and that the choices I made were based on my body's reactions.

The second surgeon looked directly into my eyes when he addressed me. He wanted to know how I felt, what I thought, what my ideas were about the procedure, my expectations, my fears. He welcomed three intense half-hour sessions with friends and family; he was as patiently abiding and informative with them as he was with me.

After lengthy consideration of the options, I chose insertion of silicone bags directly into my chestwall muscles, which were developed and stretched from years of yoga. The doc said I would be sore—a rare understatement from a Texan. I was multi-colored, from my clavicles to my waist, for weeks, and I cried that first night after the anesthesia wore off for every abused human on the face of the planet. But, the surgery accomplished in one operation what usually takes at least two, and I didn't get nauseous thanks to lengthy discussions before the operation with the compassionate anesthesiologist (not an oxymoron).

Five months later the same surgeon flensed my groin, stripping off patches of skin to make nipples with. The flesh there is just enough darker than chest flesh to create a contrast. He took two small slices, put a hole in one of them, and pulled the other one, bunched up, partially through the hole. Sounds gruesome, but it actually was the easiest and most painless of all the surgeries, and my skin healed very fast. The acquisition of nipples for me was solely aesthetic. When you lose your nipples, you lose much of the early warning system for cold; the reconstructed ones have no such sensitive temperature receptors. By this time—about five months after reconstruction—I was again doing yoga, working to encourage the rearranged muscles to do the right thing.

In the summer of '91 I stopped taking tamoxifen; it had been two years since the mastectomy and I was not aware that recurrence often occurs when it is stopped. My oncologist was reluctant, but I was persistent in wanting to be off medication.

In the spring of '92 I was standing on my head when I realized my breasts hurt: They were tender, sensitive. That's funny, I thought, what I have is silicone, not breast tissue. Wrong. The subsequent nightmare—discovery of a recurrent lump in the original site, other lumps, needle biopsy, remastectomy on the left side and removal of the implant (*ciao* cleavage) (and all this weeks before a planned three-week trip to Scotland)—is mercifully obscured by the mists of time. More than three ounces of breast tissue was removed from the left breast by another surgeon, a breast specialist this time around. (The good news is that the first surgeon has retired. The lesson is: Seek specialists.) Two lymph nodes out of the ten extracted during this fourth surgery were positive. Back on tamoxifen and six months of chemotherapy.

Menopause was finally wrought upon me during this ordeal by the combination of drugs and time. It was a bitch, and I never knew what was the specific cause of the multiple distresses I experienced. It was all I could do to get through the day and know I was one day closer to being done with the process. I vacillated between exhaustion and tenacity, a fierceness overcoming me at times that carried me through the physically debilitating effects of the chemo and untold, unnameable menopausal states of being.

Herbal allies were so important to me at this time of chemical assault from without and within. Trying to prepare a meal for my son with wave after wave of inability to confront food, the deep retching response arising, arising: Stick a thumbnail into fresh ginger, or into a lime, and repeat Mama's mantra: "Dear God Give Me Strength."

I used motherwort tincture when wombness was more than I could bear, and felt the easing of the pulling as blood spiraled inward and stopped trying to leave on a regular schedule. Nettle and more nettle infusion, the silken comfort of green nourishment, so simple, so useful, so strengthening to my nails and hair. Oatstraw infusion helped me get the goddamn situation of being treated with life-threatening chemicals into manageable perspective, helped me into more relaxed states. And the reassuring smell of slippery elm powder with maple syrup, little balls popped onto a coated tongue to just sit there, allaying nausea.

I think the most helpful of all the herbal substances that I used during those six months of chemo-assault was milk thistle seed tincture, which unfailingly dissipated the dull ache which frequently arose under my right ribs. Liver? Gall bladder? Don't know. I took it as many times a day as the spot ached, and it always brought relief. And the most helpful food for me during chemotherapy? Mama's Marrow Soup, a bone-deep brew. (The recipe is on page 312.)

An interesting aside: I often experienced nasty flashes of nausea, months after the cessation of treatment, when passing the office where my chemo had been administered. How many of our reactions in life are the result of expectation, fear, programming?

The first time through the breast labyrinth the insurance from my husband's union paid for 80 percent of everything, right through the reconstruction. I was given five years after my husband's death to continue with the union's insurance plan; I was aware that after the five years (which expired in '91) I would have to find other insurance.

Hah. There is no insurance that will cover cancer survivors until you've made it seven, or even ten years past the end of the last treatment. But my oncologist has been clever and generous in advising me which drug companies offer reductions or deferrals or elimination of fees for the drugs; and some of the laboratories have offered blood analyses at greatly reduced cost or *gratis*. I'm lucky to live near enough to the Mexican border to get tamoxifen at less than half the cost of any pharmacy on this side of the border. Nevertheless, in the year in which I had the remastectomy and chemo, my medical bills totaled over $14,000, of which I paid 100 percent.

"Always do something," said Janice Guthrie from the Health Resource, and—whether it's vitamins or Essiac or yoga or prayer or chanting or a thousand other "ors"—I need to do something that inspires, awakens, fortifies, energizes. After four surgeries, chemotherapy, and menopause, I emerged pale and enervated, seeking nothing, yearning for naught but the down comforter. I was left, two months after the last chemo treatment, directionless. I was waiting, waiting, scripting deathbed scenes, unable to find even the enthusiasm to share tea and crumpets with my best friend,

speculating whether my family would need to advise the cremato-
rium of my silicone implant so I wouldn't cause an explosion in
the oven when they reduce me to ashes . . . death by unchanneled,
uncontrolled thought.

I followed friend Sherry's suggestion that I get some help
and a good haircut. Counseling, and working out at a club owned
by a woman who also had breast cancer and was giving out passes
for a week of free classes, set me back on the lifetrack. Counseling
afforded me a repository for the parts of my cancer experience
which I was unwilling to deposit with family or friends. I began to
recover my physical being by doing low-impact aerobics, and then
moved on to yoga classes, persistence at which has rejuvenated
me with greater strength, stamina and flexibility than ever before
in my life.

I became aware of the healing power of others' love for
me after the bilateral mastectomy, lying in my hospital bed. I was
alone and feeling sorry for myself, wondering how I would ever
get through the abyss of dis-ease-ness and emerge from it alive, let
alone well. And my son! What had I put him through? Grief seemed
endless in our lives. Rather suddenly, a current coursed through
my body in wave after wave, a hum, reassuring, the physical sensation lasting for several minutes during which I was absolutely
still and at peace. I felt carried by this current, borne along on the
good wishes of loved ones. It left me refreshed and optimistic and
rested, even in that fearsome place. That feeling of buoyancy in an
ocean of love is easier and easier for me to tune into now as I
distance myself from disease. Sometimes it's just there, a thread
connecting me to a known Good, a quantifiable inoculation of hope.

The family and friends who supported, guided, helped,
and nurtured me through these experiences were the most influential factor in my rapid healing, I feel sure. The doctors said that
the incisions sealed up "remarkably" quickly, and indeed my re-
cuperation was rapid. Maybe I was a healthy specimen to begin
with, or maybe I just couldn't wait to get out of the hospital (albeit
a kind and not unpleasant one) and back to my own home and
hearth.

I figure life's about an even mix of pain and joy and all the
other dualities we've created with Mind. There are, indeed, times
when not only does nothing hurt, everything actually feels whole
and filled with light. I do what feels good as often as possible. I
utilize a lot of herbs to feel my best. Milk thistle tincture, burdock
tincture, usnea tincture; St. Joan's and wintergreen and arnica oils

to grease my pelt. I sit in hot baths and worship at the tile throne of the steamroom. I take the clues as they appear. Yoga has taught me how to feel better; from that vantage point I am able to discern and pursue what feels good, as I leave behind the statistics, the poisons, the fears, the doubts.

All along I'd been aware of and reading about the kind of cancer I am living with (infiltrating lobular) and its characteristics. For as long I could, I worked the statistics in my favor, hoping for the high end of the good news. When I gave up statistic-scanning, as I did when they were no longer so favorable, the focus turned inward. Perhaps it was the fear, the inability to face the dread within: Was it growing, were the chemicals killing those bad guys they found in the nodes, were they running amok in my lymph system? Perhaps it was just, at last, time in my life to get serious about actually doing meditation practice. Not reading about it, not talking about it, not thinking, or cogitating on meditating. Sit: Turn off the phone, evoke the power and guidance of a mantra, and don't fall asleep. Do it and discover quickly how to get beyond the business menu of the mind.

It is meditation that affords me the most equilibrium. I yearn to be doing it again, more. And I do. I find that I am so constructing my life that I may partake of this meditative window at regular intervals. It has become a glue of my well being, and I am grateful for it. Whether I cure or heal, I know that this process of cancer is part of my life. Whether it will be part of my death I can wait to find out. I have much to live for, and my life is rich with blessings. I continue, cytologically challenged, humming with the vibrations of life around and within me. Maybe some of that hum is cancer. Maybe it will eat me. Maybe I will eat it.

It's all idle spec anyway, and trying to figure it out can get you tied in knots. Better just to sit, to be, to do, doo bee doo bee doo.

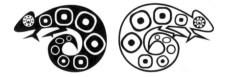

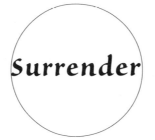

# Surrender

"The shining star in your breast has birthed sister stars who now shine forth from deep in your bones/liver/lungs. Dear GrandDaughter, be at peace. You are coming home, as we all are coming home. No matter what you are told, your time of arrival is no more certain than anyone else's.

"Now is the time to surrender. To surrender to your life. Surrender and this will nourish your health/your wholeness/your holiness. Surrender is the ultimate negation of the role of victim, for surrender is not polite and surrender is not compliant. Surrender gives in but doesn't give up. In surrender there is choice. In surrender there is power. In surrender blame cannot grow. In surrender perfection unfolds.

"Surrender to your aggression. Find your fire, find your warrior spirit. Test the mettle of your worthy opponent. Exult in the fight! Unleash your fiercest aggression. Count coup on death. But beware of judging yourself by whether or not you win the fight, oh warrior. Death, like the river, comes on. And ultimately we each enter into the flow.

"Surrender to your desire to live even as you surrender to the reality that we all must die. Surrender to your hopes, your visions, your future. Surrender to the path of life, which leads us all to death.

"Come, sit in my lap, rest your head here on my shoulder. Relax, surrender. You are not in control; you have never been in control. You did not choose cancer; cancer chose you. You do not have to surrender to cancer; you have to surrender to yourself, to your life, which now includes cancer.

"It is not death that asks for your surrender; it is life – life in all of its inexplicable, uncontrollable, ecstatic complexity. Life asks you to surrender. Life in all its wildness asks All of you."

251

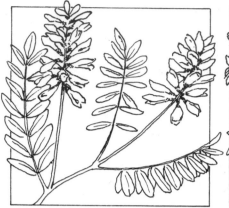

Astragalus (A. canadensis)

Chaparral (Larrea tridentata)

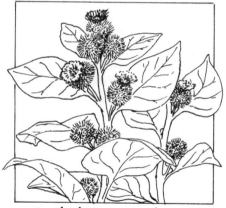

Burdock (Arctium lappa)

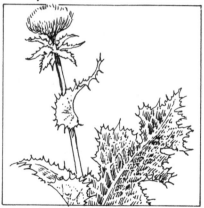

Milk thistle (Carduus marianum)

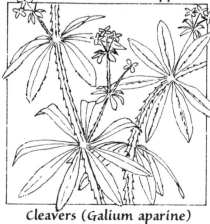

Cleavers (Galium aparine)

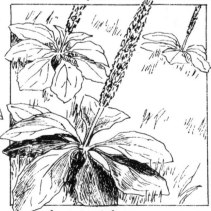

Plantain (Plantago major)

# 15.
# Late Stage Breast Cancer?

A diagnosis of late-stage metastatic cancer is something no one wants to give, or to hear, for metastatic cancer is curable only by miracles . . . *which definitely do happen.*[1]

When breast cancer metastasizes, it sheds cells which look for homes in the liver, lungs, bones, and sometimes the brain. If these shed cells grow, they can crowd out functional cells and cause death (by liver failure, inability to breathe, lack of new blood cells). No matter how large a primary breast cancer grows, it is not a threat to life—as long as it stays confined to the breast. But once it begins to invade critical organs, lifespan becomes dependent on keeping the secondary tumors as small as possible.

For some women, a diagnosis of "terminal" cancer brings up so much fear that any treatment, no matter how bizarre or damaging, seems attractive: whether it is coffee enemas three times a day, or being killed with chemotherapy and brought back to life. For some, any treatment is worthwhile if it offers a few more days to be with loved ones. For others, as for Audre Lorde and Jackie Kennedy Onassis, the diagnosis triggers a decision to "spend" the remaining time (in their communities, living and dying) rather then trying to "buy" time (in hospitals, being treated and dying).

No matter what choices you make when the diagnosis is grim, Wise Woman ways can help you enjoy every turn and each sway of your final waltz or your last tango . . . no matter how abbreviated or extended.

## Step 0. *Do Nothing*

• There's nothing to do and everything to **be**.

• Just as when you were first diagnosed with breast cancer: Stop. Frequently a sense of failure comes with a diagnosis of metastatic disease. This feeling of failure can open the door to the role of willing victim: It's easier to do whatever you're told, easy to be swept away by fear, grief, and betrayal, to go along while others decide on your treatment. **Stop**. This is not a test. This is your life. You don't have to be a victim. (Fighting the cancer can be done as a victim, if you're ready to lay down the fight but continue only because others want you to.)

Don't commit to any treatment unless it feels right to you and you feel ready for it. Now, more than ever, the best choices are the ones you feel best about, no matter what anyone else says is best for you. Many women find it helpful to take some time off to be **alone**, on retreat, doing nothing, before making treatment decisions. Others find solitude too difficult to bear.

★ The simplest **meditation**—on nothing—is the most effective. Trying to control the process of healing can be frustrating; meditating on eliminating the cancer, or any specific result, makes success elusive. Allowing the mind to be empty on a regular basis—even for a short time daily—makes room for spontaneous, out-of-the-ordinary, against-the-odds remission.

### Step 1. *Collect Information*

★ When the diagnosis is terminal, the Wise Woman Tradition suggests **the path of the heart**. The heart reminds us to be wary of those using fear tactics, and to question statistics. Orthodox therapies are more closely studied, but no more successful in prolonging life, increasing well being, and causing remission of metastasized breast cancer than the best of the non-orthodox therapies.

• Step 1 is also **"share information."** If time seems short, remember, you still have choices. You could tell your story of breast cancer to help other women. You could create a scrapbook for your family. Start a foundation. Write poetry. Patent your inventions. Become a phone-calling, letter-writing activist to help younger women avoid breast cancer. Paint, draw, sculpt, sing, photograph, sew, build. However you do it, you still have time to live artfully. It could heal you; it could show you how you are whole. You don't have to spend the last of your time and money resisting death.

**Step 2.** *Engage the Energy*

★ Women with metastasized breast cancer who attend a weekly **support group** live twice as long as women who don't.

• Spend some time talking to your death. Make plans for your future. Be here now.

• Gay Luce, founder of Seven Gates Mystery School, offers this query for all of us: "What do you need in order to die complete and happy, satisfied and smiling? Get it. Do it. Say it."

**Step 3.** *Nourish and Tonify*

★ Women dancing with metastatic cancer who want high levels of nutrients without the risks of supplements do this: Every day they eat generous helpings of carotene-rich foods, cabbage family vegetables, beans, seaweeds, and wild mushrooms. In addition, they include in their daily diet: A quart/liter of a nourishing and cancer-inhibiting infusion (e.g., **nettle, comfrey leaf, red clover, violet**, or **burdock root**); one or more large spoonfuls of a liver-strengthening, anti-tumor herbal vinegar (e.g., **dandelion, burdock, yellow dock** roots); and a dose of an anti-cancer, immune-strengthening tincture (e.g., **echinacea, poke, usnea, astragalus**, or **burdock**). *See* Materia Medica.

★ Research in Asia shows that **wild mushrooms** can slow tumor growth by 40 percent. Read more about them on page 86.

• **Carotenes** counter all phases of the cancer cascade and are as important to the woman with metastasized cancer as the one who wants to prevent it. As little as one **carrot** a day can retard the progression of cancer. In some cases and in some laboratory studies, carrots have enabled cells to return to normal, leaving no remaining trace of cancer. (More about carotenes on page 47.)

★ Foods from the **cabbage family** are exceptional sources of phytochemicals which help reverse cancer metastases. So do the lignans in **beans**.

★ Of laboratory animals with advanced breast cancer who ate the seaweed **kelp**, 95 percent lived longer than expected.

• According to Neal Barnard, M.D., a woman with metastatic breast cancer increases her risk of dying by 40 percent for every extra 1,000 grams of fat included in her diet per month.[2] The best fats for women with cancer–from strictly organic sources, please–are **flax seed oil, olive oil, nuts,** and **fatty fish.**

**Step 4.** *Stimulate and Sedate*

★ Women with liver metastases who took **evening primrose oil** (2–3 teaspoons/9–18 grams of oil or 18–36 capsules a day) reduced the size of their tumors and doubled their survival time. Although most of the women in the group had a prognosis of less than two months' life expectancy, 12 percent of the group taking

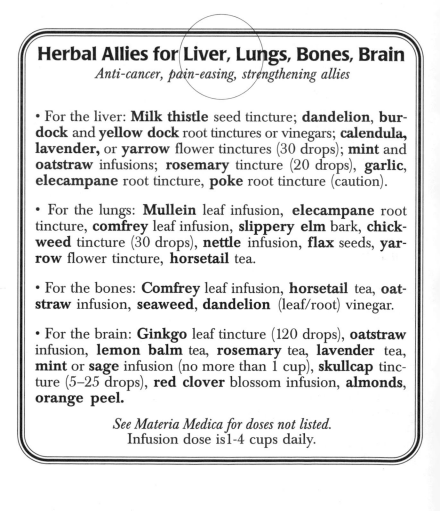

# Herbal Allies for Liver, Lungs, Bones, Brain
*Anti-cancer, pain-easing, strengthening allies*

• For the liver: **Milk thistle** seed tincture; **dandelion, burdock** and **yellow dock** root tinctures or vinegars; **calendula, lavender,** or **yarrow** flower tinctures (30 drops); **mint** and **oatstraw** infusions; **rosemary** tincture (20 drops), **garlic, elecampane** root tincture, **poke** root tincture (caution).

• For the lungs: **Mullein** leaf infusion, **elecampane** root tincture, **comfrey** leaf infusion, **slippery elm** bark, **chickweed** tincture (30 drops), **nettle** infusion, **flax** seeds, **yarrow** flower tincture, **horsetail** tea.

• For the bones: **Comfrey** leaf infusion, **horsetail** tea, **oatstraw** infusion, **seaweed, dandelion** (leaf/root) vinegar.

• For the brain: **Ginkgo** leaf tincture (120 drops), **oatstraw** infusion, **lemon balm** tea, **rosemary** tea, **lavender** tea, **mint** or **sage** infusion (no more than 1 cup), **skullcap** tincture (5–25 drops), **red clover** blossom infusion, **almonds, orange peel.**

*See Materia Medica for doses not listed.*
Infusion dose is 1-4 cups daily.

evening primrose oil was still alive three years later. Evening primrose oil is usually 9 percent GLA (gamma-linoleic acid) which has been shown to prevent the proliferation of malignant cells and to reduce the growth rate of breast cancer in rats.

• **Whole body hyperthermia** is the medical name for one of the world's oldest methods of helping those with severe illness: getting them hot, hot, hot. Native American healers use heat and the power of prayer in the Stone People's Lodge, more commonly known as the sweat lodge; in Scandinavia, the sauna is preferred. Medical literature is sprinkled with dramatic cancer cures occurring after infections which caused very high fevers, especially erysipelas. In one study, a dose of **Coley's Mixed Toxins** (given in an IV or injected directly into a solid tumor) strong enough to produce a fever of 101°F or higher within an hour, put 50 percent of those with metastases into remission. (Coley's Mixed Toxins was removed from the American Cancer Society's list of unproven remedies in 1972.)

• **Hansi** is a combination botanical and homeopathic remedy developed in Argentina by Dr. Juan Hirschmann. Of the 65,000 people with "terminal" metastases who've used it, many have had complete or partial remission.[3] Sometimes the metastases did not shrink, but the blood supply to the tumor shut down and surgery successfully removed the necrotic tumor. *See* Resources, page 261.

• Metastasized cancers can cause pain. See boxes on pages 256 and 258 for Wise Woman ways to ease it. And read *You Don't Have to Suffer: A Complete Guide to Relieving Cancer Pain for Patients and Their Families* (Resources, page 261).

**Step 5a.** *Use Supplements*

★ Coenzyme $Q_{10}$, at daily doses of 390 mg, caused complete remission of numerous metastases in the liver of a 44-year-old woman with breast cancer.[5] More information is available from Janice Guthrie of Health Resource; *see* page 261.

• In one study, those with terminal cancer who took 10 grams of **ascorbic acid** a day quadrupled their expected survival time. Critics note that all of the people in this study refused aggressive chemotherapy and speculate that that had as much to do with their increased longevity as the vitamin C.

## Dealing with Pain

• Stephen Levine's pain meditations are incredibly helpful.[4]

• Many writers note that those who reduce their pain, even if they must use large doses of pain-killers, have a better prognosis than those who stoically bear it. Pain-killing drugs are often dramatically less effective for women; don't be afraid to ask for more.

• **Skullcap** (5–10 drops fresh plant tincture) is my first choice for relieving pain as it is mildly anti-cancer. But repeated doses (several in an hour) may be very sleep-inducing. **Passion flower** (*Passiflora incarnata*) and **valerian** (*Valeriana officinalis*) root tincture are other frequently used herbal painkillers; the dose is 10–25 drops, repeated as needed. Stronger yet (and more sleep-inducing) are **hops** tea or **wild lettuce** (*Lactucca* species) sap in alcohol (10–20 drops).

• **Turkey corn** (*Corydalis formosa*) is a beautiful woodland plant whose root is tinctured and used as a painkiller in China when cancer is advanced, lymph nodes are swollen, and the skin is scaly. Dose: 5–20 drops. **Caution**: Toxic reactions can occur.

• Waiting for a delayed airplane in the Midwest, I struck up a conversation with a woman who, as chance would have it, has been doing research on cancer metastasis for several decades. "Prevent the cancer from forming blood vessels around itself and you will prevent most metastases," she told me. "Slow blood vessel growth and you slow metastatic growth."

★ **Genistein**, a phytochemical found in **chickweed, lentils,** and **tofu**, slows blood vessel growth and prevents tumors from forming new blood vessels: It is an anti-angiogenic factor. In addition to preventing metastases, anti-angiogenic factors are powerful, life-prolonging allies for women with metastatic cancer.

• A well-studied (but controversial) anti-angiogenic supplement is **shark cartilage**. Proponents claim that very, very high doses used for four to six months, can cause remission of metastatic and primary tumors, and that it extended the lives of more than half of the women with "terminal" breast cancer who took it.[6]

★ **Bromelain**, an enzyme found in pineapple, decreased lung metastases in animals—sometimes by as much as 90 percent—and primary tumors in addition to metastases in women.[7] Both dried and fresh forms were active.

**Step 5b.**  *Use Drugs*

• Several antihistamines—Claritin, Hismanal, and Atarax—and two antidepressants—Elavil and Prozac—have been shown to cause existing cancers to grow more quickly and act more aggressive.

★ When injectable **benzaldehyde** was used by those with terminal cancer in Japan, all lived longer than expected, and their tumors decreased in size or went into total remission. *See* page 47.

• An English study reported positive response within six weeks when women with advanced breast cancer took **oral thyroid extract**, 200 mg a day.

• A French M.D. reported a dramatic remission of breast cancer in a woman with an inoperable brain metastasis after she began taking 2.5 mg of **bromocriptine** three times a day.[8]

• An IV infusion of **pamidronate** can increase survival time for women with breast cancer metastasized to the bone by keeping their blood calcium levels within normal range. (Approximately half of the deaths from bone metastases are due to hypercalcemia.)

★ If you have metastasized breast cancer and chemotherapy is suggested, ask direct questions: What's the best I can expect? The worst? **It is not unusual to discover that you'll live longer (and more comfortably) if you refuse chemotherapy at this stage.** If you agreed to chemotherapy before, it may be hard to feel like you have the right to say "no" this time. But every situation is different, and what was right for you before may not be right for you now.

      Chemotherapy may be urged on you even when there is no hope that it will cure you of cancer. Why? To extend your life. (How long?) Or to try to shrink your tumor or decrease the number of tumors. (Will this shorten your life?) Or to satisfy a doctor's need for research subjects. (Who benefits?) Or to satisfy a doctor's emotional need to have something to offer you. (Is this what you want or need?) Or to "keep the patient oriented to orthodox medicine," according to Dr. Victor Richards.[9] (What might happen if you used non-orthodox treatments?)

• Most statements about the effectiveness of chemotherapy for metastatic disease refer to response rate. The response rate is the percentage of tumors which shrink partially or wholly in response to the chemotherapy. There is no study which connects tumor shrinkage with an increase in survival time, thus **response rate does not imply extended longevity**.

• **Taxol** and taxol sisters are currently the drugs of choice for the woman whose metastatic breast cancer is unresponsive to other agents. Although taxol can delay the growth of metastatic tumors, it does little to increase actual survival time. Taxol is especially toxic to bone marrow and may cause loss of sensation in the toes and fingers.

• People with "terminal" cancer are considered good guinea pigs for trials of new protocols and treatments. Maybe you'd prefer to test alternatives to orthodox treatment. If so, keep records—and work with someone who can substantiate your results—so others may benefit from your experience.

**Step 6.** *Break & Enter*

• **Autologous bone marrow transplant** (ABMT) is considered a last hope for women with metastasized breast cancer. But a review of 40 studies (published in the October 1995 *Journal of American Medical Association*) concluded that "the available data suggest that ABMT not only fails to extend the lives of women with metastatic breast cancer, but is also likely to be life shortening." The Japanese herbal formula **Juzentaihoto** (page 300) is a complementary medicine for women choosing ABMT. It nourishes the spleen, keeps the blood healthy, and accelerates recovery from injury to the bone marrow. You will also want to build powerful immunity; *see* Chapter 4.

# Resources
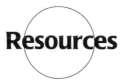

- **Hansi** information: Sasha White, PO Box 6, Boulder, CO 80306
- Health Resource, Inc., 209 Katherine Dr., Conway, AR 72032; 501-329-5272
- Patient Advocates for Advanced Cancer Treatments (PAACT), PO Box 141695, Grand Rapids, MI 49514; 616-453-1477
- *You Don't Have to Suffer,* Susan Lang, Ohio University Press, 1994

**Thinking About Death:**
- *Dealing Creatively with Death: A Manual of Death Education & Simple Burial,* Ernest Morgan, Celo, 1990
- *Death: An Anthology of Ancient Texts, Songs, Prayers, and Stories,* David Meltzer, ed., North Point Press, 1984
- *Death, The Final Stage of Growth,* Elisabeth Kubler-Ross, Simon & Schuster, 1975
- *Healing into Life and Death,* Stephen Levine, Anchor, 1987
- *How We Die,* Sherwin Nuland, M.D., Vintage, 1993
- *The Sacred Art of Dying: How the World Religions Understand Death,* Kenneth Kramer, Paulist Press, 1992
- *Who Dies? An Investigation of Conscious Living and Conscious Dying,* Stephen Levine, Doubleday, 1982
- The **Hemlock Society**, 1-800-247-7421, provides information on ending your life when you choose.
- National **Hospice** Organization, 1901 N. Moore St., Suite 901, Arlington, VA 22209; 703-243-5900; fax: 703-525-5762, will connect you with local resources for excellent end-of-life pain management and support for dying at home.
- **Choice In Dying**, 200 Varick St., New York, NY 10014-4810; 1-800-989-WILL or 212-366-5540, offers information on living wills and medical directives.
- Advance Medical Directives help you be specific about life support and other medical choices: $5 plus SASE to: Harvard Medical School Health Publications, Dept. MD-MED, PO Box 380, Boston, MA 02117.

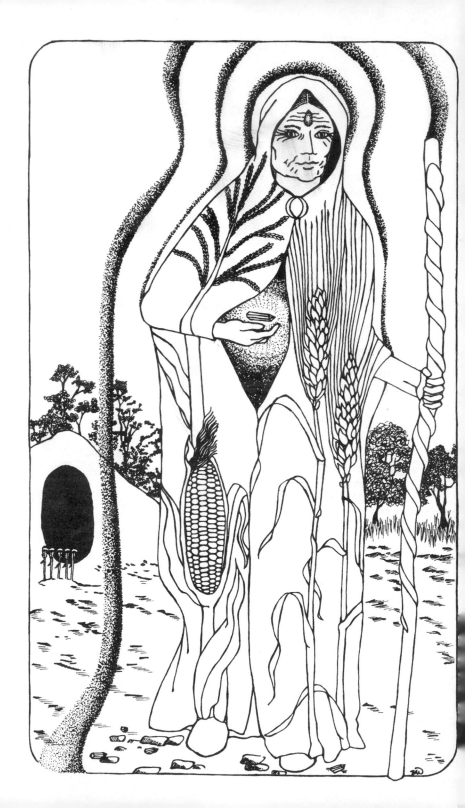

# Walk Toward Death

"You begin your walk toward death the moment you are conceived. Your life is your walk toward death. And each day your life brings you one day closer to death. Every day you have the opportunity to ask yourself: 'How will I walk today on my way to death? How will I live? By others' fears? Or by my own unique truth? In beauty, in joy, with awareness? From my heart?'

"Consciously or unconsciously, with acceptance or denial, every day you move one day nearer to your death. Is today a good day to die? Are you complete? Have you lived fully? Have you honored your dreams? Can you look death in the eye without regret?

"Death is not honorable in your dominant Western culture. You set death apart from life, portray death as if it were to be feared, as if it were opposed to life. No, precious GrandDaughter, no!

"Death and life are lovers. They are dancing partners. One does not exist without the other. Giving birth gives death, for death comes to all who are born. Death makes way for life, for is it not said that all who die will be reborn? Death and life in loving embrace; death and life dancing. For there is only the dance, only the walk, the path, your way from birth to death and back to birth again.

"Yes, GrandDaughter, your death is certain, but not predictable. Your death is known, yet it honors chaos; it neither avoids you when you would hold it off, nor arrives docilely when you call. There is no medical miracle, no right thinking, no correct eating, no magic, no saintliness, no bargain with God – or Goddess – which can avert or avoid the truth of your death.

"Your death waits patiently at the end of your path, around a bend you haven't noticed, hidden from sight. Your death. Your Way. In your own time.

"So many of your modern healers, alternative and orthodox alike, fear death. A diagnosis of cancer is made, and death becomes the enemy. Fear of death – rather than love of life – chooses the treatment. When you remember that every path ends in death, you can begin to dance with your death; your choices multiply and you find your way through the fear. You find ways to love your life without clinging. You find ways to honor your death.

"Yes, we know, death still calls forth fear in you. It is hard to honor it. Let us hold you, GrandDaughter. Rest in our gentle strength. Let us teach you to embrace your fear, to embrace the truth of your fear: with death your body ceases to be you.

"How can you honor your fear of death? Dance in the space between knowing and not knowing, between being and not being, between living and dying. We are here to hold you in your confusion. We will hold you in the midst of chaos. We will hold you safely, we will hold you close, now and whenever you call.

"We who are steeped with the wisdom of the years, we who have seen the spiraling dance of life and death, we have something to show you. Come with us now, GrandDaughter. Hold our hands and leap off the cliff. Fall with us. Give yourself to space. And look! A spiraling flow of sparkling joy catches you up and carries you off. Let go into the sensation of weightlessness, of being supported by a gently turning, vibrating spiral of particles that catch the light. A pulsing spiral with no beginning and no end. A spiral that holds you tightly, yet always allows you total freedom.

"Relax for a moment in the All. Reverberate with the silence. Let yourself move in perfection, expanding and growing, into life, into death, and, when you wish, back into life again."

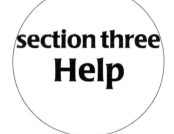

section three
# Help

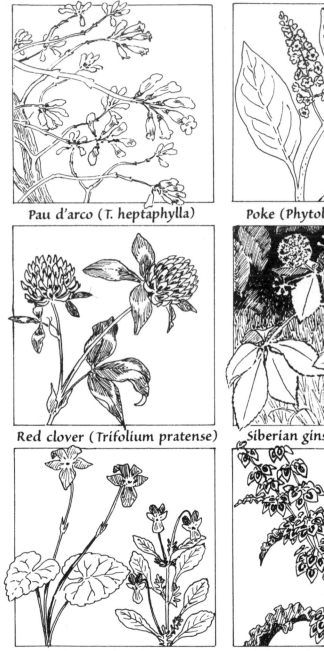

Pau d'arco (T. heptaphylla)

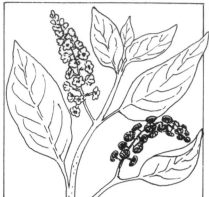

Poke (Phytolacca americana)

Red clover (Trifolium pratense)

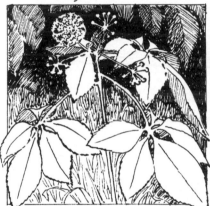

Siberian ginseng (Eleuthero)

Violet (Viola odorata)

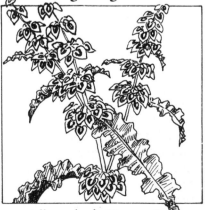

Yellow dock (Rumex)

# Materia Medica
## Herbal Allies

Here are the specifics you need to start using green allies now. Whether you want to preserve breast health, mitigate the side effects of orthodox treatments, prevent breast cancer recurrence, strengthen your immune system, or counter an early cancer, the information presented here (and in the next section) will help you help yourself to health with green allies.

Some of the plants discussed here are safe enough to be used as foods; others need to be used with caution. For greater peace of mind, use no more than two herbs a day, switching to others on different days if desired. Some herbs work well alone; others work well with partners. If you wish to make combinations, check the type of the herbs. A nourishing or tonifying herb may be combined with any other herb (even stimulating/sedating or potentially poisonous ones) as well as drugs. But if the herb is stimulating/sedating or potentially poisonous, it could be dangerous to combine it with stimulating/sedating herbs, potentially poisonous herbs, or drugs. (Type + indicates exceptional ability.) *Italicized actions are particulary strong.* **25 drops = 1 ml.**

## Astragalus
*Astragalus membranaceus, A. mongolicus, A. hoantchy*

**Other Names:** Yellow vetch, milk vetch root, Huang-qi
**Type:** Nourishing +
**Found in:** China; easily cultivated in North America; 400 species.
**Part Used:** Five-year-old, autumn-harvested roots.
**Actions & Uses:** *Enhances immune system* (restores T-cell function, increases interferon synthesis, strengthens killer cells); *invigorates,* builds rich blood; protects lungs; protects and restores bone marrow; improves appetite; *protects against stress* (protects spleen, adrenal cortex, and pituitary gland); relieves lymphedema;

lowers high blood pressure; anti-tumor; anti-inflammatory.

**Important Constituents:** Choline, betaine, glucuronic acid, linoleic and linolenic acids, phytosterols, polysaccharides, saponins, selenium and many other minerals.

**Preparation & Daily Dose:** No limit on duration of use.

    Dried root infusion: 1–4 cups.

    Cooked fresh roots: eaten freely.

    Tincture of fresh or dried root: 45–60 drops.

    Dried root: up to 2 ounces/60 grams.

**Toxicity:** None reported, even from large doses over long periods.

**Works Well With:** Echinacea, garlic.

**Results & Notes:** Life-span is significantly increased when astragalus is used as a *complementary medicine* with chemotherapy or radiation treatments, as is frequently the case in China.

**References:** 1, 7, 10, 21; illustrated on page 252.

# Burdock
### *Arctium lappa, A. minus*

**Other Names:** Gobo, Wu shih

**Type:** Tonifying +

**Found in:** Vacant lots, barnyards, roadsides, of temperate regions in Asia, Europe, and North America; easily cultivated.

**Part Used:** Fall-dug first-year roots; mature seeds.

**Actions & Uses:** *Internally–Anti-cancer, reverses pre-cancers and* in situ *cancers;* resolves chronic skin problems; fresh root binds and removes heavy metals and chemicals; *tones liver;* anti-tumor, anti-carcinogenic. *Externally–*Oil encourages growth of new hair.

**Important Constituents:** Essential oils, inulin, mucilage, phytosterols, tannins; selenium and many other minerals.

**Preparation & Daily Dose:** Use for six weeks to three years.

    Dried root infusion: 1–2 cups.

    Cooked, dried, or raw root: eaten freely.

    Fresh root vinegar: 1–4 tablespoons.

    Tincture of fresh roots or seeds: 30-250 drops.

    Infused oil of seeds: as needed on skin or scalp.

**Toxicity:** None known; extensively used.

**Works Well With:** Dandelion, red clover.

**Results & Notes:** Burdock is slow acting but miraculous. It is not unusual to take burdock regularly for 2–3 years. Literature citing burdock as a specific cure for breast cancer dates back to at least

1887 (in the Ukraine). Burdock root is a mainstay ingredient in many anti-cancer formulas (e.g., Hoxsey's Elixir, Essiac). I've seen regular use of the infusion or tincture eliminate precancerous cells and *in situ* cancers of the breast and cervix. Burdock is a highly regarded *complementary medicine,* and great preventive medicine, too.
**References:** 1, 4, 5, 6, 9, 10, 11, 21, 22, 24; illustrated on page 252.

# Chaparral
*Larrea tridentata, L. divaricata,* and other species

**Other Names:** Creosote bush, greasewood, hediondilla
**Type:** Stimulating/Sedating; Potentially Poisonous
**Found in:** Deserts of southwestern North America.
**Part Used:** Healthy leaves and stems, harvested anytime.
**Actions & Uses:** Shrinks tumors; improves energy and appetite; increases hair growth; enhances immune system; lowers blood pressure; Native American remedy against liver and lung cancers.
**Important Constituents:** Norhydroguariaretic acid (NDGA), antioxidants, camphor; selenium, zinc and many other minerals; essential oils including limonene and pinenes.
**Preparation & Daily Dose:** Used with caution for up to one year.
　　Fresh or dried herb infusion: 1–3 cups..
　　75% alcohol tincture of fresh or dried herb: 60–180 drops.
　　Dried herb: up to 14 grams.
**Toxicity:** Liver damage is possible, especially with long use.
**Works Well With:** Red clover, burdock.
**Results & Notes:** The bag was labeled: "Drink freely to prevent cancer." But I couldn't swallow more than a tiny sip of the resulting brew. It smelled like the inside of a stove pipe and tasted like dirty pipecleaners. Guess I didn't need it. That chaparral *is* drinkable is attested to by the thousands who've used the Hoxsey Elixir, which includes it, and by a breast cancer survivor who says: "The taste of the infusion wasn't great, but it felt better in my body than the tincture." Reports such as the one in *The Journal of the American Medical Association* (1995; 273: 489-90) about a woman who suffered severe liver damage after taking 2 tablets of chaparral daily for 10 months have made it increasingly difficult to buy chaparral, but it's easy to obtain if you live in the Southwest (or know someone who does) where it grows profusely.
**References:** 3, 10, 14, 21, 22; illustrated on page 252.

# Citrus
### *Citrus reticulata, C. aurantium*

**Other Names:** Bitter orange is specific, but any citrus is useful.
**Type:** Stimulating/Sedating
**Found in:** Tropical and sub-tropical regions of the world; easily cultivated where frost is rare, although *C. aurantium* will grow outdoors as far north as Baltimore, Maryland if given protection.
**Part Used:** Immature (green) peel and fruit.
**Actions & Uses:** *Relieves congestion*; reduces chest pains; heals abscesses; dissolves tumors; relieves menopausal symptoms; strengthens immune system; antiseptic, anti-cancer; traditional Chinese remedy against breast cancer.
**Important Constituents:** Antioxidants, carotenes, essential oils, flavonoids, phytoestrogens, vitamin C complex.
**Preparation & Daily Dose:** Used 3 weeks a month for 2-3 months.
      Dried peel: 3–9 grams.
      Fresh peel preserved in honey: 2 ounces/60 grams.
***Citrus Peel Honey:*** Juice several organic lemons or oranges. Drink juice. With a sharp knife, slice the peels, with clinging pulp, into slivers. Cook with an equal amount of honey on medium heat, stirring frequently, until it boils and billows up. Quickly remove from heat; pour into clean jars. Cover; cool; store in refrigerator.
**Toxicity:** None known.
**Works Well With:** Garlic, honey.
**Results & Notes:** Bitter orange is worth seeking if you need the strongest medicine, but any citrus peel can be used as a preventive.
**References:** 3, 7, 9, 10, 21

# Cleavers
### *Galium aparine*

**Other Names:** Goosegrass
**Type:** Stimulating/Sedating
**Found in:** Moist wild areas of all temperate zones worldwide; a common weed of cities, gardens, streamsides, and forest edges, notable for its tendency to cling (cleave) to other plants.
**Part Used:** Flowering or seeding plant.
**Actions & Uses:** Strengthens lymphatic circulation; eases breast congestion; *relieves breast swelling, counters lymphedema*; tonifies veins;

counters bloodclots, antispasmodic, anti-tumor.
**Important Constituents:** Anthraquinones, carotenes, coumarin, glycosides, malic acid, tannins.
**Preparation & Daily Dose:** Used without limit at low doses.
Dried herb infusion: 1–2 cups.
Tincture of fresh herb: 20–160 drops.
Fresh plant juice: 1–2 teaspoonfuls/5–10ml.
Poultice of fresh or dried herb: as needed.
**Toxicity:** Cleavers contains coumarin, a blood thinner related to the chemical drug coumadin. While thin blood decreases death from cancer, stroke, and heart disease, it increases the risk of hemorrhage during surgery. Some women report increased menstrual flow after using cleavers to relieve premenstrual breast tenderness.
**Works Well With:** Dandelion.
**Results & Notes:** Relief from breast pain and lymphedema is usually prompt using 20 drops every 15 minutes for two hours. External use also has a long-standing reputation for shrinking tumors.
**References:** 4, 6, 11, 12, 21; illustrated on page 252.

## Comfrey
*Symphytum officinale*

**Other Names:** Knitbone, boneset, heals-all, "The Comforter"
**Type:** Nourishing + (leaves); Potentially Poisonous (roots)
**Found in:** Asia Minor, Siberia, and Europe; easily cultivated.
**Part Used:** Healing properties are concentrated in leaves, leaf stalks, and flower stalks throughout the growing season, but move to the roots during cold months or when there is no green growth.
**Actions & Uses:** *Protects lungs and skin;* heals broken skin and bones; heals ligaments and tendons; rebuilds blood quickly; anti-cancer.
**Important Constituents:** Allantoin, antioxidants, carotenes, glucuronic acid, inulin, mucilage, phytosterols, rosmarinic acid, tannins; selenium, zinc, and many other minerals.
**Preparation & Daily Dose:** Leaves can be used without limit. Restrict use of roots to external treatments.
Dried leaf infusion: up to1 quart/1 liter.
Fresh or dried leaf poultice: as frequently as possible.
Infused oil of fresh roots (or leaves): used freely.
**Toxicity:** None for leaves. Internal use of comfrey root may cause congestion of the hepatic (liver) veins.
**Works Well With:** Mints.

**Results & Notes:** Superb *complementary medicine*, especially for women choosing surgery or radiation. Herbalist S. Clymer writes of numerous "uncontradicted" reports of lung cancers going into remission after treatment with nothing other than infusion of whole green comfrey leaves.
**References:** 1, 3, 4, 6, 8, 9, 10, 11, 12, 15, 17, 21, 22, 24, 25

# Dandelion
*Taraxacum officinale*

**Other Names:** Lion's Tooth, piss-in-bed
**Type:** Leaves are Nourishing +; Roots are Tonifying +
**Found in:** Greece; naturalized worldwide in temperate regions.
**Part Used:** Leaves (best tasting when weather is cold in spring and fall); fall-dug roots, 1–2 years old; flowers; entire plant.
**Actions & Uses:** *Protects, heals, and tones liver*; eases breast congestion; stops cancer promotion; relieves anemia; improves outlook; *improves digestion* and appetite, relieves food allergies; protects immune system (increases interferon production).
**Important Constituents:** Antioxidants, carotenes, coumaric acid, d-glucuronic acid, inulin, lecithin, many phytosterols, saponins, tannins; selenium, zinc, and many other minerals.
**Preparation & Daily Dose:** Prolonged use considered beneficial.
      Fresh leaves and flowers: eaten freely.
      Cooked greens: 1/2–2 cups/125–500 ml.
      Dried root infusion: 1–3 cups/250–750 ml.
      Tincture of fresh plant, including root: 15–120 drops.
      Wine of fresh flowers: no more than 6 ounces/200 ml.
      Infused oil of fresh flowers: as needed.
**Toxicity:** None.
**Works Well With:** Burdock, milk thistle, nettle.
**Results & Notes:** Dandelion is a superb ally for liver and breasts. Regular use—internally before meals and externally before sleep—helps keep breasts healthy, reverses cancerous changes, and stops promotion of oncogenes. Digestion is settled and strengthened a few minutes after taking a dose. Results in the breast tissue are slower, taking six weeks or more to become evident.
**References:** 1, 3, 4, 5, 6, 8, 9, 10, 11, 12, 21, 22, 24, 25; illus. page 32.

*"Dandelion root is . . . a possible preventive for breast cancer."*[21]
Michael Tierra, herbalist (1988)

# Echinacea
*Echinacea purpurea, E. angustifolia*

**Other Names:** Purple coneflower
**Type:** Tonifying+
**Found in:** Prairies of North America; *E. purpurea* is easily culti-vated, but retains little medicinal value when dried.
**Part Used:** Autumn-dug, five-year-old roots; whole plant in flower.
**Actions & Uses:** Anti-tumor, anti-cancer; *enhances immune system* (increases interferon, enhances macrophage activity); *raises white blood cell count*; relieves pain and swelling; *counters all infections,* especially antibiotic-resistant ones (e.g., wound infections, staph, strep, pneumonia, mastitis, blood poisoning, flu, colds, sinus/ tooth/ gum infections, abscesses); reduces side effects of chemotherapy.
**Important Constituents:** Antioxidants, many alkaloids, car-otenes, flavonoids, inulin, limonene, phenolic acid, pinenes, quer-cetin; selenium, zinc and many other minerals.
**Preparation & Daily Dose:** Up to 6 months of daily use.
    Dried root infusion: 2 cups/500 ml.
    Fresh or dried root tincture: A dose equals 1 drop for every 2 pounds/1 kilogram body weight.
• *For general immune strengthening:* A dose once or twice a week.
• *For those with cancer or chronic infection:* A dose 1-3 times a day.
• *For those with acute infection:* A dose every two hours for 1-2 days (if I don't see results in 24 hours, I get help), then every three hours for 1-2 days, then every four hours for 1-2 days, reducing to three times a day, then twice a day, then once a day for a week. If signs of infection return, I go back to a higher dose.
**Toxicity:** None.
**Works Well With:** Poke, burdock, cleavers.
**Results & Notes:** Large doses of echinacea can raise white blood cell count dramatically and within hours. Recommended as an anti-cancer and anti-infection herb for centuries, more than 200 pharmaceutical preparations made from echinacea are currently in use worldwide. Superb *complementary medicine* for women choos-ing surgery or chemotherapy. Echinacea may be used for months with continuing benefit, although many herbalists, myself included, previously suggested a break after two weeks. Echinacea and poke root combine to counter breast infections quickly and dramatically.
**References:** 1, 2, 3, 6, 9, 10, 11, 12, 21, 25

# Elecampane
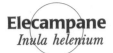
*Inula helenium*

**Other Names:** Elf dock, Helen of the Fields
**Type:** Tonifying +
**Found in:** Europe, Asia, Tibet; naturalized in mountainous, cold, wet pastures of Japan and eastern North America; easily cultivated.
**Part Used:** Fall-dug roots, at least two years old.
**Actions & Uses:** *Protects and heals lungs* (asthma, congestion, pneumonia, shortness of breath); eases breast pain and congestion; antiseptic, anti-tumor; Chinese folk remedy against breast cancer.
**Important Constituents:** Inulin, pectins, many phytosterols, resins, essential oils including azulene.
**Preparation & Daily Dose:** Restrict large doses to 6 months.
     Fresh root tincture:15–60 drops.
**Toxicity:** Large doses may be sedative; can raise/lower blood sugar.
**Works Well With:** Echinacea, calendula, honeysuckle.
**Results & Notes:** Elecampane was screened by the National Cancer Institute and found to have significant anti-tumor activity.
**References:** 1, 3, 4, 6, 9, 10, 21, 24, 25

**Essiac**: See pages 276 and 301.

**Garlic** (*Allium sativum*): This important anti-cancer herb is discussed on page 33. You may also want to read *The Healing Power of Garlic,* Bergner, Prima, 1995.

# Ginger
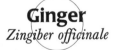
*Zingiber officinale*

**Type:** Strongly Tonifying to Stimulating/Sedating
**Found in:** Tropical Asia; widely cultivated, especially in Jamaica.
**Part Used:** Rhizomes, at least one year old.
**Actions & Uses:** *Internally*–Warming to intestines, belly, solar plexus; *anti-nausea* (especially after anesthesia); enhances immune system (increases interferon production); increases appetite, improves digestion; anti-inflammatory, anti-tumor. *Externally*–*Breaks up congestion;* circulates lymph; enhances immune response; *relieves pain;* dissolves cysts and tumors.
**Important Constituents:** Antioxidants, camphor, carotenes, lecithin, phytosterols, quercetin, selenium, zinc and other minerals,

acids (e.g., linoleic, linolenic, oxalic); volatile oils (e.g., camphene, citral, gingerol, lineol, pinenes, thujone).
**Preparation & Daily Dose:** Discontinue as symptoms abate.
Tea of fresh or dried roots: 2–4 cups.
Compress of fresh root: morning and night, *see* page 305.
Infused oil of fresh roots: as needed.
**Toxicity:** None, even with large doses for a long time, but even small amounts of ginger may increase menses and menopausal flooding and cause self-limiting flushing/sweating.
**Results & Notes:** Fresh ginger is more active than dried.
**References:** 1, 3, 4, 6, 8, 9, 10, 11, 15, 17, 21, 24, 25

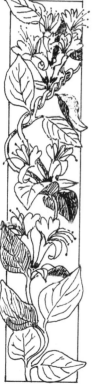

# Honeysuckle
*Lonicera japonica*

**Other Names:** Jin-yin-hua, Chinese echinacea
**Type:** Tonifying +
**Found in:** China; easily cultivated; a frequent escapee to thickets and roadsides in eastern North America.
**Part Used:** Flowerbuds harvested May/June, dried quickly in the sun without turning or handling.
**Actions & Uses:** *Counters breast cancer* and cervical cancer; enhances immune system; *rejuvenative*; anti-microbial; anti-inflammatory; antibiotic; anti-cancer; antiseptic (against *Salmonella, Pseudomonas aeruginosa, Staphylococcus aureus, Streptococcus pneumoniae, Mycobacterium tubercolis,* and many mastitis bacteria).
**Important Constituents:** Glucosides, mucilage, salicylic acid.
**Preparation & Daily Dose:** Used freely.
Dried flower tea, infusion: 1–4 cups/250–1000 ml.
Dried flowers: 9–15 grams.
**Toxicity:** No reported ill side effects from continued use or large doses. *Berries are poisonous.*
**Results & Notes:** One of the most vigorous vines known, honeysuckle is analogous to cancer in its ability to take over an area. Excellent *complementary medicine.* An injectable form is used in Chinese hospitals to counter severe infections.
**References:** 7, 10, 12, 21

# Essiac

*See* Burdock, Sheep Sorrel, Slippery Elm, Turkey Rhubarb

Most modern doctors scoff at the idea that herbs could cure cancer. Fifty years ago, a Canadian nurse, Rene Caisse, found it just as difficult to believe. But when a patient claimed to have cured herself of breast cancer with herbs from an Ojibwa medicine man, Caisse experimented with them, and eventually offered them—as Essiac (her name backwards)—to thousands of people with cancer.

Her results? Infusions and injections of Essiac prompted remission in some cases, significantly reduced pain in all cases, and often prolonged life in terminal cases.

During her life, Caisse (like any wise woman) kept changing Essiac. Since she never revealed a final formula, various authors have claimed, since her death, to have the "real" one. All contain the same four herbs: burdock, sheep sorrel, slippery elm, and turkey rhubarb.

When I first heard the story though, the medicine man suggested only two herbs. Which two? Not Turkey rhubarb. It's neither native to nor naturalized in Canada. But rhubarb's wild sister—yellow dock—has been naturalized in the New World for over 300 years and is widely used against cancer. Their actions are similiar, but where yellow dock gently tickles the intestines, rhubarb rudely stimulates them. (Slippery elm was probably added to protect the intestines from the rhubarb.) It's unlikely that one of the original herbs was sheep sorrel. Although concentrated sorrel juice has been used externally as an anti-cancer caustic, it has little value internally. The more I thought about it, the more likely it seemed that the original formula was simply burdock and yellow dock roots simmered together—primitive, not tasty, but highly effective. I call it Wessiac. Learn how to make Essiac on page 301; Wessiac on page 302.

Many women dancing with cancer told me they used some version of Essiac as *complementary medicine.*

**To learn more,** read *Calling of an Angel: The Story of Essiac* by Gary Glum, Silent Walker, 1988; or *The Essiac Report* by Richard Thomas, Alternative Treatment Information Network, 1993 (1244 Ozeta Terr., Los Angeles, CA 90069)

## Kelp

*Alaria esculenta, Nereocystis luetkeana, Laminaria* species, *Fucus* species, and many, many others

**Other Names:** Wakame, bull whip kelp, kombu, bladderwrack
**Type:** Nourishing +
**Found in:** Oceans of the world, sea coasts worldwide.
**Part Used:** Fronds, rinsed in salt water only, eaten or quickly dried.
**Actions & Uses:** *Prevents breast cancer, prevents damage from radiation and chemotherapy;* rejuvenative; *heart tonic* (lowers cholesterol, normalizes blood pressure, increases contractive force in the atria); heals skin, scalp, hair; antibiotic; antitoxic (draws heavy metals and radioactivity out of the body); anti-inflammatory; anti-cancer.
**Important Constituents:** Algin, antioxidants, fatty acids, histamine, iodine, laminine.
**Preparation & Daily Dose:** Used without limit; best eaten daily.
     Fresh or soaked seaweed: 2 ounces/60 grams.
     Dried seaweed: 1/4 ounce/7.5 grams, eaten as is or cooked.
**Toxicity:** There is no toxicity or ill effect associated with eating kelp, even in enormous quantity. The heavy metals present in some Japanese seaweeds have been shown, in human studies, to be unusable, harmless, and completely excreted in the feces.
**Works Well With:** All cooked food.
**Results & Notes:** Kelp is an anti-cancer herb without peer. Effects from lavish use can be noticed within a week, and increase as time passes. Mail order sources, page 54.
**References:** 3, 5, 10, 21; illustrated on pages 41 and 217.

## Milk Thistle

*Carduus marianum*

**Other Names:** Previously *Silybum marianum;* lady's thistle
**Type:** Tonifying +
**Found in:** Southwest Europe; naturalized in North America; easily cultivated.
**Part Used:** Ripe seeds.
**Actions & Uses:** *Protects liver,* improves digestion; increases appetite; *prevents damage from chemotherapy;* anti-cancer; eases headaches.
**Important Constituents:** Silymarin flavonoids (including silybin, silydianin, and silycristin), essential oils, fumaric acid, mucilage.

**Preparation & Daily Dose:** Taken as needed, for years.
  Tincture of fresh or dried seeds: 60-100 drops.
  80% silymarin liquid extract: $1/4$ teaspoon/1 ml.
**Toxicity:** None, even with large doses over extended periods.
**Works Well With:** Burdock, dandelion.
**Results & Notes:** Milk thistle has been used medicinally for over 2000 years. It can literally regenerate the liver. Used regularly, it protects the liver from the detrimental effects of chemotherapy, organochlorine pollution, hormones, and free radical damage by increasing glutathione (a metabolic enzyme) by 35 percent. One of the most important *complementary medicines* for women choosing chemotherapy. Best taken on an empty stomach.
**References:** 1, 3, 4, 6, 9, 10, 12, 16, 21, 25; illustrated on page 252.

# Mints
## *Laminariacea* or *Labiatae*

**Other Names: Catnip** (*Nepeta cataria*), **Ground Ivy** (*Glechoma hederacea*), **Rosemary** (*Rosmarinus officinalis*), **Self-Heal/Heal-All** (*Prunella vulgaris*), **Skullcap** (*Scutellaria lateriflora*), and all mints.
**Type:** Tonifying +; mint tinctures are Stimulating/Sedating.
**Found in:** Common in all soils, wet and dry, cultivated and wild, in temperate regions worldwide; easily grown.
**Part Used:** All mints—leaves and budding tops, late spring through late fall. Ground ivy only—fall-dug roots in addition to tops.
**Actions & Uses:** *Eases pain*; stops spasms; supports liver; eases headaches and bellyaches; stabilizes nervous system;  antibiotic; antimutagenic; anti-tumor; anti-cancer.
**Important Constituents:** Acids, antioxidants, carotenes, chlorophyll, essential oils, selenium.
**Preparation & Daily Dose:** Used without limit.
  Fresh leaves in salads and tabouli: to taste, as desired.
  Dried leaf infusion: no more than 1 quart/1 liter.
  Tincture of fresh plants: 5–30 drops as needed.
**Toxicity:** None.
**Works Well With:** Comfrey, nettles, red clover.
**Results & Notes:** All mints are exceptionally rich in calcium and other minerals. Catnip and skullcap tinctures are superb pain relievers. Self heal is exceptionally rich in antioxidants. Ground ivy roots (compress or infused oil) can check the growth of cancers.
**References:** 4, 6, 9, 10, 11, 15, 17, 21, 24; illustrated on page 40.

# Mistletoe
*Viscum album*

**Other Names:** European mistletoe (*Do not use American mistletoe.*)
**Type:** Stimulating/Sedating
**Found in:** Semiparasitic on deciduous trees in Europe, northern Asia.
**Part Used:** Leaves and young twigs collected just before berries form; best after fermentation in water.
**Actions & Uses:** *Inhibits tumors*; cytotoxic; cytostatic; enhances immune system (increases macrophages, natural killer cells, and T-cells); increases weight of thymus; tonifies heart and nerves.
**Important Constituents:** Flavonoids, lectins, polypeptides, polysaccharides, saponins, tannins, tri-terpenes, viscotoxin.
**Preparation & Daily Dose:** Used only as needed.
    Dried leaf infusion: 1–3 cups/ 250–750 ml.
    Tincture of fresh plant: 25–75 drops.
    Dried leaves: 6–18 grams.
    By injection: *see* page 158.
**Toxicity:** Large doses impair heart action; *berries are poisonous.*
**Results & Notes:** Mistletoe has been used clinically in Europe for the treatment of breast (and other) cancers since 1926. It is most effective when injected under the skin near the tumor, but the tincture is also used orally as a systemic treatment. Mistletoe is said to work by causing an inflammatory reaction which walls off the tumor, checking its growth and spread.
**References:** 1, 3, 4, 6, 9, 18, 21, 23. Illustrated on page 158.

# Nettle
*Urtica dioica, U. urens*, and other species

**Other Names:** Stinging nettle
**Type:** Nourishing +
**Found in:** Temperate lands worldwide; rich soils, vacant lots, gardens, roadsides, river banks.
**Part Used:** Leaves and stalks, harvested before flowers form.
**Actions & Uses:** *Rebuilds adrenals and kidneys*; protects lungs and liver; *rejuvenative*; enhances immune functioning; promotes hair growth; *builds blood*; improves blood clotting; improves thyroid function; Russian folk remedy against cancer.

**Important Constituents:** Acids (e.g., linoleic, linolenic), antioxidants, chlorophyll, carotenes, glucoquinines, phytosterols; selenium, silica, zinc, and other minerals; tannins, vitamin E.

**Preparation & Daily Dose:** Used without limit, for years. Best to start with 4 ounces/125 ml of infusion daily and increase slowly.

Cooked young plants eaten with broth: as desired.

Dried herb infusion: up to 1 quart/liter.

**Toxicity:** Stomach upset possible from using plants harvested when flowering. Contact with fresh nettles causes a stinging rash.

**Works Well With:** Mint.

**Results & Notes:** Superb *complementary medicine* for women choosing chemotherapy. Response is often rapid, with energy levels rising within a few days, hair growth obvious in a few weeks, and improvement in blood work seen in a week. Frequent urination may accompany the first week's use, but is self-limiting.

**References:** 1, 3, 4, 5, 6, 9, 10, 11, 12, 21, 22, 24, 25

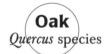

# Oak
## *Quercus* species

**Other Names:** White oak (*Quercus alba*) is most useful; red oak (*Quercus rubra*) is next best.

**Type:** Stimulating/Sedating

**Found in:** Temperate forest regions worldwide.

**Part Used:** Inner bark, collected in early spring before the leaves open; green leaves, dried, can be used when bark is not available.

**Actions & Uses:** Inhibits inflammation; *checks diarrhea*; slows profuse menses; dries skin eruptions (e.g., from lymphedema); improves blood clotting; strengthens blood vessels; checks falling hair; shrinks tumors; antiviral; antiseptic; anti-cancer.

**Important Constituents:** Acids (e.g., tannic and ellagic), antioxidants, flavonoids, quercetin, tannins; selenium, zinc, and other minerals.

**Preparation & Daily Dose:** Used 2 weeks on, 2 weeks off.

Infusion of dried inner bark: up to 1 cup/250 ml, in sips.

Infusion externally: as compress or bath; use as needed.

**Toxicity:** Overuse of tannins—such as drinking 30 or more cups of black tea a day—can cause cancer.

**Works Well With:** Comfrey leaves.

**Results & Notes:** The tannins in oak bark infusion bind to weeping sores and quickly form a "false skin" which prevents bacterial

infections, making this a very important ally for women with severe lymphedema. Oak bark generally prompts a rapid response.
**References:** 3, 6, 9, 10, 11, 12, 21, 25

# Pau D'Arco
*Tabebuia serratofolia, T. avellandedae, T. heptaphylla,* and others

**Other Names:** Lapacho, ipe roxo, taheebo
**Type:** Tonifying +
**Found in:** South America, specifically Brazil, Paraguay, Argentina, and the Andes.
**Part Used:** Dried inner bark, wood, or leaves.
**Actions & Uses:** Shrinks tumors; *enhances immune functioning* (even at extremely low doses); eliminates candida overgrowth; relieves herpes; *relieves pain;* prevents damage from chemotherapy; increases red blood cell count; anti-inflammatory; antibacterial; antifungal; anti-microbial; antiparasitic; antiviral; folk remedy against lung and breast cancers, especially to prevent metastases.
**Important Constituents:** Anthraquinones, flavonoids, lapachol, napthaquinones, quercetin, tabetuin, xyloidone.
**Preparation & Daily Dose:** Used as needed, no limit.
>    Infusion of dried leaves, wood, bark: up to 1 quart/1 liter.
>    Tincture of wood is highest in lapachol ("herbal chemo").
>    Poultice of inner bark or leaves: as desired.
**Toxicity:** Nausea and diarrhea occasionally accompany moderate doses. With very high doses, metabolic disturbances, anemia, and loss of vitamin K may occur, but are self-limiting.
**Works Well With:** Siberian ginseng, wild mushrooms, red clover, cabbage family, garlic, kelp. Native healers of the Bolivian Andes combine it in equal parts with plantain (*Plantago tomentosa*) and nettle (*Urtica flabellata*) to treat those with cancer.
**Results & Notes:** Brazilian healers say taheebo brings remission of pain in hours, remission of symptoms within a few weeks, and remission of cancer within months. Pau d'arco is a cherished herbal ally for those dealing with complications after surgery or the side effects of chemotherapy, as well as those interested in actively preventing recurrence. In laboratory tests pau d'arco suppressed tumor formation, inhibited solid tumors, and weakened or killed most cancer cells. It is unusual in that it contains two strong immune system tonics—anthraquinones and napthaquinones.
**References:** 20, 21; illustrated on page 266.

## Plantain
*Plantago major, P. lanceolata*

**Other Names:** Band-aid plant, white man's foot (Not a banana.)
**Type:** Nourishing +
**Found in:** Temperate regions worldwide; waste areas, driveways, paths, lawns, playgrounds, parks.
**Part Used:** Leaves (harvested anytime);  ripe seeds with hulls.
**Actions & Uses:** *Internally*–Seeds: anti-microbial, against thrush; Leaves: promote blood clotting, *increase iron in blood,* strengthen digestion; important Latin American folk remedy against cancer. *Externally*–Leaf poultice or oil reduces cysts, helps prevent cancer, heals skin and connective tissues, *stops itching,* prevents scars.
**Important Constituents:** Allantoin, antioxidants, chlorophyll, phytosterols, tannins, acids (e.g., chlorogenic, ascorbic, benzoic, coumaric, linoleic, linolenic, oleic, salicylic).
**Preparation & Daily Dose:**  Used without limit.
    Raw leaves: 3–20 chopped in salad.
    Dried leaf infusion: up to 1 quart/1 liter.
    Fresh leaf vinegar: 1–2 tablespoons/15–30 ml.
    Seeds cooked or soaked overnight in cold water: as needed.
    Fresh leaf oil/ointment or poultice: as needed.
**Toxicity:** None.
**Works Well With:** Calendula flowers, pau d'arco, nettle.
**Results & Notes:**  Internal response is prompt; noticeable improvement in blood iron is seen in two weeks of daily use. External response is also rapid: itching ceases, bleeding stops, pain abates, and swelling recedes in minutes. Plantain promotes quick, scarless healing from biopsies, breast surgery, and needle sticks.
**References:** 1, 3, 4, 6, 9, 10, 11, 12, 20, 21, 22, 24; illus. page 252.

## Poke
*Phytolacca americana*

**Other Names:** Cancer root, kermesberro, skookum, ink berry
**Type:** Potentially poisonous
**Found in:** Gardens (as a weed) and roadsides of northeastern North America; easily cultivated; naturalized in Europe, Australia.
**Part Used:** One- or two-year-old roots, dug after first frost, *fresh only*; berries, before frost, fresh or dried–do not chew.

**Actions & Uses:** Resolves cysts, lumps, and some *in situ* breast cancers; stimulates immune system; counters infection (especially pneumonia); protects lungs; relieves lymph congestion; antiviral; antiseptic; anti-tumor; anti-cancer. Used externally and internally.

**Important Constituents:** Acids, antioxidants, alkaloids, carotenes, phytosterols, pokeweed-antiviral-protein, saponins, tannins, resins (root only).

**Preparation & Daily Dose:** Used with caution for short periods; rarely for more than 10 months.

Tincture of fresh (not dried) root: 1–20 drops.

Fresh berry juice preserved with honey: 4 teaspoons/20ml.

Dried berries: 1–4 swallowed whole. *Seeds are poisonous.*

Oil/ointment/poultice of fresh roots: *with care.*

**Toxicity: Caution!** All parts of fresh or dried poke—except berries with unbroken seeds and well-cooked young leaves—can cause such intense vomiting, diarrhea, and pain that you don't know which end to point at the toilet. This is frequently accompanied by out-of-the-body sensations, but rarely leads to death. (I felt a little "spacey" when I swallowed two dried berries as an anti-inflammatory against joint pain one evening.) The numerous seeds are only toxic if crushed, and are too hard for children (and most adults) to break. I've read of skin rashes caused by handling fresh poke, but have never personally experienced such problems. Alkaloids in poke root tincture can accumulate in the kidneys, making extended use risky, though some people have taken doses of 15 drops a day for a year or more without apparent harm.

**Works Well With:** Echinacea.

**Results & Notes:** Poke root tincture kicks the immune system into gear incredibly fast. I've seen chronic infection of many years' standing begin to resolve after only one dose, and acute infection subside in a matter of hours. Poke's effect seems to be focused on the lymphatic and glandular tissues of the breasts, ovaries, throat, and uterus, where it reliably resolves cysts, growths, infections, and swellings. First-hand reports attest to the ability of fresh poke root poultices to burn away tumors, including breast cancers. *Phytolacca* is a standard homeopathic remedy against breast cancer. Women at high-risk of developing breast cancer may wish to follow advice from Traditional Chinese Medicine and use one drop of poke tincture daily from the beginning of May until mid-June yearly as a preventive. To be assured of a supply of poke tincture, I make it myself, as it is rarely found for sale.

**References:** 1, 3, 6, 8, 11, 12, 21, 22; illustrated on page 266.

# Red Clover
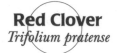
*Trifolium pratense*

**Other Names:** "The herb of immortality"
**Type:** Nourishing
**Found in:** Temperate regions worldwide; fields, roadsides, lawns.
**Part Used:** Just-opened blossoms with a few leaves clinging.
**Actions & Uses:** *Internally*—*Anti-cancer*; alkalinizes, builds blood; *helps prevent breast cancer recurrence;* anti-angiogenetic; protects liver and lungs; improves appetite; relieves constipation; eases anxiety; relieves symptoms of premature menopause, increases fertility. *Externally*—Softens, reduces breast lumps; antifungal (vinegar).
**Important Constituents:** Acids (e.g., ascorbic, chlorogenic, salicylic), allantoin, antioxidants, coumarin, flavonoids, genistein, lignans, phytoestrogens, phytosterols, resin, vitamin E; selenium, zinc, and other minerals.
**Preparation & Daily Dose:** Used without limit.
    Fresh blossoms: eaten freely.
    Infusion of dried flowers: up to 1 quart/1 liter.
    Tincture/mother tincture of fresh blossoms: 15–100 drops.
    Fresh flower vinegar: 1–4 tablespoons/15–60 ml.
    Fresh blossom oil/ointment/poultice: as often as needed.
**Toxicity:** Overconsumption of blood-thinning coumarins—present in low amounts in red clover but found in greater amounts in other clovers such as sweet clover (*Melilotus officinalis*)—can lead to breakdown of red blood cells and increase risk of hemorrhage.
**Works Well With:** Mints, dandelion, echinacea.
**Results & Notes:** Red clover belongs to a family (the legumes) renowned for anti-cancer properties. It shares with its better-studied sisters—soy, lentils, and the Chinese herb astragalus—the ability to repair damaged DNA, turn off oncogenes, and reverse precancers and *in situ* cancers. It is a widely used folk remedy against cancer. According to J. Hartwell, author of *Plants Used Against Cancer*, medical literature has reported and confirmed hundreds of cases of remission of cancer after consistent use of red clover. I personally know of several such cases. Homeopathic *Trifolium* (mother tincture) is a specific against breast cancer.
    **Alfalfa** (*Medicago sativa*), the infusion not the sprouts, is another anti-cancer legume. Dose of infusion is 1 cup/250 ml daily.
    **White clover** (*Trifolium repens*) can also be used.
**References:** 1, 3, 4, 6, 8, 10, 11, 12, 15, 17, 21, 22, 24, 25; illus. page 266.

# St. Joan's Wort
*Hypericum perforatum*

**Other Names:** St. John's wort, Klamath weed
**Type:** Tonifying +
**Found in:** Temperate regions worldwide; pastures, roadsides.
**Part Used:** Flowers in bud, flowers in bloom, flowering tops.
**Actions & Uses:** *Internally—Heals nerves, relieves pain*; inhibits cancer growth; reduces caked breasts, shrinks enlarged glands, counters swelling in breast tissues; *relieves/prevents muscle aches*, antiseptic; anti-microbial, *antiviral,* heals shingles; *antidepressant,* anti-tumor; anti-cancer. *Externally—Protects skin against radiation damage*; heals burns, cold sores, herpes sores, and shingles; relieves deep soreness in muscles, bones, and nerves; eases sciatica pain; antiviral.
**Important Constituents:** Antioxidants, alkaloids (e.g., hyperin, hypericin, pseudohypericin), carotenes, chlorophyll, essential oils including limonene and pinenes, flavonoids, phytosterols, quercetin, saponins, tannins.
**Preparation & Daily Dose:** Used without limit.
Fresh flower oil/ointment: used freely.
Tincture of fresh flowers: 25–75 drops; or as needed, as often as every 15 minutes for acute muscle spasms, headaches, pain.
**Toxicity:** Antiviral constituents in St. Joan's wort react with sunlight, occasionally causing hypersensitivity to the sun. The antiviral effect of the oil is said to be heightened by sunbathing.
**Works Well With:** Skullcap.
**Results & Notes:** If I were restricted to using only one herb, this would be it: to ease my muscles and nerves, counter infection, cheer me, and relieve aches and pains. I don't leave home without it.
**References:** 4, 6, 9, 10, 11, 12, 21, 25; illustrated on page 236.

# Sheep Sorrel
*Rumex acetosella*

**Other Names:** Sour grass, red top
**Type:** Stimulating/Sedating
**Found in:** Temperate regions worldwide; acid soils, gardens, roadsides, pastures, orchards.
**Part Used:** Leaves, stems, roots, harvested before plant flowers.
**Actions & Uses:** *Internally—*Protects against damage from chemotherapy/radiation; stops diarrhea. *Externally—*Dissolves cysts.

**Important Constituents:** Acids (ascorbic, oxalic, tartaric), anthraquinones, carotenes, coumarin, chlorophyll, hyperin, tannins.
**Preparation & Daily Dose:** No more than 40 cups tea per year.
  Tea of dried leaves: no more than 1 cup/250 ml.
  Fresh leaf poultice: as needed.
**Toxicity:** Large doses over many months can cause poisoning.
**Results & Notes:** Some sources claim a long history of use as a cancer cure; this is true of external uses, not internal. *See* Essiac.
**References:** 4, 6, 12, 22

# Siberian Ginseng
*Eleutherococcus senticosus*

**Other Names:** Eleuthero
**Type:** Nourishing +
**Found in:** Native to Russia; easily cultivated in temperate areas.
**Part Used:** Root, harvested when dormant.
**Actions & Uses:** *Protects against effects of chemicals, radiation, and stress;* enhances and strengthens immune system (stabilizes production of red cells and white cells, increases macrophage activity); protects liver, adrenals, and central nervous system (eases anxiety and tension, improves sense of well-being); *inhibits metastases;* increases endurance and stamina; anti-inflammatory; anti-cancer.
**Important Constituents:** Antioxidants, glycosides, phytosterols, selenium and other minerals.
**Preparation & Daily Dose:** Used 4 weeks out of 5, for years.
  Liquid extract of fresh root: 4–5 ml.
  Tincture of fresh or dried root: 25–80 drops.
  Powdered dried root: 1–3 grams.
**Toxicity:** Dr. I. I. Brekhman, authority on Eleuthero, states that even lengthy use of large doses is completely without side effect.
**Works Well With:** Echinacea.
**Results & Notes:** Siberian ginseng shows remarkable cancer preventive properties, and in a dose-related way. As a *complementary medicine,* it is taken one hour before and one hour after each radiation or chemotherapy treatment. Also used before and after surgery, beginning four or more days prior to surgery. Russian researchers emphatically recommend the use of Siberian ginseng in the treatment of mammary cancer, including primary tumors, recurrences, and metastases.
**References:** 1, 7, 10, 21; illustrated on page 266.

# Slippery Elm
*Ulmus fulva*

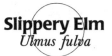

**Other Names:** Red elm
**Type:** Nourishing +
**Found in:** Deciduous forests of Central and North America, Asia.
**Part Used:** Spring-harvested inner bark.
**Actions & Uses:** *Internally*–Heals and soothes mucus surfaces of digestive, respiratory, and reproductive systems; *absorbs poisons*; stops candida overgrowth; nourishes. *Externally*–Dissolves lumps.
**Important Constituents:** Antioxidants, ascorbic acid, carotenes, cholesterol, galactose, glucose, phytosterols, phytoestrogens, proteins, tannins, vitamin B complex; selenium, zinc, and other minerals.
**Preparation & Daily Dose:** Used without limit.
  Powdered bark cooked with hot cereal: eaten freely.
  Powdered bark lozenges: eaten freely (recipe, page 301).
  Tea of 1 teaspoon/5 ml bark per cup/250 ml of water: freely.
**Toxicity:** None, even with large doses over time.
**Works Well With:** Maple syrup, oatmeal, milk.
**Results & Notes:** Slippery elm is an exceptional ally for anyone whose digestive or respiratory system is in distress. Given by the spoonful, or from a baby bottle, slippery elm dependably stops diarrhea and vomiting, and nourishes when all else fails. Mixed with milk or water, it replaces tube feeding or IV nourishment. (I agree with hospice in allowing those dying to refuse food.) As an antidote to poison, I give it by the spoonful, hourly, until all's well. Slippery elm poultices draw, soothe, and form a healing skin over wounds and burns. Superb *complementary medicine. See* Essiac.
**References:** 3, 6, 10, 11, 12, 21

# Sundew
*Drosera rotundifolia*

**Type:** Tonifying +
**Found in:** Damp, sandy soil throughout North America; rare in Europe; easily cultivated.
**Part Used:** Juice of fresh whole plant.
**Actions & Uses:** Shrinks solid tumors; treats inflammatory breast cancer; alleviates pain (especially headaches); enhances immune system (supports T-cells, T-helper cells, and macrophages); antiviral; antibiotic, antiseptic (effective against strep, staph, and pneu-

monia bacteria); protects lungs; antispasmodic; aphrodisiac; anti-tumor; anti-cancer.
**Important Constituents:** Napthaquinones.
**Preparation & Dose:** Used 6 days out of 7, perhaps for life.
    Extract (equal parts sundew juice and pure grain alcohol, plus enough distilled water to blend): 3–30 drops, 3–5 times a day.
**Toxicity:** May be irritating, start with lowest dose.
**Results & Notes:** Sundew (*Drosera*) is related to the endangered, hard-to-cultivate, but well-studied anti-cancer herb, Venus's flytrap (*Dionea*). Both are carnivorous plants and their actions are virtually identical, but sundew is active orally, while *Dionea* is injected.
**References:** 4, 6, 9, 12, 19, 21; illustrated on page 158.

## Turkey Rhubarb
*Rheum palmatum*

**Other Names:** Rhubarb, Chinese rhubarb, Turkish rhubarb
**Type:** Extremely Stimulating/Sedating, Potentially poisonous
**Found in:** Tibet and China; easily cultivated (but most garden varieties of rhubarb have slight medicinal value).
**Part Used:** Fall-dug roots.
**Actions & Uses:** *Purging laxative*; improves appetite.
**Important Constituents:** Aloe-emodins, hyperin, tannins, zinc.
**Preparation & Dose:** Used no more than 3 weeks per year.
    Cold infusion (made by soaking 1 ounce/30 grams of dried root in 16 ounces/500 ml of cold water overnight.): use no more than 3 tablespoons/45 ml a day; start with 1 tablespoon/15 ml.
**Toxicity:** Normal use is so stimulating that laxative dependence can ensue. Overdoses cause powerful painful purging diarrhea.
**Works Well With:** Ginger, slippery elm.
**Results & Notes:** Used in China for 5,000 years.
**References:** 3, 4, 6, 7, 9, 10, 21

## Valerian
*Valeriana officinalis*

**Other Names:** Fragrant valerian
**Type:** Stimulating/Sedating
**Found in:** Temperate regions worldwide; roadsides and thickets.
**Part Used:** Roots–at least 2 years old–dug after frost.

**Actions & Uses:** *Antispasmodic;* regulates involuntary nervous system; *induces sound sleep, eases anxiety,* improves ability to relax; *relieves pain* (even of migraines); lowers blood pressure; relieves intestinal pain; anti-microbial; anti-cancer.
**Important Constituents:** Acids (e.g., ascorbic, oxalic, linoleic), alkaloids, carotenes, coumarin; essential oils including azulene, camphene, and pinenes; phytosterols, quercetin, tannins, selenium.
**Preparation & Daily Dose:** Best limited to 2 weeks out of 4.
　　Tincture of fresh/dried rhizomes: 25–250 drops/1–10 ml.
**Toxicity:** Tincture of old or dried roots may disturb digestion. There is virtually no limit to the amount one can safely take for a few days; long-term use, however, can create dependency or symptoms of poisoning such as vomiting, headaches, and lethargy.
**Works Well With:** Skullcap, oatstraw, Siberian ginseng.
**Results & Notes:** Some find valerian stimulating, not relaxing. If you need valerian's power long-term, keep doses low, and take it in a cup of nerve-nourishing oatstraw infusion.
**References:** 1, 3, 6, 8, 9, 12, 17, 21, 24, 25

# Violet
*Viola odorata* and other species

**Other Names:** Fragrant violet, sweet violet, wild violet, lawn violet
**Type:** Nourishing +
**Found in:** Temperate regions worldwide; streamsides, gardens.
**Part Used:** Leaves, harvested anytime, even during flowering.
**Actions & Uses:** *Internally–Dissolves breast lumps;* protects lungs; soothing, cooling; anti-cancer. *Externally–*Eases pain and inflammation; heals mouth sores; softens skin; antifungal; *checks tumor growth.*
**Important Constituents:** Antioxidants, carotenes, essential oils, phytosterols, quercetin, salicylic acid, saponins.
**Preparation & Daily Dose:** Used without limit. **Non-toxic.**
　　Fresh leaves: in salad, as desired.
　　Dried leaf infusion: up to 1 quart/1 liter.
　　Fresh or dried leaf poultice: continuously, day and night.
**Results & Notes:** Internal and external use of violet can shrink a breast lump in a month. Violet's ability to slow cancer growth makes her an excellent ally for the woman who needs time to research her options. Homeopathic mother tincture of *Viola,* a dose of 3 drops taken 3 times a day, is a specific against breast cancer.
**References:** 3, 5, 6, 9, 10, 21, 22, 24, 25; illustrated on page 266.

## Yellow Dock
*Rumex crispus, R. obtusifolia,* and other species

**Other Names:** Dock, curly dock, patience dock, bitter dock
**Type:** Tonifying +
**Found in:** Temperate regions worldwide, even in deserts; waste areas, gardens, roadsides, orchards.
**Part Used:** Roots, at least two years old, dug after autumn frosts or very early in spring; leaves, harvested anytime; ripe seeds.
**Actions & Uses:** *Internally*–Root: *Builds healthy blood*; protects liver; antifungal (checks *Candida* overgrowth); laxative; prominent folk remedy against cancer. Seed tea: Heals mouth sores and checks diarrhea. *Externally–Dissolves lumps,* anti-tumor; antifungal.
**Important Constituents:** Anthraquinones, rumicin, chrysophanic acid, tannins.
**Preparation & Daily Dose:**  Used daily for 3–12 months.
    Tincture of fresh roots: 10–60 drops.
    Fresh root vinegar: 1–2 tablespoons/30 ml.
    Dried seed tea: no more than 1 cup/250 ml.
    Fresh root oil/ointment: liberally.
**Toxicity:** Overuse of yellow dock root can cause gastric distress or loose stools, and can lead to dependence on its laxative effects.
**Works Well With:** Dandelion, burdock, echinacea.
**Results & Notes:** Root preparations increase the iron level of the blood quickly and dramatically, and are excellent *complementary medicine* for women choosing chemotherapy. Yellow dock oil can dissolve hard lumps and help reverse *in situ* cancers.
**References:** 3, 6, 8, 11, 12, 17, 21, 22, 24, 25; illustrated, page 266.

## Plants That May Induce  Cancer

Comfrey is *not* carcinogenic, nor is sassafras (*Sassafras albidum*), but some plants–and some plant compounds such as tannins–can encourage cancer when consumed in excess.
• *Acorus americanus* • sweet flag/calamus • rootstock
• *Cynoglossum officinale* • hound's tongue • roots
• *Medicago sativa* • alfalfa • sprouts
• *Myrica cerifera* • candleberry, wax-myrtle • berry wax
• *Pteridium aquilinum* • bracken fern • roots, fiddleheads
• *Tephrosia virginiana* • goat's rue • whole plant in excess

# More Anti-Cancer Herbs

*Caution: Many of these plants are **poisonous**, even in small amounts.*

Many of these folk remedies for cancer have been scientifically validated as able to inhibit the growth of tumors, invigorate the immune system, or supply potent cytotoxic compounds. Those who've used them—usually as tinctures taken internally—report varying degrees of success. (Parts not listed may not be poisonous.) **Exercise caution.**

- *Apocynum androsaemifolium* • spreading dogbane • roots
- *Apocynum cannabinum* • dogbane, Indian hemp • whole plant
- *Aristolochia macrophylla* • Dutchman's pipe • whole plant
- *Asarum canadensis, A. europea* • wild ginger • roots
- *Asclepias syriaca* • common milkweed • roots
- *Baptisia australistinctoria* • blue false indigo, wild indigo • roots
- *Caltha palustris* • cowslip, marsh marigold • roots
- *Cheladonium majus* • celandine • sap, fresh; roots, tinctured
- *Conium maculatum* • poison hemlock • whole plant • established homeopathic remedy for women with breast cancer
- *Datura stramonium* • Jimson weed • leaves, roots, seeds
- *Gleditsia triacanthos* • honey locust • leaves
- *Hemerocallis fulva* • daylily • root • Chinese folk remedy against breast cancer • 1 cup dried root tea daily for 6 weeks
- *Physalis heterophylla* • clammy ground cherry • whole plant
- *Podophyllum peltatum* • May apple/American mandrake • roots
- *Sanguinaria canadensis* • bloodroot • fresh root tincture • homeopathic specific for women with breast cancer
- *Senecio aureus, S. jacobea, S. vulgaris* • ragwort, groundsel • roots
- *Solanum dulcamara* • bittersweet nightshade • leaves and berries • recommended by Galen (150 A.D.) against cancer
- *Solanum nigrum* • black nightshade • leaves and berries
- *Thuja occidentalis* • northern white cedar • needles, tinctured
- *Trichosanthes kirilowii* • Tian-hua-fen (roots) and Gua-lo (fruit and seeds) • used against breast cancer in China for 300 years
- *Veratrum viride* • American hellebore • rhizome
- *Yucca glauca* • Spanish bayonet • 1/2 ounce (14 grams) dried roots daily for 6–12 weeks

### Caution:
*Many of these plants are **poisonous**, even in small amounts.*

# Herbal References

1. *Encyclopedia of Natural Medicine*, M. Murray and J. Pizzorno, Prima, 1991
2. *Echinacea*, Steven Foster, Inner Traditions, 1990
3. *Energetics of Western Herbs*, Peter Holmes, Artemisia, 1989
4. *Guide to Medicinal Plants*, Schauenberg and Paris, Keats, 1977
5. *Healing Wise*, Susun Weed, Ash Tree Publishing, 1989
6. *The Herb Book*, John Lust, Bantam, 1974
7. *Herbal Emissaries*, S. Foster and Y. Chongxi, Healing Arts, 1992
8. *Herbal Healing for Women*, Rosemary Gladstar, Simon & Schuster, 1993
9. *Herbal Medicine*, R. F. Weiss, M.D., AB Arcanum, 1988
10. *The Herbs of Life*, Leslie Tierra, Crossing Press, 1992
11. *Indian Herbology*, Alma Hutchens, Merco, 1969
12. *Medicinal Plants*, Steven Foster, James Duke, Houghton Mifflin, 1990
13. *Medicinal Plants of the Mountain West*, Michael Moore, Museum of New Mexico Press, 1979
14. *Medicinal Plants of the Pacific West*, M. Moore, Red Crane, 1993
15. *Medicines from the Earth*, R. E. Schultes, Harper & Row, 1978
16. *Milk Thistle*, Christopher Hobbs, Botanica, 1992
17. *Natural Healing in Gynecology*, Rina Nissim, Pandora, 1986
18. "Natural killer and antibody-dependent cell-mediated cytotoxicity activities in Viscum album-treated breast cancer patients," Hajito and Langrein, *Oncology* 43:93-7, 1986
19. Notes from a talk by herbalist Ed Smith of HerbPharm, 1994
20. *Pau d'Arco—Immune Power from the Rain Forest*, K. Jones, Healing Arts, 1995
21. *Planetary Herbology*, Michael Tierra, Lotus, 1988
22. *Plants Used Against Cancer*, Jonathan Hartwell, Lloydia, especially vol. 31(2) June 1968; and Vol. 33(1) March 1970
23. "Recent studies on the anti-cancer activities of mistletoe and its alkaloids," Khwaja, et al., *Oncology*, 43: suppl.1; 42-50, 1986
24. *Random House Book of Herbs*, R. Phillips and Nicky Fox, 1990
25. *Therapeutic Herbalism*, David Hoffman, private printing, 1992

# Herbal Pharmacy
# Recipes

# How to Make An Herbal Infusion

Herbal infusions are my daily beverage. By using dried herbs and steeping them for long periods, I am able to extract many nutrients (especially minerals) and medicinal factors (such as phytosterols, glycosides, and starches) which extract poorly, or not at all, into teas and tinctures. Because these **nourishing** and **tonifying** infusions are protein-rich, they do not store well. Most spoil in a day or two, even if refrigerated. I drink a different infusion each day. The usual dose is 1–4 cups.

**To make an infusion** you'll need: A glass jar that holds exactly 4 cups/1 liter, a tight lid for the jar, spring or filtered water (if chlorinated water must be used, boil it for 10 minutes before proceeding), a non-aluminum pan to boil the water in, and dried herb.

**To make a leaf infusion** (e.g., nettle, violet, or comfrey): Place 1 ounce/30 grams of crushed dried herb in a quart/liter jar and fill the jar to the top with boiling water. Cap tightly and let it sit at least four hours. (I usually make my infusion before I go to sleep and let it steep overnight so it's ready to use the next day.) Strain the herb out and give it back to the earth. Drink the remaining liquid–the infusion–iced or heated, with sweetener or with salt.

**To make a root or bark infusion** (e.g., astragalus, burdock, dandelion, pau d'arco or Siberian ginseng): Place 2 ounces/60 grams of dried, cut root in a quart/liter jar and fill the jar to the top with boiling water. Cap jar tightly and let it sit at least eight hours before straining and drinking the liquid.

**To make an infusion of a flower**: For heavy blossoms like red clover, proceed as though you were using a leaf. For light blossoms, like calendula, proceed as though you were using seeds.

**To make an infusion of seeds** (e.g., burdock): Pour a cup of boiling water over a tablespoon/15 ml of seeds, cover and steep for no more than 30 minutes. Note: Infuse plantain seeds in cold water.

# How to Make An Herbal Tincture

Alcohol-based plant preparations are called tinctures or extracts. Tinctures are concentrated sources of alkaloids (powerful **tonic** and potentially **poisonous** compounds) and other phytochemicals. I prefer to make my tinctures from fresh plants, but occasionally I tincture dried roots, berries, or seeds. Tinctures last indefinitely if protected from heat, light, and evaporation. The usual dose ranges from 1–100 drops/.04–4 ml a day.

**To make an herbal tincture** you'll need: A glass jar of any size with a good-fitting lid (if you use small jars, such as baby food jars, you can make many different tinctures without spending a lot of money on alcohol), sticky labels and a waterproof pen (to label your tinctures with date and plant name), a pair of scissors or a knife, a pint or more of 100-proof vodka (or a mixture of grain alcohol and 80-proof vodka; if pure grain alcohol is used, the tincture may be too harsh), and fresh plants.

**To make a fresh root tincture** (e.g., poke, burdock, dandelion, or yellow dock): On a fine autumn day, after a frosty night, take a digging fork (not a shovel), a trowel, and a bucket or basket, and go to the nearest patch of weeds. Sit for a minute and enjoy the air, the sun, the spirit of the place, and the spirits of the plants. Use the spading fork to loosen the soil in a circle around each root that you wish to harvest. Gently pull the roots up, using the trowel as needed. Burdock and poke roots are so large that you'll have to go around many times with the spading fork. For safety, bring a separate container for each kind of root you plan to harvest, or harvest only one kind of root at a time.

At home, place the roots in water to loosen clinging soil, shake them dry, then cut into small pieces. Fill a jar right to the top with cut roots, then completely fill it with vodka. Cap tightly and affix a label with the date and the plant name. Let it sit at room temperature, but out of the sun, for at least 6 weeks, then strain out the plant material (return it to the earth or your compost pile), and bottle the liquid—your tincture.

**To make a dried root, bark, berry, or seed tincture** (e.g., astragalus, echinacea, Siberian ginseng, witch hazel, hawthorn berry, or milk thistle seeds): Fill any size jar one-quarter to one-third full of dried, cut roots or bark or whole seeds or berries (no leaves, please). Then fill the jar completely with 100-proof alcohol. Cap it well, affix your label, and store for at least six weeks before straining and using the liquid tincture. I prefer to let tinctures made from dried materials sit for three or more months, even as long as a year, before decanting and using them.

**To make a fresh leaf or flower tincture** (e.g., St. Joan's wort, red clover, calendula, chickweed, or cleavers): Pick herbs after the dew has dried, on a sunny day filled with bird song and butterflies. Bring your jar and alcohol to the plant so you can capture the fairies in your tincture. Pick individual blossoms or use scissors to cut stalky, leafy material into small pieces. Loosely pack flowers and/or leaves into your jar, then fill it to the top with 100-proof vodka. Cap tightly and affix a label. Smile at it daily for six weeks, then strain out the plants and rebottle the liquid—your tincture.

## How to Make Medicinal Herbal Vinegars

Vinegar extracts the minerals from plants better than any other medium, although more slowly than water. Medicinal herbal vinegars are **nourishing** and **tonifying**. They are always made from fresh plant material (dried mushrooms may be used) and steeped for six weeks. Medicinal herbal vinegars last for up to ten years when stored in a cool, dark place. If you use unpasteurized vinegar, harmless (but strange-looking) slimy pancakes known as vinegar mothers will grow in your bottles. Remove them before using the vinegar. The usual dose is 1 tablespoon.

**To make a medicinal herbal vinegar** you'll need: A jar of any size, waxed paper or plastic wrap, apple cider vinegar, and fresh plants. Fill your jar with fresh plant material like dandelion roots and leaves, violet leaves, red clover blossoms, or burdock roots. Add room temperature vinegar, completely covering the herbs. Place plastic or waxed paper over the jar before capping. Label it with the date and plant name. Wait six weeks, then use lavishly.

# How To Make Infused Herbal Oils/Ointments

Oil is used to extract plant components that affect the skin, under-lying nerves, blood vessels, lymphatics, fat cells, muscles, and other soft tissues. Infused herbal oils are always made from fresh plants, with the exception of calendula flowers and comfrey leaves, which are often dried for a day or two before being placed in oil. Infused herbal oils/ointments remain potent for as long as 4 years if made without heat and kept in a cool, dark place.

**To make an infused herbal oil** you'll need: A dry, large-mouthed glass jar with a good lid, labels, a waterproof marker, olive oil, and fresh plants. Infusing herbal oils ooze and make a mess; put them in a bowl or lipped tray to contain the spread of oil stains. To keep your label legible, put it on the lid rather than the side of the jar.

**To make a flower blossom oil** (e.g., calendula, dandelion, red clover, St. Joan's wort, or yarrow): On a day that is sunny, when the bees are active, whether morning or noon, pick dry—no dew, no recent rain—blossoms. Protect your flowers after you've harvested them: Shade them from the sun; put them in a basket, not a jar; work quickly. Stop frequently to attend to the blossoms you've already collected; it's better to make a small jar of oil every ten minutes than one big one in an hour. Fill your jar a little less than full with blossoms (or blossoms, stalks, and leaves), then fill it with olive oil. Use a small knife, a twig, or a chopstick to work the oil thoroughly down into the flowers. Add more and more oil until the plant matter is completely and generously covered. Cap the jar well, label it with the date and name of the plant, and store at room temperature. After six weeks, pour the oil through a cotton cloth (such as a handkerchief or a napkin) to remove the plant material. Store your infused oil in a cool, dry place (a lower cup-board or refrigerator) until ready to use or to make into ointment.

**To make a root oil** (e.g., comfrey, ginger, poke, or yellow dock): In early spring or late fall, when the leaves aren't present or aren't actively growing, harvest roots by digging around them with a spading fork and carefully lifting them free. Shake as much dirt as possible from them. Keep the tops attached. Keep them overnight in a well-ventilated but shady spot. Brush the remaining dry soil off them the next morning. Don't wash them unless they're already wet. Chop the roots into small pieces and put them into a jar. Add enough oil to cover them and have excess oil on top. Cap and label the jar; put it in a bowl. Strain promptly after six weeks.

**To make evergreen breast massage oil** (or plantain or other leaf oils): Harvest fresh needles or tips from any evergreen tree on a sunny day at any time of the year. (Harvest plantain leaves anytime they're green.) Close your eyes and let the sun shine on your eyelids after you've filled your jar with evergreen needles (or coarsely chopped plantain leaves). Pour olive oil into the jar until it coats and covers all the plant material. Use a twig or knife to help the oil permeate. Cap and label the jar. Keep it at room temperature, out of direct sunlight, for six weeks or more before using the oil or making it into an ointment.

**To make burdock seed oil**: When burdock burrs turn brown in the autumn, after frost but before too many wet or snowy days, collect a paper bag full. Roll the top of the bag closed and put it inside another strong paper bag. Jump up and down on this until the burrs are crushed. Go inside or somewhere protected from even the slightest breeze before opening the bags and pouring out the seeds, which are now freed from the burrs but mixed with millions of tiny, itchy hairs. Carefully sieve the hairs out of the seeds. (Burdock seed hairs on your skin or in your clothing cause intense itching.) Fill a jar two-thirds to three-quarters full of seeds, then fill with olive oil. Cap it well, affix a label, and let it sit for six weeks before straining. Warm this oil slightly before using it.

**Help! My infused oil smells weird and looks funny.** Most infused oils have strong smells, variously described as "like a delicatessen" or "like strong cheese." Unless the oil is bubbling or riddled with mold, a strong smell is not a problem.

Mold grows easily on herbs infusing in oil. If it's restricted to the top surface and can be removed intact (don't squeeze out excess oil), the infused oil can still be used—but only on unbroken skin. The usual causes of moldy infused oils are: The jar was wet when filled. Plant material stuck up above level of oil. The jar of infusing oil was exposed to the sun. The infusing oil was heated. The plant material was wet. The plant material was washed.

**To make an herbal ointment** you'll need: infused herbal oil, some beeswax, a grater, a source of heat, a pan, a saucer, and several very small, wide-mouthed containers. Strain your infused herbal oil and remove the plant material. Before making an ointment, let the oil sit for several days. Any water in the oil will sink to the bottom, where you can leave it as you carefully pour off the oil into a measuring cup. Grate some beeswax into very fine pieces. Pour your infused oil into a pan, and heat it on a very low flame. (A candle is sufficient). Stir in one large mounded spoonful of beeswax for every ounce/30 ml of oil. Mix well with a wooden spoon or your finger. The temperature of the oil should never be too hot for your finger. If the oil is overheated, it will spoil quickly.

When the beeswax melts into the oil, test the consistency of your ointment by dripping a little on a saucer where it will instantly solidify. If it's too loose, melt more beeswax into the oil; if it's too stiff, add more infused oil or some plain olive oil. When it's just right, pour the warm oil and beeswax into your containers and label them. Store in a cool, dark place (such as a refrigerator).

# How To Make An Herbal Poultice

Poultices, compresses, and fomentations bring the encapsulating, dissolving, and healing properties of herbs into direct (or very close) contact with the problem area. "Poultice" describes all these external applications, though technically each is slightly different. By dramatically increasing circulation of blood, lymph, and fluids into and out of a local area, poultices can dissolve lumps, check inflammation and infection, and slow or halt the growth of abnormal cells. Traditional (non-orthodox) remedies for breast lumps of all sorts, including cancer, always combine internal remedies and external remedies (poultices). *See* Materia Medica for cautions.

**To make a fresh plant poultice** (e.g., cabbage, comfrey leaf, dandelion flowers/leaves, poke root, potato, violet leaves): Grate, chop, grind, mash, chew, or cook fresh plant material until the juices flow. Apply wet herbs directly to the skin and cover with a close-fitting bandage. Repeat several times a day, using fresh plant material each time. Variations include mixing the bruised herbs with infused herbal oils, powdered clay, slippery elm, or honey.

**To make a powdered plant poultice** (e.g., slippery elm, albi, flax seed): Mix finely pulverized plants with enough warm water or herbal infusion to make a paste that will stay in place when applied. Bandage closely. *See* Powerful Poultice Powder, page 304.

**To make a dried-plant poultice** (e.g., violet, comfrey, ginger): Infuse dried plant material overnight (directions on page 294). In the morning, reheat the whole thing, then strain the herbs out of the liquid, retaining both. Apply the hot plant material directly (poultice). Or wrap it in a cloth and apply (compress). Or soak a cloth in the liquid and apply that (fomentation).

**To make a poultice with plant tinctures or oils/ointments**: Apply tincture, oil, or ointment to a clean cotton cloth, and tape it in place on the breast with surgical tape. Replace it every 8-12 hours.

# Juzentaihoto

*A Japanese Kampo formula used as primary treatment or complementary care for those choosing radiation, chemotherapy, or bone marrow transplant.*

- *Astragalus membranaceous* root
- *Angelica archangelica* root
- *Hoelen* root
- *Atractylodes* root
- *Rehmannia glutinosa* root
- *Glycyrrhiza glabra* root
- *Cnicus benedictus* root
- *Cinnamomum zylandicum* bark
- *Panax quinquefolius* root
- *Paeonia albiflora* root
- *Platycodon* herb
- *Polygonum lithospermum* herb

Combine 2 grams of each herb on the left with 3 grams of each herb on the right, infuse in a quart/liter of water or 4 ounces/125 ml alcohol. This brew is said to dissolve tumors within 2–10 weeks.

# Jason Winter's Tea
### *A best-selling modern formula*

- 1 part *Trifolium pratense* (red clover) blossoms, dried
- 1 part *Larrea tridentata* (chaparral) leaves, dried
- pinch of *Capsicum annuum* (cayenne) or *Cinnamomum* (cinnamon)

Infuse overnight one ounce of dried, mixed herbs per quart/liter of water. The dose is variable; try ¹/₂ cup/125 ml a day to start.

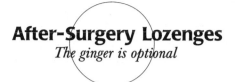

## After-Surgery Lozenges
*The ginger is optional*

• 4 parts *Ulmus fulva* (slippery elm) bark powdered
• 1 part *Zingiber officinalis* (ginger) root powdered
• Honey to mix

Mix the powders together. Slowly work honey into the mix until it becomes stiff enough to roll into balls between your palms. Coat each ball with reserved slippery elm powder. If stored in a covered tin, these lozenges will stay good for several years. They are soothing for sore throats, calming for upset stomachs, warming after the chill of the operating room, and offer a gentle bulking nudge toward resumption of intestinal movement after diarrhea, constipation, or surgery.

## Essiac, Nature's Cancer Cure
*recipe from Gary Glum*

• 6½ cups/1,625 ml *Arctium lappa* (burdock) roots, cut
• 1 pound/500 g *Rumex acetosella* (sheep sorrel) herb, powdered
• 4 ounces/125 g *Ulmus fulva* (slippery elm) bark, powdered
• 1 ounce/30 g *Rheum palmata* (turkey rhubarb) roots, powdered

Mix herbs together thoroughly. Store in an airtight container in a cool, dark place. First thing in the morning, or last thing at night, heat 2 gallons/8 liters of distilled water in a very large stainless steel pot. When it boils, add 1 cup of the mixed herbs. Cover and boil for 10 minutes. Turn off the heat; scrape the herbs off the sides and down into the water, stirring well. Cover the pot closely, push to the back of the stove, and leave it alone for 12 hours.

When the time's up, turn on the fire and reheat the brew almost to boiling, which will take about 20 minutes. Watch it closely so it doesn't actually boil. Remove the pan from the heat and pour the brew through a cheesecloth-lined colander or a fine mesh stainless steel sieve into another pot. Then transfer the hot liquid into bottles sterilized with a rinse of diluted chlorine bleach (carcinogenic) or food grade hydrogen peroxide. Cap the bottles well. Store them at room temperature only until cool, then refrigerate.

Suggested usage: Shake the bottle. A dose is 2 tablespoons/30 ml, taken at night at least two hours after dinner, and again first thing in the morning, at least five minutes before breakfast; two weeks on and two weeks off. Dilute Essiac or warm it if you like.

*See* page 276 for more on Essiac; and see Wessiac, below.

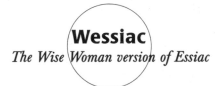

## Wessiac
*The Wise Woman version of Essiac*

1 ounce/30 grams dried *Arctium lappa* (burdock) roots, cut
¹/₂ ounce/15 grams dried *Rumex crispus* (yellow dock) roots, cut
¹/₈ ounce/3.5 grams *Ulmus fulva* (slippery elm) bark, powdered

Infuse all three herbs in 1 quart/liter boiling water for 8 hours. Strain; refrigerate liquid. Daily dose is ¹/₂ cup/125 ml, hot or cold.

Easily available, reasonably priced yellow dock replaces her difficult sisters: sheep sorrel and turkey rhubarb. Using my standard infusion technique (page 294) to make just enough brew to last for a few days eliminates the need to sterilize jars, and allows you to try Wessiac without buying pounds of herbs. (You will want to buy herbs by the pound if you're going to use Essiac or Wessiac consistently.) Because it's gentler on the intestines, Wessiac can be used daily for months. *For this deep down dirty brew I give thanks to the deep roots. Dirt is Earth; the Earth is sacred; dirty is sacred, too.*

## Yellow Salve
*A special formula from Eli Jones, M.D.–"Nothing equals it."*

Combine equal parts burgundy pitch, white pine turpentine, beeswax, mutton tallow, and olive oil in a double boiler. Heat; stir until well mixed. Cool slightly, then mix in one part Unpetroleum Jelly or Cosmoline. This salve is meant to be spread on a clean cotton cloth and applied three times a day. If more than moderate pain occurs, lessen or discontinue use.

## Hoxsey Elixir
*One of many variations. Use with caution; potentially poisonous!*

- 30 parts potassium iodide
- 4 parts *Trifolium pratense* (red clover) blossoms
- 4 parts *Glycyrrhiza glabra* (licorice) root
- 2 parts *Stillingia sylvatica* (stillingia) root
- 4 parts *Rhamnus frangula* (buckthorn) bark
- 2 parts *Phytolacca americana* (poke) root
- 2 parts *Berberis vulgaris* (barberry) bark
- 2 parts *Arctium lappa* (burdock) root
- 1 part *Xanthoxylum americanum* (prickly ash) bark
- 1 part *Rhamnus persiana* (cascara sagrada) bark

Two ounces/55 grams of the dried mixed herbs are infused overnight in one quart/liter boiling water (or tinctured for six weeks in 8 ounces/250 ml vodka) and taken 4 times daily (1 teaspoonful/5 ml or as tolerated). This classic formula has been in use for several hundred years. Variations are available already tinctured from HerbPharm (*see* Resources, page 312) and other sources.

## Hoxsey Salve
*Used to encapsulate cancer before surgery*

12 parts zinc chloride, saturated solution
12 parts antimony trisulfide
 4 parts extract* of *Sanguinaria canadensis* (bloodroot) root
* highly concentrated tincture

Combine all ingredients. This salve is meant to be applied twice a day for 2-4 weeks before surgery and once a day for 2 weeks after surgery to prevent recurrence and metastasis.. Variations of this formula have been in use for several hundred years, both as adjuncts to, and instead of, surgery. **Use with caution:** This salve can burn or injure skin.

## Black Ointment
*formula from Dr. Christopher's School of Natural Healing*

- 1 part *Larrea tridentata* (chaparral) twigs and leaves
- 1 part *Trifolium pratense* (red clover) blossoms
- 1 part *Symphytum officinale* (comfrey) root and/or leaves
- 1 part *Plantago major* or *P. lanceolata* (plantain) leaves
- 1 part *Phytolacca americana* (poke) root
- 1 part *Stellaria media* (chickweed) herb
- 1 part *Verbascum thapsus* (mullein) leaves and/or flowers

Prepare infused herbal oils with as many of these herbs as you can find fresh and in good condition. It isn't necessary to have them all. To make the ointment, melt 1 ounce/30 grams of **pine tar** into every 5 ounces of infused oil along with enough **beeswax** to make a soft ointment. It is also possible to use any of these plants (fresh or dried) to make a poultice to dissolve breast lumps.

## Powerful Poultice Powder
*A drawing application from Dr. John Christopher*

- 1 part *Ulmus fulva* (slippery elm) bark, powdered
- 1 part *Linum usitatissimum* (flax) seed, powdered
- 1 part *Lobelia inflata* (lobelia) herb in seed, powdered
- 1 part *Myrica cerifera* (bayberry) bark, powdered
- 1 part *Curcuma longa* (turmeric) root, powdered

Put 2 teaspoons/10 ml of mixed powders in a small bowl and add about 2 ounces/30 ml boiling water. Mix well and spread on a cloth, covering an area larger than the lump or inflammation. In acute situations, use a continuous poultice, applying a new one every two hours. Bathe the skin over the lump with witch hazel and warm water each time the poultice is changed.

## Ginger Compress
*Easy, effective, inexpensive, pain-relieving, and anti-inflammatory*

Grate 5 ounces/140 grams of fresh ginger root onto a clean piece
of cloth. (I use an old cloth napkin, a handkerchief, a kitchen towel,
or a clean diaper.) Gather the ends of the cloth together and secure
them with a piece of string or a rubber band. Put the bundle into a
pan with 2 quarts/2 liters water and heat to 158°F/70°C. Boiling
will destroy much of the value of the ginger, so if you don't have a
thermometer, heat only until you see bubbles forming on the bottom of the pan. Keep a low flame under the pot until the water
turns a pale yellow, 5–15 minutes. Pull the bundle out of the water, and squeeze or press it to extract all its liquid. (Add to pan.)
   Soak a small towel in the hot ginger liquid. Wring it out. (This
is hard to do; your hands will get red and hot.) When you apply
the hot wet towel, the breast skin will redden and there will be an
intense sensation of heat, but you shouldn't be in pain. Cover the
compress with layers of towels to retain the heat. When it cools,
remove it, soak it again in the hot ginger water, and reapply. Continue until the skin gets very red and warm. Repeat morning and
night. If there is no active infection, the towel and ginger water
can be used over and over again. If fresh ginger is not available,
dried ginger may be used, but will not be as effective. Fresh turmeric may be substituted for fresh ginger, but it stains everything.

## Lump Liniment
*A formula used by William Fox, M.D. in 1904*

• 2 parts tincture of *Iris versicolor* (blue flag) root
• 1 part tincture of *Trifolium pratense* (red clover) blossoms
• 1 part tincture of *Sanguinaria canadensis* (blood root) root

Shake tinctures thoroughly before using. Saturate a clean cotton
cloth with them and use it to poultice the affected area twice a day.
Caution: This liniment can stain clothing and skin. If skin irritation occurs, discontinue use.

Breast Cancer? Breast Health!

## Three-Step Anti-Cancer Plaster
*This recipe from 1855 is reputed to be from an American Indian doctor.*

**Step One**
Roast a large red onion until it's soft; mash. Mix in a small spoonful of dried, powdered *Sanguinaria canadensis* (bloodroot) and apply just enough to cover the lump. A cancerous tumor will react
with pain and discoloration (purple to black); normal areas will be
stained but otherwise unaffected. Use twice, 12 hours apart.

**Step Two**
Grate a cupful of fresh poke root and mix with: a small spoonful of
"boar's tusk root" (I'd use marshmallow root or slippery elm bark
powder instead), a small spoonful of powdered "Jamestown" (Jimson
weed, *Datura stramonium*) seeds against pain, and enough water to
wet well. Apply morning and night, every 12 hours to draw out
the tumor. Do not squeeze or force the tumor. Do not remove
scabs or other matter prematurely. If the tumor is still present
after 10 days, return to step one before continuing with step two.

**Step Three**
After the tumor has been extracted, bathe the breast frequently
with strong tea of *Chimaphila umbellata* (pipsissewa) leaves to heal
it. (I would use an infusion of comfrey or yarrow leaves instead.)

## Red Clover Tar
*Used by Dr. Samuel Thomson (1769-1843)*

Cook fresh red clover blossoms in pure water to cover in a double
boiler for one hour. Squeeze all the liquid out of the blossoms and
replace them with fresh blossoms. Cook for another hour. Squeeze
all liquid out of them, too. Over low heat, reduce the red clover
liquid to a thick tar-like juice. (This will take many hours.) Spread
your red clover tar on a gauze pad before applying to the lump.
Repeat at least twice a day. Rinse the area with dandelion tincture
between applications.

# Favorite Fast Cabbage
## Serves 1-2

*Ready to eat in 15 minutes. For variety, substitute thinly sliced kale,
collards, or Brussels sprouts for the cabbage, or add fresh ginger, fresh
burdock root, or fresh wild mushrooms. A good way to help prevent
cancer, check recurrence, and counter side effects of chemotherapy and
radiation.*

1 **onion**, sliced from top to bottom like crescent moons
1 tablespoon/15 ml **olive oil**
2 cups/500 ml finely sliced or shredded **cabbage**
1 **carrot** grated
4 ounces/120 g **seaweed**  (hijiki, sea palm fronds, or alaria)
1 tablespoon/15 ml **tamari** (soy sauce)
4 tablespoons/60 ml **sunflower seeds**

Soak seaweed in 2 cups/500 ml hot water. On low heat, saute
onion crescents in oil. When they're limp and translucent, add
the cabbage and cook another five minutes, stirring several times.
Drain seaweed. (Reserve soaking water.) Arrange the grated carrot in a circle on top of the cabbage and onion. Put seaweed in
the center of the carrot circle. Add tamari and 3–4 tablespoons/
45–60 ml of the seaweed soaking water to the skillet. Cover
tightly. Raise heat and cook until steam appears, then lower heat
and cook another five minutes, or until the vegetables are very
tender. While it finishes cooking, toast the sunflower seeds. Strew
them liberally over the dish just before serving.

## Anti-Radiation Easy Meal
*Serves 2–4*

1 cup/250 ml sliced **cabbage**
1 cup/250 ml sliced **carrots**
1–2 fresh **burdock roots** sliced
$^1/_2$ cup/125 ml soaked **seaweed**
8 ounces/240 grams fresh wild or exotic **mushrooms**
4 cups/1 liter **water** (spring water or filtered water)
fresh grated **ginger** to taste
1 cup/250 ml cooked **lentils** or beans
4 tablespoons/60 ml **miso** plus 8 tablespoons/125 ml water

Combine all ingredients except beans and miso. Bring to a boil. Lower heat and cook until carrots are tender, about 30 minutes. Add the beans. Serve, or refrigerate for later use. (This dish is equally tasty cold or warm.) Wait until just before serving to blend the warm water and miso, and add to the vegetables.

## Good Enough to Live (Not Die) For Stir-Fry
*Serves 3–4*

6–8 large cloves **garlic**, sliced thinly
1 tablespoon/15 ml **olive oil**
1 cup/250 ml fresh **shiitake**, sliced or 1 ounce/30 grams dried
2–4 fresh **yellow dock roots**
1–2 fresh **burdock roots**
1–2 fresh **dandelion roots**
1 pound/500 grams **tofu** cut in cubes
2 cups/500 ml cooked **fresh stinging nettles**
$^1/_2$ cup/125 ml **almonds**
1 tablespoon/15 ml **tamari**

Cook garlic briefly in oil at the lowest possible heat. Raise heat a little. Add mushrooms and cook for several minutes, stirring often. Slice roots thinly on the diagonal and add them to the skillet. Cook for five minutes, stirring frequently. Add tofu, nettle leaves, and some of the nettle cooking water. Cover tightly and cook at medium-high heat for five minutes. While it cooks, slice and toast almonds. To serve, pour over soba (buckwheat noodles) or brown rice, sprinkle with tamari, and garnish generously with almonds.

# Immune A-Go-Go Soup
### *Serves 6-8*

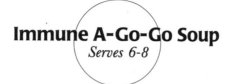

*Good enough for dinner any night, this soup is of special benefit for those in the midst of chemotherapy or radiation treatments. Variations on this soup are a regular part of my anti-cancer lifestyle.*

2 cups/500 ml **beets**, sliced
2 cups/500 ml **water** (spring water or filtered water)
1 cup/250 ml dried **seaweed** (2 cups/500 ml after soaking)
6 cups/1500 ml **cabbage**, thinly sliced
3 **onions**, sliced from top to bottom (like crescent moons)
4 tablespoons/60 ml **olive oil**
1 teaspoon/5 ml **sea salt**
10–20 cloves **garlic**, sliced
1 thumb's worth of **ginger**, sliced
4 ounces/120 grams fresh shiitake, reishii, or wild **mushrooms**
     or 1 ounce/30 grams dried mushrooms
2 cups/500 ml **carrots**, sliced
8–12 cups/2–3 liters **water** (spring water or filtered water)
1 ounce/30 grams **dried Siberian ginseng root**, whole or cut
     optional: **organic chicken**, any amount
     optional: 1 cup/250 ml **cooked brown rice**

Cover beets with water; cook until tender, about 20 minutes. Meanwhile, soak seaweed in hot water. On a low fire, saute the cabbage and onion in olive oil until limp, 5–10 minutes. Add salt, garlic, ginger, mushrooms, carrots, cooked beets and their cooking water, seaweed and its soaking water (watch out for grit at the bottom), and Siberian ginseng. Stir well. Add chicken and/or rice. Add water. Cover the pot tightly and raise the heat to high. As soon as the soup boils, reduce the heat. Simmer for 1 hour. Let it rest for several hours or overnight. Reheat before serving. Don't worry about leftovers. The taste of this soup improves as it ages.

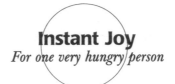

# Instant Joy
*For one very hungry person*

*Part of Joy Craddick's no-more-cancer lifestyle, this dish is simple, nutritionally complete, and takes only seven minutes to prepare.*

2 cups/500 ml **water** (spring water or filtered water)
1 organic **carrot**, grated
1 ounce/30 grams organic **ginger**, grated
1 cup/250 ml organic **broccoli** and/or cauliflower florets
handful of **kelp** or other tasty quick-cooking seaweed
2–4 fresh shiitake or reishii or wild **mushrooms**, sliced
1 "brick" organic **brown rice ramen noodles**
**Tofu**, organic only, as desired
2–3 tablespoons/30–45 ml **miso**
2 tablespoons/30 ml **brown rice vinegar**
**sea salt** to taste

While water comes to a boil, prepare vegetables. Add noodles, tofu, seaweed, mushrooms, and vegetables to water, cover, and cook 2–5 minutes or to taste. Mash miso and vinegar with a fork in your bowl, add soup, and enjoy: Instant Joy!

# Garlic Toast Country Style
*Serves 1*

2 slices organic **whole wheat bread**
4 cloves organic **garlic**, minced
2 tablespoons/30ml **olive oil**

Put bread in a cast iron skillet and toast one side while you mix the oil and minced garlic together. Turn the bread; spoon garlic and oil thickly onto the toasted sides. Continue to cook until the second side is toasted. Eat without delay. For city-style garlic toast, use a regular toaster and spoon garlic mixed with oil on the toast; or spoon garlic and oil on your bread and toast it in a toaster oven. *Mama mia!* Eat it for breakfast!

# Quark and Flax
*Dr. Johanna Budwig's Oil-Protein Treatment*

*Used to counter fatigue, reduce recurrences, and encourage complete remission of cancer, by itself or in conjunction with other treatments. Also used to prevent radiation- and chemotherapy-induced cancers. Current research shows flax oil particularly effective against cancers of the breast.*

100 grams/3.5 ounces **quark***
40 grams/1.5 ounces **fresh flax oil**
25 grams/1 ounce nonfat organic **milk**

Mix quark and oil, adding only enough milk to blend the mixture. Eat immediately or refrigerate in a dark, tightly closed container.

This recipe makes the minimum amount that needs to be consumed per day, but start with small amounts and increase gradually to counter the tendency of flax oil to loosen the bowels. Discontinue use if you experience severe diarrhea.

The mixture can be left plain or seasoned: Add honey and fruit for a sweet variation, or herbs and garlic for a zesty variation. Eat it alone or use it as a topping for bread, grains, granola, vegetables, or baked potatoes.

* If quark is not sold in your area, you can use nonfat cottage cheese, or make your own quark. It's easy. Line a colander or kitchen sieve with a loosely woven cotton cloth (such as a large handkerchief, a clean piece of old sheeting, or several layers of cheesecloth). Place the cloth-lined colander in a large bowl and pour a quart of nonfat or organic yogurt into it. Cover it loosely with plastic and let sit at room temperature for 12–24 hours. The yogurt will separate into a spreadable cheese (the quark) and a liquid (the whey, which has dripped into the bowl). Using a rubber spatula, scrape the quark off the cloth, and store it in a glass container in the refrigerator. It will stay fresh for 7–10 days. (I use the whey as the cooking liquid for rice or millet; yum!)

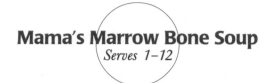

## Mama's Marrow Bone Soup
*Serves 1–12*

8–10 two-inch marrow bones (from pure cows only! This is the
very marrow of their being, becoming yours . . .)
2 onions, chopped
lots of garlic cloves, whole or sliced
handful of celery tops, chopped
4 carrots, chopped
1 teaspoon/5 ml kosher salt
seasoning herbs of your choice (thyme, rosemary, marjoram)
2 cups/500 ml cooked barley (or rice or millet or corn)

Cover the bones with water; bring to a boil. Simmer, skimming
gray matter from the top frequently. After an hour, add remaining
ingredients (except grain) and simmer another hour and a half,
covered. Remove bones; poke the marrow out of their centers.
Puree remaining soup in a Foley mill, blender, or food processor.
Chill puree and marrow separately overnight. Remove any fat
from the puree. Reheat puree, adding marrow and cooked grain.

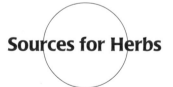

## Sources for Herbs

- *See* page 75 for more mail-order resources.
- **Avena Botanicals** (see page 75). Whole **milk thistle** seeds.
- **Blessed Herbs,**109 Barre Plains Rd, Oakham, MA 01068
- **Frontier**, Box 299, Norway, IA 52318; 1-800-669-3275. Excellent wholesale source for dried herbs, tinctures, oils.
- **Green Terrestrial**, 1449 Warm Brook Rd, Arlington,VT,05250 Nourishing dried herbs; complete line of tinctures, oils.
- **HerbPharm**, PO Box 116, Williams, OR 97544; 503-846-6262; fax: 503-846-6112. Tinctures include *sundew, poke,* and *mistletoe.*
- **Herbalist and Alchemist**, PO Box 553, Broadway, NJ 08808; 908-689-9020.Tinctures include *astragalus, orange,* and *schisandra.*
- **Mt. Rose Herbs**, PO Box 2000, Redway, CA 95560; 1-800-879-3337. Castor oil, clay, tinctures, dried herbs, infused oils.

# Organizations That Offer Help

**African American Breast Cancer Alliance**
1 W. Lake St., Apt. 423, Minneapolis, MN 55408; 612-644-7119
Information, support groups, advocacy.

**Arlin J. Brown Information Center**
PO Box 251, Fort Belvoir, VA 22060; 703-752-9511
Information, newsletter on non-toxic cancer therapies.

**American Holistic Medical Association**
4101 Lake Boone Trail, Suite 201, Raleigh, NC 27607; 919-787-5181
Patient advocacy, referrals, help with complementary approaches.
National Referral Directory: $8.

**American Self-Help Clearinghouse**
25 W. 43rd St., NY, NY 10036-7406
SASE for list of support groups in your area.

**Breast Cancer Action**
1280 Columbus Ave., Suite 204, San Francisco, CA 94133;
415-922-8279; fax-415-922-3253
Breast cancer survivors promoting prevention of breast cancer.

**Breast Cancer Action Group**
PO Box 5605, Burlington, VT 05402-5605; 802-863-3507
Dedicated to nurturing and empowering women to use creative
expression to share their experiences with breast cancer.

**Cancer Information Service** of National Cancer Institute (NCI)
800-4-CANCER
Very orthodox, up-to-date, free information, including PDQ.

**The Center for Medical Consumers**
237 Thompson St., NY, NY 10012; 212-674-7105
Free medical library; open to the public.

313

### Commonweal Cancer Help Program
PO Box 316, Bolinas, CA 94924; 415-868-0970
Retreat center helping those with cancer; extensive library.

### Consumers' Health & Medical Information Center
PO Box 390, Clearwater, FL 33517
Reports on standard, alternative, and late-breaking treatments.

### Cancer Support and Education Center
275 Elliot Dr., Menlo Park, CA 94025; 415-327-6166
Cancer Self-Help Intensives help you maximize inner resources.

### ECaP: Exceptional Cancer Patients
300 Plaza Middlesex, Middletown, CT 06457; 203-343-5950
Highly recommended. Information, books, lists of support/help organizations in your area. Founded by Bernie Siegel, M.D.

### Elisabeth Kubler-Ross Center
33613 North 83rd St., Scottsdale, AZ 85262
Highly recommended 5-day program, "Life, Death & Transition."

### Foundation for Advancement in Cancer Therapies (FACT)
PO Box 1242, Old Chelsea Station, NY, NY 10113; 212-741-2790
"Total-person approach," prevention, and non-toxic therapies.

### Health Reference Center
1-800-227-8431
A commercial data base of 4,000 publications.

### Health Resource, Inc.
209 Katherine Dr., Conway, AR 72032; 501-329-5272
Individual, in-depth research; including Medline search, book excerpts, medical articles, alternative and holistic reports.

### Health Training and Research Center
PO Box 7237, Little Rock, AR 72217; 501-663-5369
Refers practitioners trained in the Simonton approach to cancer.

### Lesbian Community Cancer Project
4753 N. Broadway, Ste. 602, Chicago, IL 60640; 312-561-4662; fax: 312-561-1830
Information, support groups, advocacy, direct care, library.

# Help    315

**Linus Pauling Institute**
440 Page Mill Rd., Palo Alto, CA 94306; 415-327-4064

**Mary-Helen Mautner Project for Lesbians with Cancer**
1707 L St. NW, Suite 1060, Washington, DC 20036; 202-332-5536
Direct services for lesbians, their partners and caregivers.

**Medline**
Data base of 3,600 medical journals, updated weekly, including a separate cancer data base called CANCERLIT; accessible through computer, modem, and a $30 software package (available from Grateful Med, 1-800-638-8480)

**National Alliance of Breast Cancer Organizations**
9 East 37th St., 10th Fl., NY, NY 10016-2822

**National Breast Cancer Coalition**
PO Box 66373, Washington, DC 20035; 202-296-7477

**National Breast Cancer Foundation**
PO Box 130707, Houston, TX 77219-0707
Information kit on BSE; pushes mammograms for young women.

**National Coalition for Cancer Survivorship**
1010 Wayne Ave., 5th Fl., Silver Spring, MD 21910; 301-650-8868

**National Coalition of Feminist and Lesbian Cancer Projects**
1707 L St. NW, Suite 1060, Washington, DC 20036
Offers a manual on "How to Start a Local Cancer Organization."

**National Women's Health Network**
514 10th St. NW, #400, Washington, DC 20004; 202-628-7814

**People Against Cancer**
PO Box 10, Otho, IA 50560; 1-800-662-2623; fax: 515-972-4415
Information on patient advocate alternative therapies; videos.

**Planetree Health Resource Center**
415-923-3680
In-depth report including Medline, book excerpts, standard and alternative treatment options, and contact with others who have the same condition/$100. Medline search/$35. PDQ search/$25.

**Public Citizen Health Research Group**
200 P St. NW, Washington, DC 20036; 202-833-3000

**Rosenthal Center for Alternative/Complementary Medicine**, College of Physicians & Surgeons, Columbia University, NY, NY 10032; 212-305-4755; fax: 212-305-1495

**SHARE, Self-Help for Women with Breast Cancer**
Free support services and hotlines: Spanish (212-719-4454), Chinese (718-296-7108), and English (212-382-2111).

**Susan Komen Breast Cancer Foundation**
1-800-I'M AWARE
Information on risk assessment.

**WomenCARE**
PO Box 944, Santa Cruz, CA 95061; 408-457-2273
Information, advocacy, resources, education, support groups, newsletter.

**Women's Cancer Resource Center**
3023 Shattuck, Berkeley, CA 94705; 510-548-9272
Newsletter, advocacy, support groups, information, referrals, hotline.

**Women's Community Cancer Project**
46 Pleasant St., Cambridge, MA, 02139; 617-354-9888
Advocacy, support groups, information, referrals.

**Y-ME** National Breast Cancer Organization, Inc.
212 W. Van Buren St., 4th Fl., Chicago, IL 60607; 312-986-8338
Hotlines: 1-800-221-2141 (9-5 weekdays); 312-986-8228 (24 hours)
Information, referrals, emotional support; wig and prosthesis bank; network for breast cancer survivors with silicone implants.

# Breast Cancer Risk Assessment

Your risk of developing breast cancer is probably far less than you think, and most likely far less than the widely publicized 1 in 8, which is the lifetime risk of a white woman who lives to be 95 years old. (Female life expectancy in the United States is 79 years.)

• In an eight-year study of 90,000 women at the Harvard School of Public Health, only 1.6 percent developed breast cancer.

• In a National Cancer Institute study of 284,780 women who got annual breast exams and mammograms for five years, only 1.6 percent developed breast cancer.

• Your risk varies as you vary the time factor. Risk in any given year is always less than lifetime risk. (The chart on page 326 shows lifetime risk.)

• From birth to age 40, the average white woman's risk of developing breast cancer is 1 percent, or one in a hundred. Information on risk is heavily white-biased. Women of color are at less risk of developing breast cancer, but at four times greater risk of dying from it than white women.

This questionnaire includes the widest possible range of factors affecting the risk of developing breast cancer: unvalidated (but likely) as well as scientifically validated risk factors. For explanations of these factors, see Chapter 1, "Can Breast Cancer Be Prevented?" beginning on page 3.

**Scoring**: Make two columns, one for risk increases and one for risk reductions. Write the appropriate number in each column as you answer each statement. Then see page 326.

317

# Breast Cancer Risk Assessment Questions

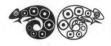

**1. I gave birth to my first child before the age of 20.**
Risk reduction = 120 minus your current age.

**2. I delayed my childbearing. I never gave birth.**
Risk increase for women who have never given birth = +55.
Or, risk increases +1 for every year older than 20 you were
when you first gave birth, up to age 30; then +2 a year.

**3. I miscarried or aborted my first pregnancy.**
Risk = 0

**4. I spent at least 13 months pregnant or lactating.**
Risk reduction = 6 plus 1 for each additional 3 months, up to a
total of 20

**5. I breast-fed my baby for 3 or more months.**
Risk reduction = 6 if you're under 50; 1 if you are 55 or older.

**6. I used birth control pills before my first pregnancy.**
Risk increase +10

**7. I used birth control pills before the age of 20 and had
never been pregnant.**
Risk increase +15

**8. I used birth control pills after my first pregnancy.**
Risk increase 0, first five years, +1 for every five years thereafter.

**9. I used high-dose birth control pills (common in the 60s).**
Risk increase +10 for one year, +1 for additional years.

**10. I used birth control pills for 10 years before pregnancy.**
Risk increase +2 for every year before the age of 35, and +1 for
every year more than 10 that you took the Pill.

**11. I began menstruating before the age of 16.**
Risk increase +2 for each year younger when you bled monthly.

**12. When I was 25–30 years old, my menstrual cycles were 25–30 days apart.**
Risk increase +2 for each day shorter than 25 or longer than 30.

**13. I continued to have menses past the age of 55.**
Risk increase +1 for each year older

**14. I menstruated for more than 40 years.**
Risk increase +10

**15. My ovaries were surgically removed.**
Risk reduction = 1 for every year younger than 50 at the time of the surgery, unless you took hormone replacement.

**16. My uterus was surgically removed.**
Risk increase 0 to +10

**17. I've used estrogen replacement.**
Risk increase +1 for every year up to 9 years; then +2 per year.

**18. I've used hormone replacement** (estrogen and progesterone).
Risk increase +2 for every year up to 6 years; then +4 per year.

**19. I took DES (diethylstilbestrol).**
Risk increase +14

**20. My mother took DES.**
Risk increase +5

**21. My mother, grandmother, or sister had breast cancer.**
Your risk of breast cancer increases with each of the following:
• My mother had breast cancer  = +15 to +18
• My only sister had breast cancer  = +23
• My mother *and* a close relative had breast cancer = +25
• Any of the above were pre-menopausal = +5 more
• The cancer was bilateral (in both breasts) = +5 more
• Cancer was multiple, multifocal, or rare = +5 more
*The older the mother when diagnosed, the lower the risk for the daughter.*

**22. My waist-to-hip ratio is above .81.**
(*Divide waist measure by hip measure to get ratio.*)
Risk increase +50, plus +5 for every extra .03 points up to +70

**23. My ancestors are Caucasian and I have light skin.**
Risk increase +10 to +30, depending on how fair you are.

**24. I am taller than 5'3" and weigh more than 154 pounds.**
Risk increase +5 for every inch taller, up to +35

**25. I am a full-figured earth goddess.** (40 percent or more over average weight for my height.)
Risk increase +15

**26. I take:** *cimetidine* (ulcer medication), *beta-blockers* (high blood pressure drugs), *Prozac* or *Elavil* (antidepressants), *antihistamines.*
Risk increase +5 for each

**27. I have severe asthma.**
Risk increase +5

**28. I have severe allergies or hay fever.**
Risk increase +9

**29. My immune system is constantly under stress.**
**I have chronic fatigue syndrome (CFIDS).**
**I had mononucleosis.**
**I have very frequent infections.**
**My gums and teeth often hurt.**
**I have lots of vaginal and bladder infections.**
**I have chronic sinus problems.**
Risk increase +3 for each "yes" answer.

**30. I eat an even-caloried diet** (total calories do not exceed actual needs; body weight stays steady) **that is 30 percent or less fat, and that fat is organic and non-hydrogenated.**
Risk =0

**31. I eat a high-calorie diet** (total calories exceed actual needs) **that is 30 percent or more fat, and those fats contain residues of farm chemicals and/or are hydrogenated.**
Risk increase +40

**32. Most of the water I drink is chlorinated.**
Risk increase +5

**33. I usually shower in chlorinated water.**
Risk increase +10

34. I swim or soak in chlorinated water an hour a week.
Risk increase +10

35. I don't think that my food choices can affect my health.
Risk increase +15

36. I eat commercial meat, eggs, or milk products every day.
Risk increase +25

37. I eat mostly organically grown food.
Risk decrease = 8

38. My mother and father ate mostly organic food.
Risk decrease = 20

39. So did my grandparents.
Risk decrease = 50

40. I eat 3 or more servings of whole grains daily.
Risk decrease = 10

41. I eat 3 cups of fruit/vegetables a day (excluding juices).
I eat some member of the cabbage family 5 times a week.
Risk decrease = 15 if yes to one; = 40 if yes to both.

42. I eat less than one serving per day of vitamin A-rich food.
Risk increase +25

43. I eat tofu, tamari, miso, tempeh, or dried beans, or drink
red clover infusion 4 or more times a week.
Risk decrease = 10 (= 20 for pre-menopausal women or those
using hormone replacement)

44. I eat iodine-rich foods, like fish and seaweed, regularly.
Risk may decrease or increase by 5

45. I am hyperthyroid.
Risk decrease = 5

46. I am hypothyroid.
Risk increase +5

47. I am a vegetarian.
Risk decrease = 20

### 48. My breasts have been exposed to ionizing radiation.
*Damage from radiation exposure accumulates over your lifetime.*
• Atomic bomb survivor (35 rads at epicenter): increase up to + 35
• Mammogram (0.5-1 rad): increase + 1 per exposure of each breast.
*One mammogram can double a 35-year-old woman's breast cancer risk.*
• Diagnostic x-rays for scoliosis (1.5 - 3 rads): increase +3  per exposure
• Fluoroscopy (7.5 rads each): increase +5 for each
• Radiation treatment (8,000 rads): increase +10 each
*The younger you are when your breasts are exposed to radiation, the greater your risk.*

### 49. I lived in Nevada during the years 1951-1963.
Risk increase +50 minus your age in 1951; and +2 for every year you lived in Nevada. *Example: You were 4 in 1951 and lived in Nevada for 5 years. 50 - 4 =  46 + (2 x 5) = +56*

### 50. I lived in North America during the years 1946-1963.
Risk +1 for every year in that time span.

### 51. I live within 50 miles of a nuclear reactor or nuclear storage site.
Risk increase +60 minus the distance, in miles, to the nearest nuclear facility. *Example: You live 22 miles from a site; your risk is 60 - 22 =  +38.*

### 52. I work in the petroleum or chemical industry.
### I live near a hazardous waste site.
### I live or work on a non-organic farm.
Risk increase +1 per question for every year this is true.

### 53. I live along a major highway.
### I regularly handle oil, gasoline, or petrochemicals.
### My home is heated with oil.
Risk increase +1 per question for every year this is true.

### 54. I live near high-voltage power lines.
### I live near a radio, TV, or microwave tower.
### I use a TV or computer monitor more than 20 hours weekly.
### I use a hair dryer daily.
### I sleep with an electric blanket or on a heated water bed.
### I sleep with my head within 12 inches of an electric clock.
Risk increase +1 per year for each "yes"

**55. I have been exposed to dioxin.** (*You probably have.*)
Risk increase +10

**56. I  smoke commercial cigarettes regularly.**
Risk increase +20,  and +2 for each year of smoking

**57. I smoke organic tobacco or other plants.**
Risk increase: pipe = 0; rolled in paper +5

**58. I drink alcohol occasionally.**
Risk increase +2 for the first four drinks per month; +1 for extras

**59. I drink daily.**
Risk increase +10 for one drink a day , +20 for two drinks a day.

**60. I am a teacher, librarian, or religious worker.**
Risk increase +3

**61. I am a lesbian.**
Risk increase up to +30

**62. There is light in my bedroom all night.**
   **I often stay up late with electric lights on.**
Risk +10 for each "yes"

**63. I sleep outside, away from electricity.**
Risk decrease = 1 per year that you spend two nights out.

**64. I regularly use sunscreen on all exposed parts of my body.**
Risk increase +10

**65. I'm outside (without contacts or glasses) 5 minutes a day.**
Risk decrease = 1 for every year this is true

**66. I have or had cysts in my breasts.**
Risk increase 0

**67. I have or had fibrocystic breast disease.**
Risk increase 0

**68. I have had sclerosing adenosis, apocrine metaplasia,**
   **duct ectasia, lipoma, fat necrosis, or mastitis.**
Risk increase 0

**69. I've had a suspicious lump in my breast biopsied.**
Risk increase 0 if tissue is normal.
Risk increase +15 if tissue shows hyperplasia/proliferative change *without* atypical cells.
Risk increase +25 if tissue shows atypical hyperplasia.

**70. I have regular mammograms.**
Risk increase +40 if premenopausal; +1 for each mammographic series done after menopause.

**71. I do breast self-massage or breast self-exam regularly.**
Risk decrease = 10

**72. I use an anti-perspirant or chemical deodorant regularly.**
**I nearly always shave the hair from my armpits.**
Risk increase +3 for each "yes"

**73. I wear a bra more than 12 hours a day.**
**My bra leaves red marks or indentations on my skin.**
**I wear an underwire bra.**
Risk increase +5 for each "yes"

**74. I exercise for at least 20 minutes, three times a week.**
Risk decrease = 30 if "yes" from ages 12–18.
Risk decrease = 1 for every year of "yes" after age 18.

**75. I feel resentful frequently.**
**I chew on my feelings.**
**I don't feel appreciated.**
**I usually feel unheard; no one listens to me.**
**I don't have anyone I can really talk to honestly.**
**What others want is more important than what I want.**
Risk increase +10 for each "yes"

**76. I'm willing to get angry, but I'm not easily upset.**
**I don't hold grudges.**
**I accept and love myself no matter how I feel.**
**I have ways to acknowledge my "difficult" emotions.**
**I have ways to be with my pain and anger.**
**I know what I need and want, and I am willing to ask for it.**
Risk reduction = 10 for each "yes"

**77. I set aside regular time to relax and get in touch with my feelings and desires.**
Risk reduction = 20

**78. My beloved died unexpectedly within the past 5 years.**
Risk increase +25 to +50

**Scoring**: Add all your risk increases. Add all your risk reductions. If your risk increase total is greater than your risk reduction total, you are at greater risk of getting breast cancer than the average woman your age. See #1 below. If your risk reduction total is greater than your risk increase total, you have less risk of getting breast cancer than the average woman your age. See #2 below.

#1. Subtract reduction total from increase total. Multiply the result by .01 (or move the decimal two places to the left). Add 1. This is your risk number. On page 326 find the age closest to yours. Replace the 1 in "1 out of ..." with your number; that's your risk.

Example: Amy's risk reduction total was 58. Her risk increase total was 116. The difference (116 – 58 = 58) multiplied by .01 is .58; her risk is .58 + 1 = 1.58. She is 35 years old. Her risk of developing breast cancer in the next 5 years is 1.58 out of 622.

Divide the number of women at risk (in this example 622) by your risk number (1.58) to express your risk as "1 out of . . ." (622 divided by 1.58 = 394.) Amy's risk is 1 out of 394.

#2. Subtract increase total from reduction total. Multiply the result by .01 (or move the decimal two places to the left) and add 1. This is your risk number. On page 326 find the age closest to yours. Multiply your score by the number of women at risk (number after "1 in . . .") to find your lower risk.

Example: Sue's risk reduction total is 246. Her risk increase total is 100. The difference (246 – 100 = 146) multiplied by .01 is 1.46. Her risk is 1.46 + 1 = 2.46. She is 35 years old. The number after "1 in . . ." is 622. Sue multiplies 622 by 2.46 (= 1530). Her risk is 1 out of 1530. (The risk number is also the percentage of risk decrease; Sue is 146 percent less likely than the average woman her age to develop breast cancer in her lifetime.)

Note: A 100 percent decrease means you are only half as likely as average to develop breast cancer. This survey helps you estimate your risk of *developing* breast cancer, not your risk of *dying* from it.

# What's My Breast Cancer Risk?

Age 25 = 1 in 19,608 (.005%)

Age 30 =  1 in 2,525 (.04%)

Age 35 = 1 in 622 (.16%)

Age 40 = 1 in 217 (.5%)

Age 45 = 1 in 93 (1%)

Age 50 = 1 in 50 (2%)

Age 55 = 1 in 33 (3%)

Age 60 = 1 in 24 (4%)

Age 65 = 1 in 17 (6%)

**Median age for developing breast cancer (USA): 69**

Age 70 = 1 in 14 (7%)

Age 75 = 1 in 11 (9%) of all white women
    1 in 14 (7%) of all African-American women
    1 in 16 (6%) of all Chinese-American women
    1 in 40 (2.5%) of all Native American women

**Average female lifespan in USA (1990): 79 years.**

Age 80 = 1 in 10 (10%)

Age 85 = 1 in 9 (11%)

Age 95 = 1 in 8 (12.5%)

data from N.C.I.

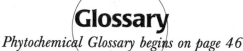

# Glossary

*Phytochemical Glossary begins on page 46*

**adaptogen:** helps one adapt to stress, pollution, and radiation without the usual health consequences.

**adenocarcinoma:** cancer originating in gland-forming tissues, such as the breasts.

**adjuvant:** treatment used to increase effectiveness of another treatment. Radiation and chemotherapy are adjuvants to surgery.

**adrenal:** gland whose cortex produces hormones (e.g., adrenalin, cortisone) in reaction to stress.

**alkaloid:** the active drug-like or poisonous principle in plants, e.g., caffeine, nicotine, heroin, cocaine.

**angiogenesis:** blood vessel growth.

**aneuploid:** an abnormal number of chromosomes.

**anti-angiogenesis:** prevents new blood vessel growth and so inhibits cancer metastasis.

**antibacterial:** inhibits or kills bacteria, including the bacteria in our gut that help us assimilate nutrients.

**antibiotic:** "against life"; a powerful antibacterial, e.g., penicillin.

**antibody:** immunoglobulin molecule made by lymph tissues to repel specific threats to the body, e.g., cancer, viral infection.

**anti-cancer:** prevents or stops the initiation, promotion, or progression of cancer.

**antifungal:** remedies or prevents fungal infections, e.g., thrush, candida.

**anti-inflammatory:** reduces inflammation.

**anti-microbial:** "against microbes"; antibiotic or antibacterial.

**antimutagenic:** prevents or remedies mutation of cellular DNA.

**antiseptic:** kills or inhibits growth of disease- and infection-causing bacteria. *Compare* antibacterial.

**antispasmodic:** stops spasms and cramps, especially in intestines, muscles, and nerves.

**antithrombotic:** prevents blood clots (thromboses).

**antitumor:** shrinks tumors.

**antiviral:** remedies viral infections, e.g., HIV, herpes, Epstein-Barr.

**aphrodisiac:** increases sexual energy and appetite.

**aspiration:** suction; a hollow needle aspirates fluid or cells from a lump.

**atypical cells:** mildly abnormal cells. All bodies have some.

**atypical hyperplasia:** lots of abnormal cells; precancerous; frequently reversed without invasive treatment.

**axillary node dissection:** surgical removal of lymph nodes in armpit.

**basophil:** a white blood cell; initiates inflammation and helps damaged tissues heal.

**benign:** non-cancerous.

**bilateral:** both sides; both breasts.

**biopsy:** removal of tissue, usually through aspiration or surgery.

*excisional biopsy*—removes the entire lump. (*See* lumpectomy.)

*incisional biopsy*—cuts into and removes part of a lump.

*needle localization biopsy*—removes suspicious tissues and calcifications guided by marker needles or dye.

*stereotactic biopsy*—removes tissue guided by continuous x-rays.

**bone marrow:** soft inner core of the bones where blood cells are created.

**bone scan:** a test using high-dose radiation to look for bone shadows which might indicate metastases.

**breast-sparing surgery:** does not remove the breast. *See* lumpectomy.

**calcifications:** small calcium deposits visible in a mammogram; sometimes indicative of cancer.

**cancer:** extremely abnormal unchecked cellular growth. About 300 types occur in humans.

**carcinogen:** initiates or promotes cancer.

**carcinoma:** cancer originating in epithelial tissues, e.g., skin, glands, the lining of internal organs; the most common type of cancer.

**cell:** basic unit of biological growth in all living organisms.

**chemotherapy:** use of drugs to kill cancer cells throughout the body.

**chromosomes:** structures that contain genes made of DNA.

**clear margins:** no cancer cells on the edge of or around a removed tumor.

**clinical study:** a review of records of people (sometimes very few) with a particular disease.

**clinical trial:** an experiment using people. *Compare* laboratory study.

**clotting time:** time required for platelets in blood to form a clot.

**CMF:** chemotherapy regime of cyclophosphamide, methotrexate, and fluorouracil (5-FU).

**complementary medicine:** remedy known by long use or clinical trial to be safe used as an adjuvant to orthodox treatments.

**contraindicated:** not to be used.

**contralateral:** the other side.

**cyst:** a fluid-filled sac or fibrous growth; benign.

**cystosarcoma phylloides:** a rare type of breast tumor.

**cytotoxic:** lethal to cells.

**cytostatic:** inhibits or stops the growth of cells.

**DCIS:** *see* ductal carcinoma in situ

**DDE** and **DDT:** organochlorine pesticides now banned in the United States, but still used in Mexico.

**DES:** diethylstilbestrol, synthetic form of estrogen; previously given to pregnant women; now used against metastasized breast cancer.

**diploid:** normal number of chromosomes.

**DNA:** deoxyribonucleic acid; the brain of the cell; genetic information wrapped in a double spiral. Damaged DNA (from free radicals, radiation, chemicals, or inheritance) initiates cancer.

**doubling time:** how long it takes a group of cells to double in number.

**duct:** a narrow tube through which material is released; breast ducts connect the lobules with the nipple.

**ductal carcinoma in situ:** mass of atypical cells with a clear boundary confined to a duct; reversible without invasive treatment according to breast specialist, S. Love, M.D.

**edema:** swelling caused by fluid build up between the cells.

**emetic:** causes vomiting.

**encapsulate:** form a wall around.

**endometrium:** tissue lining the uterus which becomes filled with blood each month of the fertile years, releasing into menstrual bleeding.

**eosinophils:** white blood cells which eat parasites and foreign organisms.

**ER status:** estrogen receptor status; may be positive or negative. ER-positive cancers are more responsive to treatment.

# Glossary

329

**escharotic:** a caustic, either acid or alkaline, that destroys tissues; external chemotherapy.

**estrogens:** hormones made by a woman's ovaries, adrenals, fat cells, and placenta, e.g., estradiol, estrone; many breast cancers are promoted by estrogen or estrogen-mimicking organochlorines; phytoestrogens can counter this.

**estrogen metabolism:** complex bodily processes which change and utilize estrogens; phytoestrogen metabolism protects against the harmful effects of other estrogens.

**estrogen receptor:** special site on a cell that allows estrogen to enter.

**fibroadenoma:** harmless fibrous tumor of the breast.

**fibrocystic disease:** fear-inducing term for benign lumps in the breasts.

**fluoroscopy:** high-dose x-ray (radiation) used in an examination, not to take a picture.

**free radical:** oxygen molecules with unpaired electrons which disrupt normal cellular functions. Produced in the body by radiation, cigarette smoke, smog, and rancid fats. Free radicals damage DNA. Anti-oxidants eliminate them.

**genes:** biological units, composed of DNA, that control an individual's physical and biochemical traits.

**hematoma:** blood pooled in soft tissues; a common side effect of surgery that can be painful, weakening, and an entry for infection.

**hepatotoxin:** liver poison.

**heterogeneous:** different things; several types of abnormal cells.

**homeopathy:** "like treats like"; health care system where infinitesimal amounts of herbs and elements are used as remedies.

**homeopathic mother tincture:** an herbal tincture; usually diluted into a homeopathic remedy.

**hyper-:** too much, going too fast; *hyperthyroid* speeds up metabolism.

**hyperplasia:** excessive growth of cells, abnormal but not cancerous.

**hypo-:** too little, going too slow; *hypothyroid* produces too few hormones and slows down metabolism.

**immune system:** network of cells and cell products that defends the body against bacteria, viruses, parasites, and cancer.

**immunoglobulins:** IgA, IgD, IgE, IgG, and IgM are antibodies which are active throughout the body.

*in situ:* "in the original site"; contained completely within the tissue of origin; not invasive or infiltrating.

**infiltrating breast cancer:** cancer that has grown out of the tissue of its origin and into the immediately surrounding tissues; not aggressive.

**infiltrating ductal carcinoma:** a common type of breast cancer; originating in a duct, it has grown into the surrounding tissues.

**initiation:** event that damages the DNA, turns on oncogenes, and starts the cancer cascade.

**interferon:** protein produced by the immune system; inhibits viral multiplication and activates T-cells.

**intraductal:** within the duct.

**intraductal papilloma:** benign tumor in the lining of a breast duct.

**inulin:** type of plant sugar.

**invasive breast cancer:** cancer growing beyond the tissues of origin; like infiltrating, *not aggressive.*

**kidneys:** organs which filter chemicals and waste from the blood.

**laboratory study:** an experiment using cell cultures or animals (in breast cancer studies, usually mice).

**LCIS:** *see* lobular carcinoma in situ

**liver:** the body's recycling center; this large organ performs functions critical to digestion, utilization of hormones, and removal of chemicals from the body.

**lobular carcinoma in situ:** cancer cells in a breast lobule; sign of possible later breast cancer in either breast in 17 percent of women, but rarely invasive or metastasizing.

**lobules:** milk-producing breast tissues.

**local recurrence:** cancer of the same type as previously diagnosed, appearing in the same tissues after removal of a primary tumor; commonly at the surgical incision site.

**lumpectomy:** breast surgery which removes a lump, usually with some normal-looking tissue all around it. (*See* clear margin.) Types include:

  *wide-excisional lumpectomy*–removes a very wide margin of breast tissues along with the lump.

  *segmental mastectomy*–removes a wedge of tissue including the lump.

  *quadrectomy*–removes a quarter of the breast and one or more lumps.

  *partial mastectomy*–removes up to half the breast.

**lymph fluid:** a thin, clear liquid originating in many organs and tissues; it circulates among the cells and through the lymphatic vessels.

**lymph nodes, lymph glands:** tissues that circulate and filter lymph; found throughout the body, but especially in the neck, armpit, abdomen, and groin; part of the immune system. Metastasizing cancer cells may collect in the lymph nodes.

**lymph node dissection:** surgical removal of lymph nodes; may accompany a biopsy, lumpectomy, or mastectomy; may cause lymphedema.

**lymphatic system:** a vast, complex system of capillaries, thin vessels, calces, ducts, nodes, and organs which forms a continuous network throughout the body, protecting and maintaining the fluid environment. Includes tonsils, thymus, and spleen.

**lymphedema:** swelling caused by build up of lymph fluid from damage to or removal of lymph nodes.

**lymphocytes:** unique white blood cells (e.g., T-cells, B-cells) tailor-made to seek out specific viruses and tumor cells; lifespan, ten years.

**macrophage:** any large cell that can surround and digest foreign substances in the body; found in the liver, spleen, and loose connective tissues. *Compare to* phagocyte.

**malignant:** cancerous.

**mastalgia** or **mastopexy:** pain in the breast.

**mastitis:** breast infection.

**mammogram:** picture of the breast taken with x-rays.

  *screening mammogram*–two views of each breast, or four x-rays, are taken to look for unsuspected cancers.

  *diagnostic mammogram*–unlimited number of x-rays taken when breast cancer is suspected.

  *digital mammogram*–a less radioactive way to picture breast tissues with sensitive light detectors.

**mass:** a group of cells.

**mastectomy:** surgical removal of a breast. Types include:

  *partial mastectomy*–lumpectomy.

  *complete* or *total mastectomy*–removes all breast tissues including skin.

  *modified mastectomy*–removes all breast tissues, some lymph nodes.

  *radical mastectomy*–removes all breast tissues, all lymph nodes, and all the muscles of the chest wall.

*prophylactic subcutaneous mastectomy*–removes all breast tissues, leaving skin and chest muscles, when no breast cancer is present.

**melatonin:** anti-cancer hormone produced in the dark by the pineal.

**menarche:** first menstrual period.

**menopause:** permanent cessation of menstruation.

**menses:** menstrual flow of blood.

**metabolic:** refering to metabolism.

**metabolism:** organic chemical process that take place in the body liberating nutrients and energy.

**metastatic recurrence:** breast cancer growing somewhere other than the breast or lymph nodes.

**metastasis** (sing.), **metastases** (pl.): cancer of the same type as the primary cancer growing at a distant site other than the lymph nodes.

**metastasize:** spread of a cancer to a distant site; breast cancer commonly metastasizes to liver, lungs, or bones (sometimes brain).

**micro-metastases:** "undetectably" small metastases, even individual cancer cells.

**monocytes:** white blood cells that consume dead cells and debris.

**mucilage:** gluey, sticky substance.

**necrosis:** tissue death. Some tumors contain necrotic tissues. Some necrotic tissues attract calcium.

**neoplasia:** more abnormal than hyperplasia; tumor cells are neoplastic; may be benign or malignant.

**neutrophil:** white blood cell that counters infection; pus consists almost entirely of neutrophils.

**node status:** positive (= presence) or negative (= absence) for cancer cells found in the lymph nodes.

**nourishing:** provides nutrients.

**oncogene:** a normal gene which, when damaged or turned on, initiates cancer; 100 currently known.

**oncogenesis:** process of initiation and growth of a tumor through biological, chemical, or physical actions; turning on of oncogenes.

**oncologist:** cancer doctor.

**oophorectomy:** surgical removal of one or both ovaries; female castration.

**orthodox treatments:** currently accepted treatments for breast cancer, including local treatments (surgery, radiation) and systemic treatments (chemotherapy, hormones).

**oxidation:** a destructive cellular process in which the amount of oxygen is increased or a free radical is formed.

**palliative:** soothes or relieves but does not cure.

**palpate:** feel with the fingers.

**phagocytes:** cells that can surround, eat, and digest small living things and cell wastes; some are fixed to one place, and some, like white blood cells, are free to move.

**phyto-:** "plant."

**phytochemical:** natural chemical made by plants.

**phytoestrogen:** plant "estrogen."

**phytosterol:** plant hormone.

**platelets:** thrombocytes, a blood component that stops bleeding and repairs blood vessels; lifespan, ten days.

**poultice:** a soft, hot substance applied directly to the body or a lump. Herbal poultices are made of chewed fresh herbs, cooked fresh or dried herbs; herbal oils, ointments, and tinctures; or powdered herbs.

**primary cancer:** first cancerous mass. *Compare to* recurrence.

**prognosis:** a doctor's prediction of the likely outcome of a disease.

**promotion:** events which allow initiated cancer cells to elude the immune system and nourish themselves enough to begin to grow.

**prophylactic:** preventive.

**protocol:** custom; a program of scientific inquiry designed to answer a specific question; particular dosages and combinations of chemotherapeutic drugs.

**purgative:** produces rapid, usually painful, emptying of the bowels.

**rad:** abbreviation for radiation-absorbed dose; the basic unit of taken-in dose of ionizing radiation.

**reconstruction, breast:** surgical procedures used to create breast-like shapes, e.g., silicone and saline implants, tram-flaps, skin grafts, and shaping of the other breast.

**recurrence:** return of cancer after it is believed to be gone.

**red blood cells** (erythrocytes): each makes a complete circuit of the body every 30 seconds, exchanging carbon dioxide for oxygen. Lifespan, 4 months.

**rejuvenative:** an agent that restores the vigor of youth.

**rem:** abbreviation for roentgen equivalent man. A dose of radiation that causes in humans the same effect as one unit of x-rays. Half of those exposed to 500 rems die.

**remission:** shrinkage of a tumor or disappearance of detectable cancer.

**rhizome:** a specialized plant stem growing underground which resembles a fleshy root.

**side effect:** undesired result.

**silicone:** inorganic material used in breast reconstruction which can cause health problems.

**soy products:** foods made from soy beans: e.g., tofu, miso, tamari, tempeh, soy milk, and vegetable protein.

**species:** different types of the same kind of plant.

**spleen:** gland that produces lymph cells; part of the immune system.

**S-phase fraction:** percentage of cancer cells reproducing at a given time.

**staging:** cancer classification system based on size of primary tumor, lymph node involvement, and presence or absence of metastases.

**stem cells:** produced in the bone marrow; the source of all red blood cells, platelets, and white blood cells.

**subcutaneous:** beneath the skin.

**synergistic:** parts working together in such a way that the whole is more effective than the sum of the parts.

**systemic treatment:** in orthodox medicine—remedy used internally to kill cancer cells throughout the body and prevent metastases; in wholistic medicine—remedy used internally to strengthen the organism in order to slow or reverse the cancer process.

**T-cells:** specialized lymphocytes that eat cancer cells; e.g., suppressor T-cells, helper T-cells, and N-K (natural killer) cells.

**tamoxifen:** a hormone-like drug which blocks the uptake of estrogen.

**tissue:** body structure made up of similar cells; e.g., breast tissue, muscle tissue, fat tissue.

**tonify:** improve functional ability.

**tumor:** a benign or malignant mass of abnormal cells.

**virus:** a tiny organism that can only grow in the cells of another animal. More than 200 human diseases are caused by viral infections.

**white blood cells** (leukocytes): lymphocytes, basophils, eosinophils, monocytes, and neutrophils that eat bacteria, parasites, viruses, and damaged or abnormal cells.

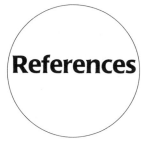

# References

## Chapter 1. Can Breast Cancer Be Prevented?

1. *The Truth About Breast Cancer*, Claire Hoy, Stoddart, 1995
2. *Dr. Susan Love's Breast Book*, Susan Love, Addison-Wesley, 1990
3. *Understanding Breast Cancer Risk*, Pat Kelly, Temple University, 1991
4. *New England Journal of Medicine* 328:176, 1993
5. "Women Who Breastfeed," Jennifer Chris, *American Health*, April 1994
6. "More About that 1 in 8 Breast Cancer Statistic," *Health Facts*, May 1993
7. "Breast Cancer and Pesticides," *Soil and Health*, January 1994
8. "The Other Reward of Exercise," Harriet Brown, *Health*, July 1994
9. "Menstrual cycles may affect cancer risk," J. Raloff, *Science News*, January 7, 1995
10. Menstruation and Reproductive History Study, Elizabeth Whelan, report in *American Journal of Epidemiology*, December 15, 1994
11. "Soybeans and Breast Cancer," Wanda Gardner, *Nutrition & Dietary Consultant*, September 1993
12. "Broccoli inhibits cancer—mostly," *Science News*, December 1994 (442)
13. "EcoCancers," *Science News*, July 3, 1993 (10-13)
14. *Estrogen and Breast Cancer: A Warning to Women*, Carol Ann Rinzler, Macmillan, 1993
15. "Progestin fails to cut breast cancer risk," *Science News*, June 17, 1995
16. "Breast Cancer: Risk and Prevention," *MidLife Woman*, Vol. 2, No. 5, 1993
17. "EcoCancers," *Science News*, July 3, 1993 (10-13)
18. "Breast cancer: environmental factors," *Lancet*, October 10, 1992 (904)
19. "The Environmental Link to Breast Cancer," *Ms*, May/June 1993
20. "Breast Cancer and Pollutants," Michele Turk, *American Health*, July/August 1994
21. National Women's Health Network News, May/June 1990
22. "Pill Ups Cancer Risk in Young Women," *Science News*, June 10, 1995
23. "Oral Contraceptive Use and Breast Cancer Risk in Young Women," *Lancet*, 1989 (973-982)
24. "Breast Cancer Risk Factors: Are They Taken Too Seriously?" *Health Facts*, September 1993
25. "Breast Cancer: A Reassuring Look at Your Odds," *Health*, January 1993
26. "Vital Signs," *Health*, October 1993
27. University of Texas *Lifetime Health Letter*, October 1992

28. "Breast Cancer and Body Shape," *Annals of Internal Medicine,* 112, 1990 (182-186)
29. "Breast cancer risk and DDT: No verdict yet," K. A. Fackelmann, *Science News,* April 23, 1994
30. *The Journey Beyond Breast Cancer, Taking an Active Role in Prevention, Diagnosis, and Your Own Healing,* Virginia Soffa, Healing Arts, 1994
31. "Pollutants Linked to Breast Cancer," Andrew Weil, M.D., *Natural Health,* November/December 1993
32. "Breast Cancer Coverup," *Mother Jones* special, May/June 1994
33. "This fat may aid spread of breast cancer," J. Raloff, *Science News,* November 1994 (421)
34. *Journal of the National Cancer Institute,* 87: 110, 1995
35. "Breast Cancer: A Formula for Prevention," *American Health,* May 1990
36. "Role of the Antioxidants in Cancer Prevention and Treatment," *Townsend Letter for Doctors,* October 1993
37. "New risks for meat eaters," G. Matino, *Science News,* 146, July 16, 1994
38. "Additional source of dietary 'estrogens'," J. Raloff, *Science News,* June 3, 1995
39. "Do Antihistamines Spur Cancer Growth?," K. A. Fackelmann, *Science News,* May 21, 1994 (324)
39A. "Epstein-Barr Virus Link to Breast Cancer," *Science News,* March 14, 1995
40. "Thyroid: Misconceptions," R. Peat, *Townsend Letter for Doctors,* November 1993
41. *Informed Woman's Guide to Breast Health,* Kerry McGinn, Bull, 1992
42. "Fibrocystic Breast Disease . . . Or Is It?" Tori Hudson, N.D., *Townsend Letter for Doctors,* May 1994
43. *Preventing Breast Cancer: The Story of a Major, Proven, Preventable Cause,* J. Gofman, Committee for Nuclear Responsibility, 1995
44. "Study shows risk in low-level radiation," Dr. Alice Stewart, *American Journal of Industrial Medicine,* March 1994
45. "Public Testimony Before Texas Officials: Breast Cancer and Radiation," Feb. 22, 1994
46. "Breast Cancer: Evidence for a Relation to Fission Products in the Diet," Sternglass and Gould, *Int. J. Health Services,* Vol 3, No. 4, 1993
47. "Increases in Breast Cancer Mortality Near U.S. Nuclear Reactors," *Natural Health,* November/December 1993 (19)
48. "Evaluation of the Potential Carcinogenicity of Electromagnetic Fields," EPA draft report, 1991
49. "Electromagnetic Fields," *Popular Science,* December 1991(89)
50. *Currents of Death: Power Lines and the Attempt to Cover Up Their Threat to Your Heath,* P. Brodeur, Simon & Schuster, 1989
51. "Electromagnetic Fields and Male Breast Cancer," *The Lancet,* December 1990 (336)
52. Health Report, *Time,* June 27, 1994
53. "Do EMFs Pose Breast Cancer Risk?," K. A. Fackelmann, *Science News,* June 18, 1994 (388)

54. "Cigarettes tied to fatal breast cancer," and "Fatal breast cancer and smoking," *Science News,* June 4, 1994
55. "Alcohol and the breast," *Journal of the National Cancer Institute,* 85:692, 722, 1993
56. Letter from Graham Colditz, M.D., Ph.D., Assoc. Prof. of Medicine, Harvard Med. School, published in *Mother Jones,* July/August 1994
57. "Lesbians and Breast Cancer," *The Advocate,* 1993
58. *Health and Light,* John Ott, Pocketbooks (Ariel), 1973
59. *Dressed To Kill: The Link Between Breast Cancer and Bras,* Donna Grismaijer, Avery, 1995
60. "Exercising reduces breast cancer risk," J. Raloff, *Science News,* October 1, 1994
61. *The Type C Connection,* Dr. Lydia Temoshok, Random House, 1991
62. "Vitamin E: A cancer warning," *Science News,* April 29, 1995 (271)
63. "Faulty Math Heightens Fears of Breast Cancer," Sandra Blakeslee, *New York Times,* March 15, 1992

## Chapter 2. Can Food Prevent Cancer?

1. "Epidemiological Correlations Between Diet and Cancer Frequency," P. Correa, *Cancer Research,* 41: 3685-3690, 1981
2. *Herbal and Nutritional Strategies for Treating Cancer: Focus on Breast Cancer,* Donald Yance Jr, CNMH, American Herbalist Guild, 1995
3. *Healing with Food,* Melvyn Werbach, M.D., Harper, 1993
4. *Natural Health, Natural Medicine,* A. Weil, M.D., Houghton Mifflin, 1990
5. *Organic Garden Medicine,* Dr. Jean Valnet, Erbonia, 1975
6. *The Food Pharmacy,* Jean Carper, Bantam, 1988
7. "Phytochemicals: Plants Against Cancer," David Schardt, *Nutrition Action Newsletter,* April 1994
8. "The Significance of Diet in Cancer Prevention," R.W. Bradford and H.W. Allen, Bradford Research monograph, 1994
9. "Pesticides and polychlorinated biphenyl residues in human breast lipids, and their relation to breast cancer, " Falck, et al., *Archives of Environmental Health,* 47:143-6, 1992
10. *Cancer Prevention and Nutritional Therapies,* R. A. Passwater, Keats, 1994
11. *Encyclopedia of Fruits, Vegetables, Nuts, and Seeds for Healthful Living,* Joseph Kadans, Parker, 1973
12. *Cereal Grass: Nature's Greatest Health Gift,* R. L. Siebold, ed., Keats, 1994
13. *A Cancer Therapy,* Max Gerson, M.D., Station Hill, 1990
14. "Lignans in Flaxseed and Breast Carcinogenesis," Lilian Thompson and M. Serraino, Dept. of Nutritional Sciences, Univ. of Toronto, 1989
15. *Staying Healthy With Nutrition,* E. Haas, M.D., Celestial Arts, 1992
16. *Of People and Plants,* Maurice Messegue, Healing Arts Press, 1993
17. "Garlic fights nitrosamine formation . . . as do tomatoes and other produce," *Science News,* Vol. 145, February 1994
18. "Fighting Cancer Without Fat," Bonnie Liebman, *Nutrition Action Newsletter,* June 1993

19. "This fat may fight cancer in several ways," J. Raloff, *Science News*, March 19, 1994

20. *Flax Oil as a True Aid Against Arthritis, Heart Infarction, Cancer, and Other Diseases*, Dr. Johanna Budwig, Apple, 1992

20a. "Organic Foods Have More Minerals," David Steinman, *Natural Health*, September/October 1993

21. *Breast Cancer and the Environment: The Chlorine Connection*, Joe Thornton, Greenpeace, 1992 (both editions)

22. "The Consumption of Seaweed as a Protective Factor in the Etiology of Breast Cancer," J. Teas, *Medical Hypotheses*, 7:(5)601-613, 1981

23. "Soybean Isoflavones Lower Risk of Degenerative Diseases," Morton Walker, *Townsend Letter for Doctors*, August/September 1994

23a. "Soy May Ward Off Breast Cancer," Debra Weisenthal, *Vegetarian Times*, June 1995

24. "Tea for 250 Million," Bonnie Liebman, *Nutrition Action Newsletter*, November 1994 (*Cancer Research*, 52: 3875, 1992 and *Journal of National Cancer Institute*, 85: 1038, 1993)

25. "Antitumor activity exhibited by orally administered extract from fruit body of *Grifolia frondosa*," *Chem. Pharm. Bull.* 36: 1819-27, 1988

26. "Lentinan as a Model for the Efficacy of Immunomodulators in Cancer," G. Chihara, *Townsend Letter for Doctors*, April 1994

27. "Antitumor Activity of Yogurt Components," G. V. Reddy, *Journal of Food Products*, 46: 8-11, 1983

28. "Top 10 Phytochemicals of 1994," Prevention Nutrition Consultants, *American Health*, July/August 1994

29. "Polyphenols & Bioflavonoids: The Medicines of Tomorrow," Brian Leibovitz, *Townsend Letter for Doctors*, April 1994

30. "Does Fiber-Rich Food Containing Animal Lignan Precursors Protect Against Breast Cancer?" H. Adlercreutz, *Gastroenterology*, Vol. 86:4, 1984

31. "The Diet That May Save Your Life," National Women's Health Network, *Ms.*, May/June 1993

32. *Beating Cancer With Nutrition*, Pat Quinlan, Ph.D, Nutrition Times Press, 1994 (Includes clinically proven nutritional strategies used by people in all stages of cancer.)

33. *Fats That Heal, Fats That Kill*, Udo Erasmus, Alive Books, 1994

34. *Proc. Amer. Assoc. Cancer Research*, 34:555, 1993

35. "Laetrile," Michael Culbert, *Townsend Letter For Doctors*, June 1995

36. "Origin of lignans in mammals and identification of a precursor from plants," M. Axelson et al., *Nature*, August 1982

37. *Oxford Book of Food Plants*, Masefield et al., Oxford Univ. Press, 1969

38. *Vitamins and Minerals in the Prevention and Treatment of Cancer*, Maryce Jacobs, CRC Press, 1994

39. "Foods Can Be Potent Cancer-Fighting Weapons," University of Texas *Lifetime Health Letter*, Vol. 4:12, December 1992

40. "Dodging Cancer with Diet," Bonnie Liebman, *Nutrition Action*, January/February 1995

## Chapter 3. Taking Our Breasts into Our Own Hands
1. *Breast Self-Examination,* A. R. Milan, M.D., Workman, 1980
2. "Breast Self-Exam, A New Approach," American Cancer Society, 1990
3. Herbal references, *see* page 292.

## Chapter 4. Building Powerful Immunity
1. "Epstein-Barr Virus Link to Breast Cancer," *Science News,* March 14, 1995
2. *The Body Victorious,* Lennart Nilsson, Dell, 1987
3. *Healing and the Mind,* Bill Moyers, Doubleday, 1993
4. *Vibrational Medicine,* Richard Gerber, M.D., Bear & Co., 1988
5. *Pranic Healing,* Choa Kok Sui, Weiser, 1990
6. *Your Body Believes Every Word You Say,* Barbara Levine, Aslan, 1991
7. *Healing Words,* Larry Dossey, Harper, 1994
8. *The Complete Book of Essential Oils and Aromatherapy,* Valerie Ann Worwood, New World Library, 1991
9. For an excellent overview of the immune system, with many scientific references on immune-enhancing plants, see *Encyclopedia of Natural Medicine,* M. Murray and J. Pizzorno, Prima, 1991.
10. *Herbal Emissaries,* Steven Foster and Yue Chongxi, Healing Arts, 1992
11. For a sampling of some of the thousands of scientific studies on ginseng, read *Herbal Tonic Therapies,* Daniel Mowrey, Keats, 1993.
12. *Ginseng, A Concise Handbook,* James Duke, Reference Publications, 1991
13. "Immunostimulating polysaccharides of higher plants," Wagner, Proksch, et al., *Arzneim-Forsch,* 1985(35)
14. *Double the Power of Your Immune System,* John Heinerman, Parker, 1991
15. *Mending the Body, Mending the Mind,* Joan Borysenko, Bantam, 1988
16. *Gateway to Inner Space,* Christian Ratsch, ed., Prism/Avery, 1989
17. *Plants of the Gods, Origins of Hallucinogenic Use,* R. E. Schultes, A. Hoffmann, Inner Traditions, 1979
18. *Sacred Mirrors,* Alex Grey, Inner Traditions, 1990
19. *Vine of the Soul,* R. E. Schultes, R. Raffauf, Synergetic Press, 1992

## Chapter 5. Mammograms—Who Needs Them?
1. "Experts Weigh Benefits of Mammography," *Science News,* March 6, 1993
2. "Mammography-Discovered Cancer," *Health Facts,* September 1993
3. *The New Our Bodies, Ourselves,* Boston Women's Health Book Collective, Simon & Schuster, 1995
4. "Facts About Mammography" (excerpt from a report by the National Women's Health Network), *Ms.,* May/June 1993
5. "Take Charge of Your Body: A Woman's Guide to Health," Carolyn DeMarco, M.D., Last Laugh Inc., 1989
6. "The Other Side of Mammography," *Thumper,* July 1987
7. "Breast Cancer Update," *HealthFacts,* November 1993
8. "Facts About Mammography," *Ms.,* May/June 1993
9. *Paradox and Healing,* M. Greenwood and P. Nun, Paradox, 1992

10. "Facts About Mammography," *Ms.*, May/June 1993
11. "New Questions about Mammograms," Ellen Hodgson Brown, *Whole Life Times*, October 1994
12. "Breast Cancer Radiates Doubts," Dr. S. Epstein, *New York Times*, January 28, 1992
13. "Breast Cancer and Mammography," Rosalie Bertell, *Mothering*, Summer 1992
14. "Mammogram Alert," Diana Hunt, *EastWest*, September 1991
15. Cancer cells are initiated when DNA damage turns on oncogenes, but "cancer" doesn't start until one of those cells is promoted, that is, escapes consumption by the immune system and absorbs enough nourishment to reproduce (and reproduce and reproduce).
16. *McDougall's Medicine: A Challenging Second Opinion*, John McDougall, M.D., New Win, 1985
17. "Mammogram Alert," Diana Hunt, *EastWest*, September 1991
18. *McDougall's Medicine*, John McDougall, M.D., New Win, 1985
19. "Cost of Treatment in Perspective," J. Kelley, M.D., *Southern Medical Journal*, 199: 83
20. "Better Breast Test," Karen Schmidt, *Science News*, June 19, 1993
21. "Improving Mammography," W. Conkling, *American Health*, June 1995
22. "Sharper Focus on the Breast," *Newsweek*, May 10, 1993
23. Files of Keyawis Kaplan, library of the Surgeon General of Canada

## Chapter 6. There's a Lump In My Breast
1. "What to Do about Breast Lumps," Christiane Northrup, M.D., and Susan S. Lowy, *East/West*, May 1986
2. *Keeping Abreast: Breast Changes That Are NOT Cancer*, Terry McGinn, Bull, 1987
3. "New Hope for Women with Cystic Breast Disease," Carolyn DeMarco, M.D., 1989
4. "Why Call It a Disease When It's Not?," *University of California at Berkeley Health Letter*, May 1991
5. *Breast Cancer*, Mary Eades, M.D., Bantam, 1991
6. *If You Find A Lump in Your Breast . . .*, Martha McLean, Bull, 1986
7. *For Women of All Ages: A Gynecologist's Guide to Modern Female Health Care*, Sheldon Cherry, M.D., Macmillan, 1979
8. "Breast Cancer News," Tori Hudson, N.D., *Townsend Letter for Doctors*, April 1995 (*Medical Tribune*, January 5, 1995)
9. *Keeping Abreast*, Terry McGinn, Bull, 1987
10. *The Breast Cancer Handbook; Taking Control After You've Found A Lump*, Joan Seirsky & Barbara Balaban, Harper, 1993
11. *Alternative Health Care for Women*, Patsy Westcott and Leyardia Black, N.D., Healing Arts Press, 1987
12. *Cancer Salves and Suppositories*, Ingrid Naiman, Seventh Ray, 1994
13. *Breast Cancer, What You Should Know (But May Not Be Told) About Prevention and Treatment*, Steve Austin and Cathy Hitchcock, Prima, 1994

14. "Questions and Answers About Breast Lumps," U. S. Dept. of Health and Human Services Publication 92-2401, NCI, May 1992
15. "Does Early Detection Harm or Help?" Ellen Hodgson Brown, *Whole Life Times*, October 1994
16. "Complications Associated with Needle Localization Biopsy of the Breast," W. Rappaport, M.D., et al., *J. Surg. Gyn. & Ob.*, April 1991
17. "Role of Tru-Cut Needle Biopsy in the Diagnosis of Carcinoma of the Breast," J. D. Cusick, M.D., et al., *J. Surg. Gyn. & Ob.*, May 1990
18. "Role of Aspiration Cytologic Examination in the Diagnosis of Carcinoma of the Breast," P. G. Horgan, et al., *J. Surg. Gyn. & Ob.*, April 1991
19. "Biopsy of the Breast for Mammographically Detected Lesions," D. Franceschi, M.D., et. al., *J. Surg, Gyn. & Ob.*, December 1990 (449-455)
20. "Prospective Study of Double Diagnosis of Nonpalpable Breast Lesions," K. Dowlatshahi, M.D., et. al., *J. Surg, Gyn & Ob.*, February 1991 (121-124)
21. "Breast Biopsies," *Harvard Women's Health Watch News*, February 1994

## Chapter 7. What Is Breast Cancer?

1. "Growth factor predicts cancer's spread," KA Fackelmann, *Science News*, Volume 145, March 5, 1994

## Chapter 8. The Diagnosis Is Cancer

1. "Management of Screen Detected Ductal Carcinoma In Situ of the Female Breast," R. Carpenter, et. al., *Br. J. Surg.*, 1989:76 (564-567)
2. "Axillary Lymphadenectomy for Intraductal Carcinoma of the Breast," M. J. Silverstein, M.D., et. al., *J. Surg. Gyn. & Ob.* 1991, 172:3 (211-214)
3. *Peace, Love, and Healing*, Bernie Siegel, M.D., Harper & Row, 1989
4. *How Can I Help?*, Ram Dass and Paul Gorman, Knopf, 1985
5. *Prevention and Treatment of Carcinoma in Traditional Chinese Medicine*, Jia Kun (trans. Bai Yong Quan), Commercial Press, 1985
6. *Beating Cancer with Nutrition*, P. Quinlan, Nutrition Times Press, 1994
7. Private correspondence with Carolyn Dean, M.D., and notes from a workshop given by Jeffrey Bland, M.D.
8. *The Truth About Breast Cancer*, Claire Hoy, Stoddart, 1995 (254-255)
9. *Breast Cancer: What You Should Know (But May Not Be Told)*, Steve Austin and Cathy Hitchcock, Prima, 1994
10. "Partial and complete regression of breast cancer in relation to coenzyme Q10," Lockwood, et al., *Biochem. Biophys. Res. Comm.*, 1994, 199 (1504-1508)
11. "Supplements of the Scientists," T. Adler, *Science News*, April 22, 1995
12. "Ascorbic acid as a therapeutic agent in cancer," E. Cameron and L. Pauling, *J. Intl. Acad. Prev. Med.*, 1978:5 (1)
13. *National Health Federation Bulletin*, H. W. Manner, 1977, 23:10 (1-3)
14. "4, 6-0-benzylidene-D-glucopyranose in the treatment of solid malignant tumors," Tatsumura, et al., *Brit. J. of Cancer*, 1990:62
15. "Drug of Darkness, Can a pineal hormone head off everything from breast cancer to aging?," J. Raloff, *Science News*, May 13, 1995 (300-301)
16. *Diet & Health*, National Research Council, Nat'l Academy Press, 1989

17. "Profile of Helmut Keller M.D.," M. Walker, *Raum & Zeit,* February 1991
18. *Persecution and Trial of Gaston Naessens,* Christopher Bird, Kramer, 1989
19. *Imagery in Healing,* Jeanne Achterberg, Shambhala, 1985
20. "Reduction of local tumor recurrence by primary excision with the $CO_2$ laser," Lanzafame, et al., *Lasers Surg. Med.,* 1985:2 (142-143)
21. "CO2 Laser in Breast Surgery," V. Ansanelli, *Research for Life,* 1988
22. "Axillary Lymphadenectomy for Intraductal Carcinoma of the Breast," M. J. Silverstein, M.D., et. al., *J. Surg. Gyn. & Ob.,* 172:3 (211-214), 1991
23. "Breast Cancer," Harris, et al., *New Eng. J. Med.,* 1992, 327:6 (391)

## Chapter 9. Choosing Breast Surgery?

1. "A Reappraisal of Prophylactic Mastectomy," Irene Wapnir, et al., *J. Surg. Gyn. & Ob.,* 171:2 (171-180), 1990
2. "Breast Cancer Surgery: Taking Time to Choose," Virginia Soffa, *National Women's Health Network,* September/October 1991
3. "Trends in Conserving Treatment of Invasive Carcinoma of the Breast," G. Marie Swanson, et al., *J. Surg. Gyn. & Ob.,* 171:6 (465-471), 1990 "All carcinoma of the breast 4 centimeters or smaller with negative nodes treated by partial mastectomy and radiation have equivalent disease-free survival time compared with modified radical mastectomy."
4. "Axillary Lymphadenectomy for Intraductal Carcinoma of the Breast," Melvin Silverstein, M.D., et al., *J. Surg. Gyn. & Ob.,* 172:3 (211-214), 1991
5. *J. Natl. Cancer Inst.* 1989; 320 (822-8)
6. *The Surgery Book.,* R.M. Youngson, M.D., St. Martin's Press, 1993.
7. "Breast Cancer: Redefining Acceptable," Karen Henry, *Ms,* September/October 1992
8. *Tree,* Deena Metzger, PO Box 186, Topanga, CA 90290 (also poster)
9. "Subcutaneous mastectomy is not a prophylaxis against carcinoma of the breast," L. Humphrey, *American Journal of Surgery,* 1983 (311-12)
10. "We would rarely recommend prophylactic mastectomy," M. Osborne and J. Bayle, *Primary Care & Cancer,* 1988 (25-31)
11. "Reappraisal of Prophylactic Mastectomy," *J. Surg. Gyn. & Ob.,* 1990, 171:2
12. "After Breast Cancer Surgery," *Johns Hopkins Letter,* 1994/5
13. "Lymphedema: The Seemingly Forgotten Complication," Margaret Farncombe, M.D., Gail Daniels, R.P.T., and Lisa Cross, M.D., 1993
14. "Lymphedema–An Overview," Saskia Thiadens, R.N., and Marlys Witte, M.D., *National Lymphedema Newsletter,* July 1992
15. "Use of stinkhorn mushroom and celandine in treatment of cancer in Latvia," Josef Gurvich, *Townsend Letter for Doctors,* October 1994.
16. *Up Front: Sex and the Post-Mastectomy Woman,* L. Dackman, Viking, 1990

## Chapter 10. Preventing Breast Cancer Recurrence

1. "Less Aggressive Follow-up Testing for Breast Cancer Recurrence," *Health Facts,* August 1994 (studies published in *JAMA,* 25 May 1994)
2. "The Value of Symptom Directed Evaluation in the Surveillance for Recurrence of Carcinoma of the Breast," L. D. West, M.D., et al., *J. Surg, Gyn. & Ob.,* 172(3), 191-196, 1991

# References  341

3. "Breast Cancer Patients' Survival," U.S. General Accounting Office, PO Box 6015, Gaithersburg, MD 20877

4. *Questioning Chemotherapy*, Ralph Moss, Equinox, 1994

4a. *Health Facts*, August 1994 (studies published in *JAMA*, 25 May 1994)

5. *American Health*, January/February 1994 (11-12)

6. *Love, Medicine, and Miracles*, Bernie Siegel, M.D., Harper & Row, 1986

7. *The Heroic Path*, Angela Trafford, Blue Dolphin, 1993

8. *Affirmations, Meditations, and Encouragements for Women Living with Breast Cancer*, Linda Dackman, Harper, 1991

9. *Pathwork of Self Transformation*, Eva Pierrakos, Bantam, 1990

10. *Meeting the Shadow, The Hidden Power of the Dark Side of Human Nature*, Connie Zweig and J. Abrams, eds., Tarcher, 1991

11. *Prescription for Nutritional Healing*, J. Balch, M.D., Avery, 1990

12. *See* L. Humphrey, *American Journal of Surgery*, 1983 (311-12); also M. Osborne and J. Bayle, *Primary Care & Cancer*, 1988 (25-31)

13. "Wide Local Excision as the Sole Primary Treatment in Elderly Patients with Carcinoma of the Breast," M. Reed, et al., *Br. J. Surg.*, 1989, 76: 898-900

14. *Challenging the Breast Cancer Legacy: A Program of Emotional Support for Women at Risk*, Renee Royak-Schaler and B. Benderly, Harper Collins, 1992

15. *Science News*, December 19, 1992 and March 5, 1994

## Chapter 11. Choosing Tamoxifen?

1. "Study reaffirms tamoxifen's dark side," T. Adler, *Sci. News*, June 4, 1994 (356)

2. "Studies spark tamoxifen controversy," *Sci. News*, February 26, 1994 (133)

3. *Tamoxifen & Breast Cancer*, M. DeGregorio and Valerie Wiebe, Yale University Press, 1994

4. "Tamoxifen Citrate Warning," *FDA Medical Bulletin*, May 1994

5. *Tamoxifen & Breast Cancer*, DeGregorio and V. Wiebe, Yale Univ., 1994

6. *Patient No More*, Sharon Batt, Gynergy, 1994

7. National Institute of Health Consensus Development Conference Statement: Treatment of Early Stage Breast Cancer, June 18-21, 1990 (current)

8. *Tamoxifen & Breast Cancer*, DeGregorio and V. Wiebe, Yale Univ., 1994

9. *Patient No More*, Sharon Batt, Gynergy, 1994

10. "Study reaffirms tamoxifen's dark side," T. Adler, *Sci. News*, June 4, 1994 (356)

11. "Studies spark tamoxifen controversy," *Sci. News*, February 26, 1994 (133)

12. *Ibid.*

13. "Tamoxifen Citrate Warning," *FDA Medical Bulletin*, May 1994

14. "Study reaffirms tamoxifen's dark side," T. Adler, *Sci. News*, June 4, 1994 (356)

15. "Studies spark tamoxifen controversy," *Sci. News*, February 26, 1994 (133)

16. *The Truth About Breast Cancer*, Clair Hoy, Stoddart, 1995

## Chapter 12. Choosing Radiation Therapy?

1. "Decreased survival related to irradiation postoperatively in early operable breast cancer," J. Stjernsward, *The Lancet*, November 30, 1974

2. "Is beta-carotene a radiation protectant?," *Sci. News*, February 19, 1994

3. *Radiation and Human Health*, J.W. Gofman, Pantheon, 1981

4. "Radiation: An Amazing Recovery," *Patient No More*, Sharon Batt, Gynergy, 1994

5. *Fighting Radiation and Chemical Pollutants with Foods, Herbs, and Vitamins*, Steven Schechter, N.D., Vitality Ink, 1991

6. "Adjuvant Use of Phytomedicines with Chemo- and Radiation Therapy," Ikehara Kawamura, et al., *Microbial Infections*, Plenum Press, 1992

## Chapter 13. Choosing Chemotherapy?

1. *Breast Cancer: What You Should Know (But May Not Be Told) About Prevention, Diagnosis and Treatment*, S. Austin and C. Hitchcock, Prima, 1994

2. "Lymph node removal may be unnecessary," Norma Peterson, *Breast Cancer Action Newsletter*, no. 29, April 1995

3. "Breast Cancer Patients' Survival," GAO, POBox 6015, Gaithersburg, MD 20877

4. "How American Oncologists Treat Breast Cancer," D. Belanger, et al., *J. Clin. Oncology*, 9(1), 7-16, January 1991

5. "High risk of therapy-related leukemia," M. Andersson, et al., *Cancer*, 65(11), 2460-4, June 1, 1990

6. *Breast Cancer Handbook*, Joan Swirsky, Barbara Balaban, Harper, 1994

7. "Power Foods: Looking at how nutrients may fight cancer," Tina Adler, *Science News*, April 22, 1995

8. "Body Clock," Lori Miller Kase, *American Health*, July/August 1993

9. "Putting the Pressure on Nausea," Lisa McGrath, *Amer. Health, op cit.*

10. "The Medical Use of Marijuana," Rick Doblin, *Maps* 5(1), Summer 1994 (*Townsend Letter For Doctors*, June 1995)

11. *Breast Cancer*, Rose Kushner, Harcourt, Brace & Jovanovich, 1975

12. *Chocolate to Morphine, Understanding Mind-Active Drugs*, Andrew Weil, M.D., and Winifred Rosen, Houghton Mifflin, 1983

13. *Menopausal Years, The Wise Woman Way*, Susun Weed, Ash Tree, 1992

14. *Sacred Land, Sacred Sex*, Dolores LaChapelle, Finn Hill Arts, 1988

## Chapter 14. No references

## Chapter 15. Late Stage Breast Cancer?

1. *Spontaneous Remission, An Annotated Bibliography*, Brendan O'Regan and C. Hirshberg, Institute of Noetic Sciences, 1993 (esp. pages 159-160)

2. Letter to *On the Issues*, Fall 1994

3. "Hansi," Rennie Davis, *New Science News*, 3:1, Fall 1993

4. *A Gradual Awakening*, Stephen Levine, Anchor Doubleday, 1979

5. "Progress on Therapy of Breast Cancer with Vitamin $Q_{10}$," Lockwood, et al., *Biochem. & Biophys. Research*, July 6, 1995 (172-177)

6. Dr. I. W. Lane, author of *Sharks Don't Get Cancer*, in *Townsend Letter for Doctors*, June 1994

7. *Botanical Influences on Illness—A Sourcebook of Clinical Research*, M. Werbach, M.D., amd M. Murray, N.D., Third Line, 1994

8. *The Lancet*, October 3, 1981

9. *Grace and Grit*, Ken Wilber, Shambhala, 1991 (44)

# Index

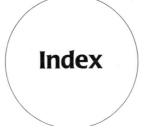

**343**

*Eleutherococcus, see* Siberian ginseng
ellagic acid 34, 43, **46**
endometrial 42, 202, 206
energy xviii, xix, 22, 59, 60, 116,
  139, 140, 144, 191, 195, 205, 207,
  208, 221, 240, 241, 248, 280
    center (chakra) 81, 216
    healing 67, 146, 178, 185
    increases 84, 85, 218, 219, 229,
      239, 269
    life force 55, 191, 216
enokidake (*Flammulina velutipes*)
  44, 87
enzyme 7, 14, 27, 29, 35, 39, 48,
  49, 154, 156, 179, 180, 278
Epstein-Barr virus 15, 79
*Equisetum arvense see* horsetail herb
essential fatty acids xxi, 48
essential oil 81, 119, 120, 197, 214,
  232, 268, 269, 270, 274, 277, 278,
  285, 289
    dangers of 63-64
Essiac 176, 248, 269, 274, **276, 301**
estradiol 6, 7, 8, 10, 14, 23, 24, 201
estrogen 6, 7, 10, 14, 15, 21, 23, 32,
  49, 116, 122
*Eupatorium perfoliatum see* boneset
evening primrose (*Oenothera biennis*)
  48, 121, 256
evergreen oil **64**, 75, 116, 298
exercise xv, xvi, xvii, 6, 9, 23, 89,
  93, 185, 210, 218, 220, 204, 205, 240
exhaustion 125, 209, 232, **239**, 247

**F**allout 4, 18, 24, 97
false negative 94, 124, 126
false positive 94, 126, 198
fasting 32, 148, 153, 154
fat necrosis 16, 108, 110
fatigue 175, 177, **218**, 202, 228, 239
fatty acids 29, 36, 37, 39, 42, 45,
  121, 149, 277
fear 146, 151, 170, 189, 191, 241, 248
    of death 253, 263-264
    of cancer x, 109, 111, 114
    dealing with 143, 163-165, 232
    as power 105

feelings 4, 23, 80, 140, 146, **163-
  165**, 170, 189, 192, 208, 246
fennel (*Foeniculum vulgare*) xxi, 50,
  205, 240, 241
fenugreek (*Trigonella foenum-graecum*)
  xxi, 67
fertile/fertility 17, 109, 122, 136, 284
fever 180, 224, 231, 232, 257
fibroadenoma 108, 110
fibroblast growth factors 135
fibrocystic 16, 108, 109
fish 25, 48, 149, 242, 256
*Flammuina velutipes* 44
flavones 33, 40, 42, 49
flavonoids 30, 34, 38, 40, 43, **48-
  49**, 51, 270, 273, 277, 279, 280, 281,
  284, 285
flax seed (*Linum usitatissimum*) **32,**
  36, **37**, 48, 50, 67, 118, 121, 300, 304
    oil 25, 37, 149, 256, 311
flower essences 81, 164, **166**
folic acid 28, 30, 31, 34, 35, 36,
  39, 42, 43, 44, **49**, 53, 154, 187
folk remedy 152, 274, 279, 281, 282,
  284, 290
foxglove (*Digitalis*) xxii, 186, 198
free radical 27, 38, 47, 50, 51, 67,
  155, 156, 278
fucus (*Fucus versiculosis*) 148, 241, 277

**G**alium aparine, *see* cleavers
*Ganoderma* species 44, 86, 87
*Gaultheria, see* wintergreen
garlic (*Allium sativum*) xv, xxi, 25,
  **33**, 38, 46, 49, 50, 52, 53, 84, 87,
  90, 97, 196, 204, 210, 212, 224,
  256, 268, 270, 274, 281, 308, 309,
  310, 311, 312
gene/genetic 8, 9, 16, 142, 155
genistein 28, 29, 35, 43, 49, 258, 284
germanium 33, 47, 49, 84, 154, 155,
  197
Gerson, Max 16, 32, 35, 38, 154
ginger (*Zingiber officinalis*) xxii, 34,
  41, 104, 115, 118, 120, 148, 177, 215,
  247, 274, 275, 288, 297, 300,
  301, 305, 307, 308, 309, 310

baseline 96
diagnostic 93, 124
dangers 96, **97-98**
mortality increase 95
postmenopausal 97, 101
radiation dose from **18**, 97, 98
screening 17, 93-103, 144
shadow on 107, 108, **110**, 123
timing of 102
manganese 53, 155
Manual Lymph Drainage 184
marijuana (*Cannabis sativa*) xxii, 48,
92, 165, 210, 216, **233**, 242, 244
marjoram (*Origanum*) xxii, 64, 312
marshmallow (*Althaea officinalis*)
xxi, 67, 306
massage xv, xvi, 116, 149, 184, 185,
191, 195, 215, 217
mastectomy 104, 124, 137, 159, 180,
198, 247, 248
bilateral 144, 249
complete 172, 174
modified 144
radical 162, 172, 173, 181
simple 162
mastitis 16, 273, 275
May apple (*Podophyllum*) xxii, 186,
291
*Medicago sativa see* alfalfa
meditate/meditation xvi, 81, 195,
241, 250, 254, 258
*Melaleuca see* tea tree
melatonin 13, 15, 20, 21, 22, 25,
81, 154, 156, 162
*Melilotus officinalis* (sweet clover)
284
melphalan 224, 229, 231, 235, 239
memory 177, 224
menarche 6, 192
menopause /menopausal 5, 6, 7, 24,
37, 96, 114, 117, 146, 192, 202, 240,
241, 247, 248, 270, 275
induced 228, **240**, 284
menses/menstrual cycle 5, 6, 7, 13,
96, 122, 173, 195, 240, 271, 275, 280
abnormal bleeding 202, 206, 224
metabolism 197, 241

metastasis/metastases 38, 99, 137,
161, 162, 172, 195, 253, 257
blocks 27, 149, 152, 176, 286
in brain 194, 259
and chemotherapy 226, 260
diagnosing 111, 135
increases 12, 154
in liver 194, 246
prevents 48, 148, 281, 303
reduces 39, 49, 146, 160, 255
Methotrexate 224, 229, 231, 234,
235, 239
micro-calcifications 79, 108, 110
microscopic cellular changes/can-
cers 69, 196
microwave 10, 15, 19, 24, 160
migraine 289
milk 12, 13, 42, 56, 149
from cows/goats 11, 15, 18, 34,
45, 148, 214, 287, 311
glands, relieve impacted 63
milk thistle (*Carduus marianum*) xxi,
53, 177, 202, 205, 212, 224, 228,
229, 240, 248, 249, 256, 272, **277**,
296, 312
minerals 148, 187, 215, 220, 234
extracting 294, 296
dangers of supplements 155
sources of xxi, **53**, 86, 268, 269,
271, 272, 273, 274, 278, 280,
284, 286, 287
mint xxii, 53, 121, 215, 219, 256,
271, **278**, 280, 284
miso 42, 84, 97, 102, 127, 210, 211,
212, 217, 237, 308, 310
mistletoe (*Viscum album*) xxii, 67,
158, 167, **279**, 312
mitomycin 224, 229, 231, 234, 235,
238, 239
moon 58, 72, 76, 149, 307, 309
motherwort (*Leonurus cardiaca*) xxi,
xxii, 89, 117, 118, 123, 165, 202,
210, 224, 240, 241, 242, 247
mouth, dry/sore 31, 66, 67, 235,
236, 246, 289, 290
mucilage 268, 271, 275, 277
mucinous carcinoma 136

radiation, protects against (cont.)
102, 211, 212, 213, 219, 221,
268, 272, 277, 286, 300, 307,
309, 311
    therapeutic 91, 188, **209-222**
radioactive 93, 100, 101
    isotopes 41, 96, 102, 212, 211
rash 61, 183, 185, 231, 280, 283
raspberry (*Rubus idaeus*) xxi, 117
reconstruction 173, 174, 175, 247
recurrence 67, 135, 141, 153, 162,
175, 181, **191-198**, 214, 240, 247, 286
    against 30, 33, 39, 43, 149,
        160, 196, 197, 201, 307, 311
    anxiety about 172
    -free survival 145
    likelihood markers 194
    metastatic 193, 194, 198
    prevents xvii, 28, 29, 34, 35,
        41, 42, 46, 50, 51, 65, 79, 148,
        156, 158, 193, 195-198, 201,
        209, 214, 219, 267, 281, 284
    risks 194, 195, 196, 203
    simple 172, 193, 195, 198, 209
red blood cells 31, 84, 202, 234,
238, 281, 284, 286
red clover (*Trifolium pratense*) xix,
xxi, 7, 14, 25, 36, 46, 50, 51, 53,
65, 116, 121, 147, 148, 196, 203, 204,
206, 215, 255, 256, 268, 269, 278,
281, **284**, 294, 296, 297, 300, 303,
304, 305, 306
    red clover blossom oil **65**, 75
redroot (*Ceanothus americanus*) xxi,
118
regenerate 84, 86, 220, 228
rehmannia (R*ehmannia glutinosa*) 300
reishii (*Ganoderma lucidum*) 44, **86-
87**, 88, 212, 230, 309, 310
rejuvenate xi, 249, 275, 277, 279
relax/relaxation xv, xvii, 57, 60, 63,
122, 125, 142, 163, 177, 205, 233,
248, 289
remission 23, 144, 149, 152, 155,
156, 157, 159, 234, 257, 259, 272,
276, 281, 284, 311
resins in plants 274, 283, 284

respiratory 156, 287
retina 205
revitalize 86, 233
*Rhammus* species 303
rhubarb, *see* turkey rhubarb
*Rincinus communis, see* castor oil
Roman chamomile (*Anthemis nobilis*)
120, 214
rose geranium (*Pelargonium*) 81, 120
rosemary (*Rosmarinus officinalis*) xxii,
40, 47, 51, 64, 81, 97, 153, 256, **278**
*Rubus idaeus, see* raspberry
*Rumex* species, *see* yellow dock

Sage (*Salvia officinalis*) xxii, 40, 50,
51, 53, 90, 236, 256
salicylic acid 275, 282, 284, 289
*Salix* species, *see* willow
*Salvia lyrata, see* cancerweed
saponins 11, 42, 49, **51**, 268, 272,
279, 283, 285, 289
scalp 64, 66, **216**, **239**, 268, 277
    nourishing 61, 217
scar 61, 110, 121, 127, 174, 175, 180,
185, 188, 189, 210, 213
    from biopsy 16, 126
    minimize 63, **178**, **179**, 282
schisandra (*Schisandra chinensis*) xxi,
229, 312
sciatica 66, 285
sclerosing adenosis 16, 108
*Scutellaria lateriflora see* skullcap
seaweed xv, xxi, 9, 16, 18, **41**, 46, 53,
84, **54**, 90, 96, 102, 117, 127, 148,
155, 179, 210, 211, 212, 217, 222, 224,
232, 238, 241, 242, 255, 256, 277,
307, 308, 309, 310
sedative 91, 122, 274
selenium xxi, **51-52**, 84, 90, 122, 154,
156, 212, 214
    benefits 14, 25, 47, 224, 228
    dangers 157, 197
    food sources 33, 34, 38, 41, 42,
        44, 53
    herbal sources 268, 269, 271, 272,
        273, 274, 278, 280, 284, 286,
        287, 289

*Verbascum thapsus, see* mullein
vinblastine 224, 229, 234, 235, 238, 239
vincristine 224, 229, 234, 238, 239
victim 141, 165, 254
vinegar, herbal xv, xvi, 26, 28, 34, 39, 87, 120, 148, 155, 202, 204, 205, 212, 237, 238, 255, **296**, 310
violet (*Viola*) xxi, 36, 46, 47, 104, 115, 116, 147, 148, 180, 210, 215, 220, 255, 294, 289, 296, 299, 300
    leaf poultice 115, 245
virus/viral 87, 88, 90, 180, 181
    infection, chronic 15
    inhibits 44, 152
*Viscum album, see* mistletoe
vision quest 145, 167
visualization 147, 151
vitality 87, 105, 148, 199
vitamins xxi, **53**, 248
vitamin A 14, 47, 53, 84, 91, 122, 154, 155, 156, 187, 197
vitamin B₆ 53, 91
vitamin B₁₇ 28, 53, 154, 156
vitamin C 14, 25, 33, 34, 39, 40, 47, 53, 84, 122, 154, 155, 156, 167, 176, 180, 187, 197, 204, 211, 228, 234, 270
vitamin D 22, 25, 40, 51, 53, 87, 154
vitamin E 14, 25, 33, 37, 43, 47, 53, 67, 84, 121, 154, 157, 176, 180, 197, 204, 211, 224, 228, 280, 284
vitamin K 53, 281
*Vitex agnus-castus see* chaste tree
*Volvariella volvacea* 44
vomit 37, 177, 202, **231**, 232, 233, 234, 283, 287, 289

**W**arfarin 46, 204
water retention 116, 224, 228
weight 4, 9, 13, 29, 122, 197, 202, 240, 241, 273
wheat grass 31, 44, 219, 239
white blood cell 80, 84, 90, 202, **229**, 231, 238, 286
    count 91, 228, 273
    production 88, 152, 230

wild lettuce (*Lactucca* species) xxii, 258
wild mushrooms xxi, **44-45**, 49, 84, 86, 196, 237, 255, 281, 307, 309, 310
wild yam (*Dioscorea*) xxi, 7, 122
willow (*Salix*) xxii, 46, 204, 210
wintergreen (*Gaultheria procumbens*) xxii, 204, 210, 249
Wise Healer Within xi, 5, 57, 60, 69, 72, 80, **82-83**, 113, 143, 193, 211
Women's Cancer Resource Center 110
witch hazel (*Hamamelis virginiana*) 178, 214, 224, 304
wounds x, 63, 212, 238, 287
    healing **178**

**X**-rays 17, 24, 42, 69, 93, 97, 98, 111, 126, 127, 207, 208, 211
*Xanthoxylum americanum* 303

**Y**ance, Donnie 15, 67, 118
yarrow (*Achillea millefolium*) 67, 90, 185, 213, 224, 256, 297, 306
    yarrow flower oil **67**, 75
yeast infection 237
yellow dock (*Rumex* species) xxi, 53, 67, 154, 176, 180, 205, 219, 228, 238, 255, 256, 276, **290**, 295, 297, 302, 308
    root oil **67**, 75, 290
yoga xv, 25, 116, 179, 182, 185, 204, 206, 220, 236, 247, 248, 249, 250
yogurt xv, 32, **45**, 53, 148, 155, 176, 210, 214, 232, 2334, 237, 311
Yogurt Fruit Freeze 215

**Z**hu ling (*Polyporus*) 44, **87**, 88
zinc 53, 90, 175, 176, 179, 188, 215, 269, 271, 272, 273, 274, 280, 284, 287, 288
*Zingiber officinale, see* ginger

5-Flu 224, 229, 231, 234, 235, 239
714X **157**, 167